616.994
C215ba
2003

A Ca
Sour
for Nurses

616.994
A cancer
nurses
57835
D0254401
WITHDRAWN

Eighth Edition

Edited by

Claudette G. Varricchio, DSN, RN, FAAN
Chief, Office of Extramural Programs
National Institute of Nursing Research
National Institutes of Health

Associate Editors

Terri B. Ades, MS, APRN-BC, AOCN
Director, Cancer Information
Health Promotions
American Cancer Society

Pamela S. Hinds, PhD, RN, CS
Director of Nursing Research
St. Jude Children's Research Hospital

Margaret Pierce, RN, CS, MPH, MS, AOCN
Assistant Professor
University of Tennessee

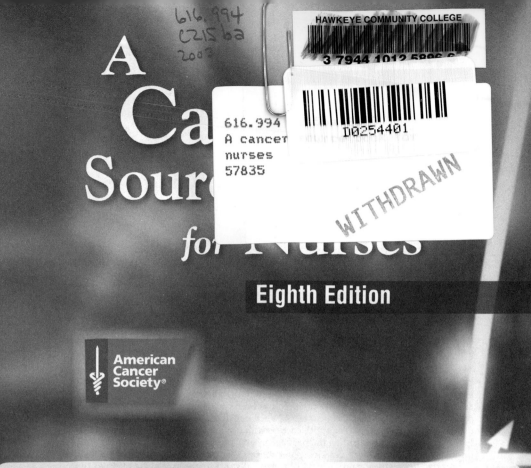

JONES AND BARTLETT PUBLISHERS
Sudbury, Massachusetts
BOSTON TORONTO LONDON SINGAPORE

057835

World Headquarters
Jones and Bartlett Publishers
40 Tall Pine Drive
Sudbury, MA 01776
978-443-5000
info@jbpub.com
www.jbpub.com

Jones and Bartlett Publishers Canada
2406 Nikanna Road
Mississauga, ON L5C 2W6
CANADA

Jones and Bartlett Publishers International
Barb House, Barb Mews
London W6 7PA
UK

Copyright © 2004 by Jones and Bartlett Publishers, Inc.

All rights reserved. No part of the material protected by this copyright may be reproduced or utilized in any form, electronic or mechanical, including photocopying, recording, or by any information storage and retrieval system, without written permission from the copyright owner.

The authors, editor, and publisher have made every effort to provide accurate information. However, they are not responsible for errors, omissions, or for any outcomes related to the use of the contents of this book, and take no responsibility for the use of the products described. The drug information presented has been derived from reference sources, recently published data, and pharmaceutical tests. When consideration is being given to use of any drug in the clinical setting, the health care provider or reader is responsible for determining FDA status of the drug, reading the package insert, and prescribing information for the most up-to-date recommendations on dose, precautions, and contraindications and determining the appropriate usage for the product. This is especially important in the case of drugs that are new or seldom used.

Production Credits
Acquisitions Editor: Penny M. Glynn
Production Manager: Amy Rose
Senior Production Editor: Linda S. DeBruyn
Associate Production Editor: Karen C. Ferreira
Editorial Assistant: Amy Sibley
Marketing Manager: Edward McKenna
Manufacturing Buyer: Amy Bacus
Cover Design: Bret Kerr
Interior Design: Shepherd Incorporated
Composition: Shepherd Incorporated
Printing and Binding: Malloy Lithographing

Library of Congress Cataloging-in-Publication Data
A cancer source book for nurses.— 8th ed. / editor, Claudette G. Varricchio ; associate editors, Terri B. Ades, Pamela S. Hinds, Margaret Pierce.
p. ; cm.
Includes bibliographical references and index. ISBN 0-7637-3276-1 1. Cancer-Nursing.
[DNLM: 1. Neoplasms-nursing. 2. Oncologic Nursing-methods. WY 156
C2198 2003] I. Varricchio, Claudette G., 1940-
RC266.C3564 2003
616.99'40231—dc22
2003026076

Printed in the United States of America
08 07 06 05 04 10 9 8 7 6 5 4 3 2 1

Contents

About the Editors

Editor

Claudette G. Varricchio, DSN, RN, FAAN

Varricchio is Chief, Office of Extramural Programs at the National Institute for Nursing Research at the National Institutes of Health. She spent 12 years at the National Cancer Institute, managing an area of research that includes symptom management, quality of life, survivorship, and end of life. She has published and served as editor and reviewer for many publications addressing these topics. Her previous experiences included a faculty position in an oncology nursing clinical specialty program and clinical practice in radiation therapy. She has served on many national committees of the American Cancer Society that addressed nursing issues, pain, and quality of life initiatives for the Society and served as an editor for the seventh edition of *A Cancer Source Book for Nurses.*

Associate Editors

Terri B. Ades, MS, APRN-BC, AOCN

Ades has been with the American Cancer Society for 14 years and holds the position of Director of Cancer Information. She has served as an editor for the sixth and seventh editions of *A Cancer Source Book for Nurses,* along with numerous other American Cancer Society publications, including two editions of *A Guide to Cancer Drugs.* When joining the American Cancer Society, Ades brought 12 years of clinical experience working with adults and children with cancer. Her oncology experiences included positions at the Medical College of Georgia, Indiana University Medical Center in Indianapolis, the Medical University of South Carolina in Charleston, and the University of Alabama in Birmingham.

Pamela S. Hinds, PhD, RN, CS

Hinds is the Director of Nursing Research and Full Member at St. Jude Children's Research Hospital. She is currently the lead investigator on two multisite studies about fatigue in pediatric oncology patients and one end-of-life communication study, and she is a co-principal investigator on a national study on quality of life in pediatric oncology patients. She serves on the Nursing Study Section for NINR/NIH and is the co-chair of the Nursing Research Committee for the Children's Oncology Group.

Margaret Pierce, RN, CS, MPH, MS, AOCN

Pierce teaches both undergraduate and graduate nursing at the University of Tennessee and is also a Family Nurse Practitioner. She has over 20 years experience in oncology nursing as a clinician and educator. She is a volunteer for the American Cancer Society and has served on the National Board of Directors. She served as an editor for the seventh edition of *A Cancer Source Book for Nurses.*

Preface

About the American Cancer Society

The American Cancer Society is the nationwide community-based voluntary health organization dedicated to eliminating cancer as a major health problem by preventing cancer, saving lives, and diminishing suffering from cancer, through research, education, advocacy, and service. As one means of fulfilling this mission, the Society has established a long history of anticipating and responding to the educational needs of professional nurses who are involved in providing care to people with cancer.

About This Book

Often referred to as *The Source Book,* this work has evolved from a book by a physician who provided the "basic knowledge of facts about cancer" to a book written *by* nurses *for* nurses.

The first edition of *A Cancer Source Book for Nurses* was published by the American Cancer Society in 1950. At that time, oncology care was provided by public health nurses in the home. Usually, the patient was dying. Since then, the field of oncology has burgeoned, and there are now more than nine million cancer survivors. Nurses in every practice setting are involved in providing care to such survivors, to individuals with cancer, and to those at risk for cancer: the family nurse practitioner providing primary health care to the woman with a history of breast cancer; the home care nurse visiting the man recovering from a radical prostatectomy; the pediatric ambulatory nurse evaluating a little one with bruising and bleeding; the staff nurse providing supportive care to the cancer patient with pain; and the nursing student making a first, tentative visit to a patient with cancer.

This new edition of *A Cancer Source Book for Nurses* was written for them and for other health care professionals. It presents clear information and easy-to-access resources so that a generalist nurse may provide safe, competent care to a person with cancer, including being able to respond to patient and family questions about care.

About the Eighth Edition

A quick, practical, and comprehensive reference appropriate for generalist nurses, nursing students, and other health professionals, the eighth edition covers the continuum in oncology care: what is known today about cancer and how to reduce one's cancer risk; early detection tests to diagnose potentially curable cancers; current treatment modalities, including information on new and specialized therapies;

advances in symptom control; and issues related to survivorship, recurrence, and end of life. In addition to information on the most common cancers and treatments, specific strategies for nursing care have been detailed by nurse specialists experienced in providing care to people with cancer.

For individuals who would like more in-depth reading, a bibliography is provided at the end of each chapter, along with a list of helpful resources such as contact information for professional organizations and free patient education materials.

Changes for the eighth edition include coverage of the latest understanding of the biology of cancer, expanded pediatric oncology information, more chapters related to symptoms, expanded coverage of underserved populations and the delivery of culturally competent care, and a more comprehensive glossary.

Acknowledgments

The American Cancer Society is grateful to the authors, reviewers, and editors for their generous contribution of time and the expertise, talent, and leadership they shared. We believe that this eighth edition reflects their commitment to the fields of oncology and nursing and to the well-being of all people with cancer. Without them, this book could not have been written.

In addition, many nurses provided their expertise to this book by reviewing chapters for accuracy and relevance to practice and the target audience. Their valuable suggestions and careful reviews added immeasurably to the final text. The time they gave is greatly appreciated.

Elizabeth Ann Coleman
Genevieve Foley
Janice Phillips
Sandra Million Underwood
Linda Sarna
Robbie Norville
Janice Post-White
Casey Hooke
Lona Roll
Donna Berry
Leslie Schover
Ki Moore
Marguerite Schlay
Laura Hilderley
Mary Gullatte
Susan Bauer-Wu
Karen Hassey Dow
Susan McMillan
Kathy Kelly
Theresa Koetters
Cynthia King
Kathi Mooney
April Frederick

List of Contributors

Terri Ades, MS, APRN-BC, AOCN
Director of Cancer Information
American Cancer Society
Atlanta, GA

Carol Reed Ash, RN, EdD, FAAN
Eminent Scholar and Professor
University of Florida College of Nursing
Gainesville, FL

Andrea Barsevick, DNSc, RN, AOCN
Director of Nursing Research
Fox Chase Cancer Center
Philadelphia, PA

Margaret Barton-Burke, PhD, RN
Assistant Professor in Nursing and Medicine
University of Massachusetts—Worcester, MA
and
Clinical Nurse Specialist
University of Massachusetts Memorial Medical Center
Worcester, MA

Susan Bauer-Wu, DNSc, RN
Director, The Phyllis F. Cantor Center
Dana-Farber Cancer Institute
Instructor of Medicine, Harvard Medical School
Boston, MA

Anne E. Belcher, PhD, RN, AOCN, FAAN
Senior Associate Dean for Academic Affairs
The Johns Hopkins University School of Nursing
Baltimore, MD

Catherine M. Bender, PhD, RN
Assistant Professor
University of Pittsburgh School of Nursing
Pittsburgh, PA

Deborah Berg, RN, BSN
Oncology Education Manager
Aventis Oncology
Derry, NH

Jean K. Brown, RN, PhD, FAAN
Associate Professor in Nursing
and
Associate Dean for Academic Affairs
University at Buffalo School of Nursing, The State University of New York at Buffalo
Buffalo, NY

Susan Budds, MSN, RN, AOCN
Oncology Clinical Nurse Specialist
Edward Hospital
Naperville, IL

Linda Casey
Administrator
Radiation/Oncology Services
Tampa Veterans Administration Hospital
Tampa, FL

Cynthia Chernecky, RN, PhD, CNS, AOCN
Professor, Department of Nursing Science
Medical College of Georgia School of Nursing
Augusta, GA

Jane Clark, PhD, RN, AOCN, APRN-BC
Independent Oncology Nursing Consultant
Decatur, GA

Mary E. Cooley, PhD, CRNP, CS
Nurse Scientist
Dana Farber Cancer Institute
The Phyllis F. Cantor Center
Research in Nursing and Patient Care Services
Boston, MA

Margaret H. Crighton, MSN, RN
Doctoral Student
John A. Hartford Foundation Building
Academic Geriatric Nursing Capacity Scholar
American Cancer Society Doctoral Scholar
University of Pennsylvania School of Nursing
Philadelphia, PA

Deena Damsky Dell, MSN, RN, BC, AOCN
Clinical Nurse Specialist/Clinical Educator
Fox Chase Cancer Center
Philadelphia, PA

Andrea M. Denicoff, RN, MS, CANP
Coordination of Palliative Care Initiatives
National Cancer Institute
National Institutes of Health
Bethesda, MD

Karen Hassey Dow, PhD, RN, FAAN
Professor
University of Central Florida School of Nursing
Orlando, FL

Deborah Fleming, MS, RN
Clinical Nurse Specialist
Brandon Regional Hospital
Brandon, FL

Marilyn Frank-Stromborg, EdD, JD, ANP, FAAN
Distinguished Research Professor and Chair
Northern Illinois University
School of Nursing
DeKalb, IL

Janese Gaddis, RN, MSN, OCN
Senior Staff Nurse
Ambulatory Oncology Center
Georgia Cancer Center for Excellence
Grady Health System
Atlanta, GA

Robin Gemmill, RN, MSN
City of Hope National Medical Center
Duarte, CA

Mary Magee Gullatte, RN, MN, ANP, AOCN
Director of Nursing
Oncology and Transplant Inpatient
Services and Oncology Data Center
Emory University Hospital, Crawford Long Hospital and Winship Cancer Institute
Atlanta, GA

Marilyn Haas, PhD, RN, CNS, ANP-C
Nurse Practitioner
Mountain Radiation Oncology
Asheville, NC

Keri Hockett, ARNP, MSN, AOCN
Sarasota Memorial Hospital
Sarasota, FL

Genevieve Hollis, MSN, RN-CRNP, AOCN
Associate Director, Adult Oncology Nurse Practitioner Program
University of Pennsylvania School of Nursing
Philadelphia, PA

Mary Casey Hooke, RN, MSN,CNS, CON
Clinical Nurse Specialist
Hematology/Oncology
Children's Hospitals and Clinics of Minneapolis and St. Paul
Minneapolis, MN

Lorraine M. Hutson, MS, ARNP, OCN
Nurse Practitioner, Comprehensive Breast Program
H. Lee Moffitt Cancer Center and Research Institute
University of South Florida
Tampa, FL

Adonica Jones, MSN, RN
Clinical Coordinator
Oncology Nursing Services
Emory University Hospital
Atlanta, GA

Katherine Patterson Kelly, RN, MN, CPON
Clinical Nurse Specialist
Pediatric Hematology/Oncology
Children's Hospital
University of Missouri Health Care
Columbia, MO

Cynthia R. King, PhD, NP, MSN, RN, FAAN
Program Director for Nursing Research
Wake Forest University Baptist Medical Center
Winston-Salem, NC

Belinda Mandrell, MSN, RN, PNP
Pediatric Nurse Practitioner
St. Jude Children's Research Hospital
Memphis, TN

Virginia R. Martin, RN, MSN, AOCN
Clinical Director Ambulatory Care
Fox Chase Cancer Center
Philadelphia, PA

Kathleen H. Mooney, PhD, RN, AOCN, FAAN
Professor
University of Utah
Salt Lake City, UT

Jamie S. Myers, RN, MN, AOCN
Oncology Clinical Nurse Specialist/Nurse Manager
The Cancer Institute
Kansas City, MO

Madeline O'Connor, PhD, RN
Director, Research Management
Division of Stem Cell and Gene Therapy
St. Jude Children's Research Hospital
Memphis, TN

Kathleen M. O'Leary, RN, MSN
Director, Care Coordination
Department of Nursing
Penn State Milton S. Hershey Medical Center
Hershey, PA

Ann O'Mara, RN, PhD, AOCN
Program Director
National Cancer Institute
National Institutes of Health
Bethesda, MD

Maureen E. O'Rourke, RN, PhD
Associate Clinical Professor of Nursing
University of North Carolina, Greensboro
and
Adjunct Assistant Professor of Medicine
Hematology Oncology
Wake Forest University School of Medicine
Winston-Salem, NC

Shirley Otis-Green, MSW, ACSW, OSW-C, LCSW
Research Specialist
Nursing Research and Education Department
City of Hope National Medical Center
Duarte, CA

Jeannie V. Pasacreta, PhD, APRN
Associate Professor
Columbia University School of Nursing
New York, NY

Janice Phillips, PhD, RN, FAAN
Program Director
National Institute for Nursing Research
Bethesda, MD

Janice Post-White, RN, PhD, FAAN
Adjunct Associate Professor
University of Minnesota, School of Nursing
Research Consultant in CAM
Minneapolis, MN

Ann Reiner, RN, MN, OCN
Program Director, Cancer Services
Director of Outreach and Education
Oregon Health and Science University
Cancer Institute
Portland, OR

Michele Rhiner, RN, MSN, NP, CHPN
Patient Coordinator/Department Manager
Supportive Care, Pain and Palliative Medicine
City of Hope National Medical Center
Duarte, CA

Kimberly Rohan, MS, RN, AOCN
Director Outpatient Oncology Services
Edward Hospital
Naperville, IL

Lona Roll, RN, MSN
Clinical Nurse Specialist
Pediatric Hematology/Oncology
The Howard A. Britton, MD Children's Cancer and Blood Disorders Center
Christus Santa Rosa Children's Hospital
San Antonio, TX

Neal Slatkin, MD, DABPM
Director
Supportive Care, Pain and Palliative Medicine
City of Hope National Medical Center
Duarte, CA

Ellen Lavoie Smith, MS, APRN-BC, AOCN
Director, Advanced Practice Nursing
Department of Hematology/Oncology
Dartmouth Hitchcock Medical Center
Lebanon, NH

Janet H. Van Cleave, MSN, ACNP-CS, AOCN
Acute Care Nurse Practitioner
The Mount Sinai Medical Center
Oncology Care Center
New York, NY

Claudette G. Varricchio, DSN, RN, FAAN
Chief, Office of Extramural Programs
National Institute for Nursing Research
Bethesda, MD

Debby Volker, PhD, RN, AOCN
Associate Professor
University of Texas at Austin
School of Nursing
Austin, TX

Shanita Williams-Brown, PhD, MPH, APRN-BC
Cancer Prevention Fellow
National Cancer Institute
Division of Cancer Control and Population Sciences Surveillance
Research Program Cancer Statistics Branch
Bethesda, MD

M. Linda Workman, PhD, RN, FAAN
Gertrude Perkins Oliva Professor of Oncology
Frances Payne Bolton School of Nursing
Case Western Reserve University
Cleveland, OH

Linda H. Yoder, RN, MBA, PhD, AOCN
Associate Professor
Graduate School of Nursing
Uniformed Services University of the Health Sciences
Bethesda, MD

Stacey Young-McCaughan, RN, PhD, AOCN
Colonel, U. S. Army Nurse Corps
Chief, Evidence-Based Practice, U.S. Army Medical Command
Fort Sam Houston, TX

UNIT I

Introduction to Cancer Nursing

Carol Reed Ash

What is *A Cancer Source Book for Nurses* and how do you use such a book? A source book is a place to find answers. It is a document about a specific topic, such as history or literature. When talking about cancer nursing, it is a document, or a collection of chapters, that helps nurses everywhere understand the many aspects of the disease cancer and find answers to questions.

Cancer is a very complex disease. It is impossible for any one nurse to know everything there is to know about it. What each nurse needs to know is how to find answers and, more importantly, where to find them. The source must be accurate, reliable, easy to use and understandable. That's the *purpose* of *A Cancer Source Book for Nurses*.

Not everyone is a cancer nurse, but all nurses need to know something about the disease. There are very few nurses whose lives have not been touched in some way by this disease. Perhaps someone you cared for or a family member, a friend, a colleague, or a neighbor, or perhaps a friend of a friend has asked for your advice. It doesn't matter. What does matter is that you, the nurse, regardless of what kind of nursing you do, or how and when you are asked, will be trusted to provide guidance and recommendations. As the health field continues to change, so, too, will the many roles and disciplines within which nursing will practice and continue to change. You may be a nurse practitioner, a clinical specialist, a teacher, an administrator, a researcher, or a student, or you may work in primary care or perhaps the operating room or any one of the many different areas nurses practice in today. Individuals who are frightened and searching for answers and assurances see a nurse, not a special kind of nurse, but a nurse they trust and someone who can help them. *A Cancer Source Book for Nurses* will help you be that nurse who provides the right answers. It will also help you help other health professionals who need to know about some particular aspect of the disease.

■ The Cancer Picture

What are the challenges? The death rate from all cancers combined is declining, as it is for the four most prevalent cancers: breast, colon and rectum, lung and bronchus, and prostate. There are encouraging increased efforts in cancer prevention, early detection, treatment, and symptom control for many forms of cancer. The increased efforts and results are very positive and provide hope, because there is increased quality of life for many after treatment of the disease. However, there is also the reality that the efforts and results will actually increase the number of people who live longer with the disease. With more people living longer, the impact of treatment and the resulting long-term effects of those treatments will generate the need for new information to help and support individuals and their families.

The cancer picture is also changing to reflect greater emphasis on cancer prevention and early detection. What are the challenges in encouraging people to change behaviors, stop smoking, eat healthier diets, practice sun protection behaviors, exercise to reduce weight, and live a healthier life style? How can you help people understand that there are things that they can do to help themselves? There is a lot of information available about what to do, but many people do not fully understand it and therefore do not take advantage of the opportunity. How will you help people deal with the fear that prevents them from developing a healthier lifestyle or seeking help when they suspect that something is wrong?

Understanding a diagnosis of cancer and deciding what to do about it are some of the most frightening experiences a patient and his or her family will have. They will try to make sense of the information that they have received and will seek more information. They will also worry about how they are going to manage treatment and all that occurs in the course of treatment and follow-up care. What will happen to them is uncertain and causes a great deal of anxiety. Each individual will have their own set of problems, depending on the diagnosis and the support system available. The most important adjustments each patient must make are to the element of change and the physical, psychological, and social changes that will take place.

■ Patient Profile

What will your cancer patients look like? Who are they? Identities of our patient population are changing and are projected to change even more. They will be very different tomorrow from what we see today. We know that people of advanced age will dominate. Cancer is a disease of the aging, occurring predominantly in older persons. The number of persons aged 65 years and older with cancer is projected to double. Therefore, the need for understanding the disease and its treatment and providing answers and assistance to all who know or care for the patient with cancer will double as well. Care will be more complex because of the chronic diseases associated with the aging process that many will already be living with. Cancer is frequently seen as an acute disease. In an acute phase an individual is seen as being ill and in treatment. However, there is often a continuum of cancer care that may span many years for the individual from diagnosis through follow-up and may also span issues of survivorship to possibly palliation and end-of-life care.

Our population is also becoming more diversified, with increasing numbers of African Americans, Asian Americans, Hispanics, and Native Americans making up our culture. Each group needs to be understood for the differences they present in incidence, prevalence, and mortality from cancer. They also need to be understood for the way in which each culture interprets and responds to a diagnosis and treatment. This will greatly influence the way we design and offer cancer education and care.

■ What Each Nurse Needs To Know

All nurses need to know some basic information. The language of every disease is different. Cancer, because it is so many different diseases and because it involves so many different aspects of care, requires knowledge that begins with signs and symptoms and sometimes continues through treatment to death. Think about what you know about the disease called cancer.

What is cancer? What are the risk factors for the different cancers? What can you do to help someone understand what he or she could be doing to help themselves for the future? You need to know the signs and symptoms of the different cancers and how to guide someone about checkups. What if a friend asks you about a strange-looking mole, or a lump in the breast, or complains of shortness of breath or increased fatigue? That friend needs to be directed for appropriate assessment and care, and you need to help your friend understand why. The fright that many people feel when concerned about having cancer can often be eased when you help them understand that there are positive steps to take. There are enormous opportunities to help people understand that what they do in their everyday life, if changed, could help them avoid a cancer diagnosis as they become one of the aging population. Your presence at a community function, or a church meeting, or an athletic event with your children will often generate questions that you can find answers to in *A Cancer Source Book for Nurses.*

■ Why Specialize in Oncology?

There are many opportunities for nurses to specialize in cancer care, just as there are for nurses to work in so many other specialty areas, such as critical care, pediatrics, and neurology/neurosurgery. Cancer is a rapidly changing field that offers a challenge to all who work in it. You may choose acute care, special units in hospitals or ambulatory care facilities, primary care practices, or specialties in chemotherapy, radiation therapy, surgery, or genetics. You may choose to be an educator, researcher, clinician, advanced practitioner, or administrator. You may also collaborate with other health care practitioners to create a new and exciting role. Because the field of cancer is so broad and the science is constantly emerging, being a part of that environment is exciting.

Oncology nurses are on the front line of getting new information to patients, providing support through the continuum of care and working with families to understand and assist with whatever needs to be done. Oncology nurses help disseminate new information and help all nurses put into practice what is being learned every day. It is an exciting field that offers many rewards, both personally and professionally. When someone changes personal behavior to promote a healthier lifestyle, you feel good about it. When people are quickly diagnosed and treated because you helped them understand what they need to do, you feel good about what you do. And you are rewarded every day for the interpersonal relationships you share with patients, families, and colleagues.

Where Will You Practice?

The choices of where oncology nurses practice are endless. As the care for patients with cancer changes, so, too, do the places where care is provided. Much more care is offered outside the hospital, away from acute care settings. Hospital stays are shorter, and more diagnostic work is completed in an outpatient or satellite setting before hospital admission. More care is provided in the home setting, increasing the need for families and friends to learn how to support the patient. With technology so far-reaching and the delivery of diagnosis and treatment consultations now possible via the Internet, there are few places in the world where cancer care cannot be addressed. Education, too, can be delivered throughout the world via web-based and distance education. Where you will practice is your choice. Whatever the choice, it will be exciting and rewarding.

■ Where Do You Get Help?

A Cancer Source Book for Nurses will provide many answers to your questions. There are also numerous national, regional, state, and local organizations that offer assistance to both professional and consumer. While you are seeking information, your patient may be also. Many web sites, although certainly not all, provide accurate, reliable, and easy-to-use information for all.

Information is also available from professional literature, not only the nursing literature, which has specialty journals in cancer nursing, but also from multidisciplinary journals and books. We live in a world today where interdisciplinary collaboration is necessary to provide the best possible care to people. As Florence Nightingale so appropriately stated, "What nursing has to do is to put the patient in the best possible condition for nature to act upon him" (Skeat, 1980). In today's world, that means working together for the most positive outcome possible for anyone touched by the disease cancer. Many programs and printed materials are also available from our national agencies, and each has a web site that provides extensive information for both consumer and professional. These include the American Cancer Society (*www.cancer.org*), the Centers for Disease Control and Prevention (*www.cdc.gov*), the National Cancer Institute (*www.cancer.gov*), and the Oncology Nursing Society (*www.ons.org*). All of these sites provide information about the different diseases of cancer, treatment options and clinical trials, current research, and consumer issues. For additional help and to locate specific information for patients and professionals, the American Cancer Society can be contacted at 800-ACS-2345.

The American Cancer Society (ACS) is an example of how these national agencies can help you. The ACS is a nationwide, community-based voluntary health organization dedicated to eliminating cancer as a major health problem by preventing cancer, saving lives, and diminishing suffering from cancer, through research, education, advocacy, and service. The ACS is headquartered in Atlanta, Georgia, with state divisions and more than 3,400 local units in communities throughout the United States. It is the largest source of private, nonprofit cancer research funds in the United States.

■ Cancer Information

Providing the public with accurate, up-to-date information on cancer is a priority of the ACS. The society provides information on all aspects of cancer through a variety of channels, including printed materials, consumer books, professional journals, a toll-free national cancer information center, and a web site. Materials can be ordered on the web site, by contacting your local division or unit or by calling the toll-free National Cancer Information Center.

By calling 800-ACS-2345, people facing cancer can have access to clear, reliable information to help them understand their disease and make informed decisions about their care. Trained cancer information specialists are available 24 hours a day, 7 days a week to answer questions about cancer, link callers with resources in their communities, and provide information on local events. Calls are answered in English and Spanish. The center also includes an email response center for those who wish to contact the society via email. The society's web site at *www.cancer.org* provides the same in-depth information as that provided through the cancer information center. Information is also available in Spanish.

Cancer Prevention

The society's prevention programs focus on controlling tobacco use, educating about the relationship between diet and physical activity and cancer, promoting coordinated comprehensive school health education, and reducing the risk of skin cancer. Programs are designed to help adults and children make wise decisions about their health.

Early Detection and Treatment

Through the dissemination of its early cancer detection guidelines and its cancer detection and advocacy programs, the society also seeks to ensure that cancer is diagnosed at the earliest possible stage, when there is the greatest chance for successful treatment.

Patient Services

A variety of patient service programs are available to patients and their families. Some of the society's patient service programs follow.

Cancer Survivors Network The Cancer Survivors Network is an interactive electronic support service created by and for cancer survivors and their families. In the privacy of their own homes, they can access the free service either by telephone or the Internet 24 hours a day, 7 days a week. Both the telephone and the Web site contain approximately 150 hours of prerecorded personal stories and discussions among survivors or family caregivers. Additionally, the web community has many interactive features designed to help users find and connect with one another to share experiences and support. Interested parties my log in at *www.cancer.org* or call toll free at 877-333-4673 (HOPE).

Reach to Recovery "Reach to Recovery" is an ACS program designed to help people cope with their breast cancer experience. This program has provided more than 30 years of service in the fight against breast cancer. "Reach to Recovery" volunteers are breast cancer survivors who are trained to offer support at various points along the breast cancer continuum: diagnosis; decision making about treatment; dealing with treatment and its side effects; returning to a full, active life; or confronting any long-term effects, including a possible recurrence of the disease.

tlc A service offering of the Society, "tlc" is a "magalog" designed to provide needed medical information and special products for women newly diagnosed with breast cancer and breast cancer survivors. The magalog features articles that focus on medical questions specific to breast cancer, and also has a question and answer section. "tlc" features a variety of hats, caps, turbans, hairpieces, swimwear, bras, prostheses, and breast forms. Many of these products are appropriate for any woman experiencing treatment-related hair loss. Free copies are available by calling 800-850-9445.

Look Good . . . Feel Better In partnership with the Cosmetic, Toiletry and Fragrance Association Foundation and the National Cosmetology Association, this free program is designed to teach women beauty techniques to help restore their appearance and self-image during chemotherapy and radiation treatments.

Man to Man This group program provides information about prostate cancer and related issues for men and their partners in a supportive atmosphere. Some areas offer "Side by Side," a group program for the partners of men with prostate cancer and/or a visitation program in which a trained prostate cancer survivor provides support to a man who is newly diagnosed with prostate cancer.

Children's Camps In some areas, the society sponsors camps for children who have, or have had, cancer. These camps are equipped to handle the special needs of children undergoing treatment.

Hope Lodge Housing is provided in some areas through funds raised specifically to purchase a dwelling to house patients during their treatment; 17 such lodges are in operation.

I Can Cope This patient and family cancer education program consists of a series of classes, often held at a local hospital. Doctors, nurses, social workers, and community representatives provide information about cancer diagnosis and treatment, as well as assistance in coping with the challenges of a cancer diagnosis.

Research

The research program consists of three components: extramural grants, intramural epidemiology and surveillance research, and the intramural behavioral research center. Scholarships for nursing education are available for graduate study. Information about the society's research program and applications is available at *www.cancer.org*.

Advocacy and Public Policy

The society strives to advocate for and strengthen our nation's laws and regulations in a way that will:

- Increase investments for cancer research, prevention, early detection, and care
- Increase access to quality cancer care, screening, prevention, and awareness efforts
- Reduce health disparities among minorities and the medically underserved
- Reduce and prevent suffering from tobacco-related illness

Volunteering

Everyone can get involved in the activities of the ACS. Whether a nurse, a patient, a family member, or someone interested in volunteering time, there is something for everyone to do in support of cancer patients and their families. There are numerous fundraising events, such as "Relay for Life," "Making Strides Against Breast Cancer," and the "Coaches vs Cancer" basketball event. Many volunteers are needed to make these events a success, and they are fun to be a part of. There are also volunteer opportunities that include everything from information fairs for the community to support groups and cancer prevention and screening clinics.

Whatever your question, or that of your patients, the ACS and other national organizations can provide answers and assistance.

Bibliography

A helping hand: The resource guide for people with cancer (4th ed.). (2002). New York: Cancer Care, Inc.

Bednash, G. (2001). *Ask a nurse: From home remedies to hospital care.* New York: Simon & Schuster Source.

Dochterman, J., & Grace, H. (2001). *Current issues in nursing* (6th ed.). St. Louis: Mosby.

Perry, K., & Burgess, M. (2002). *Communication in cancer care.* Malden, MA: BPS Blackwell.

Simmonds, M. A. (2003). Cancer statistics, 2003: Further decrease in mortality rate, increase in persons living with cancer. *CA: A Cancer Journal for Clinicians, 53,* 4.

Skeat, M. (1980). *Notes on nursing.* Edinburgh: Churchill Livingstone.

Stewart, B., & Kleihues, P. (Eds.). (2003) *World cancer report. World Health Organization.* Lyon: IARC Press.

UNIT II

Overview of Cancer

Claudette G. Varricchio

This overview of cancer biology and epidemiology serves as an introduction and basis for the cancer information presented in the remainder of this book. An understanding of the biology and pathophysiology of cancer in general will provide a better understanding of the natural history of a specific cancer and of the choice of treatment for that cancer. This knowledge is also needed to understand the derivation of screening guidelines and surveillance for the early detection of cancer or of recurrence of the disease after treatment.

Epidemiology is the science by which the incidence and occurrence of specific cancers are identified in the population as a whole or in targeted subsets of the population. Knowing the cancer incidence in a given group provides the basis for exploring and identifying risk factors for that group. This, in turn, helps us identify, design, and test prevention interventions and screening guidelines that target these common cancers. Chapter 3 builds on the incidence and risk factor information presented in Chapter 2 to discuss the state of knowledge of early-detection recommendations for specific groups. The site-specific cancer chapters build on this information.

The chapters related to treatment approaches, specific cancers, and symptom management assume that the nursing approach will include culturally competent care. Culturally competent care goes beyond awareness of minority differences in cancer incidence and risk factors and beyond the gene/environment interaction. The nurse must be aware of the ethnic/cultural differences in the individual that could influence his or her risk for cancer or influence acceptance of risk-reduction behaviors. Cultural and ethnic differences are individual specific and are influenced by the level of acculturation to the majority culture and adherence to the original culture's health practices and beliefs. All of these factors influence an individual's risk for cancer and response to recommendations for early detection and adherence to treatment regimens.

Complementary and alternative approaches to the management of cancer and symptoms have been highlighted because of the increased use of these products among people with cancer and their families; this could be particularly significant because in some instances, the patients and families do not acknowledge the use of these approaches to health care–providers. The effectiveness of many of these products has not been established, and neither has their safety for general use. Even less is known about the possible interaction of complementary and alternative medicine products with standard cancer therapies. Information is provided in Chapter 5 to help you guide your patients through the process of deciding whether to continue or stop the use of complementary and alternative medicine during their cancer therapy.

As you read about specific cancers, therapies, and symptoms, referring back to this overview group of chapters will improve your understanding of the approaches to treatment and symptom management described throughout this book.

CHAPTER

1

The Biology of Cancer

M. Linda Workman

Although cancer is classified by organ system, it is actually a disease of cells. The human body contains many differentiated cell types, each with a unique structure and a unique function contributing to normal total-body physiologic functioning. Every malignancy arises from one cell or a group of cells that were originally normal but have been altered at the gene level in some way. The end result of the change, or transformation, is the loss of some or all of the cells' normal characteristics and the expression of abnormal characteristics. The changes that take place affect the cell's appearance, its function, its surface membrane, and its growth characteristics.

Cancer is a type of abnormal cell growth. Growth of most cells and tissues is expected during childhood. Some cells, such as those located in tissues where constant damage or wear is likely, continue to grow by mitosis (cell division) throughout a person's lifespan. This growth is needed to replace dead cells and normally occurs in the skin, hair follicles, bone marrow, mucous membranes, and linings of organs such as the lungs, stomach, intestines, bladder, and uterus. Cells in these tissues retain the ability to divide throughout the life span. This normal growth is well controlled to ensure that only the right number of cells is always present in any tissue or organ.

Some tissues and organs stop growing by cell division after development is complete. For example, skeletal muscle cells no longer divide after fetal life; the number of skeletal muscle cells is fixed at birth. Muscles increase in size as a person grows because each cell gets larger, but the number of muscle cells does not increase. This type of growth

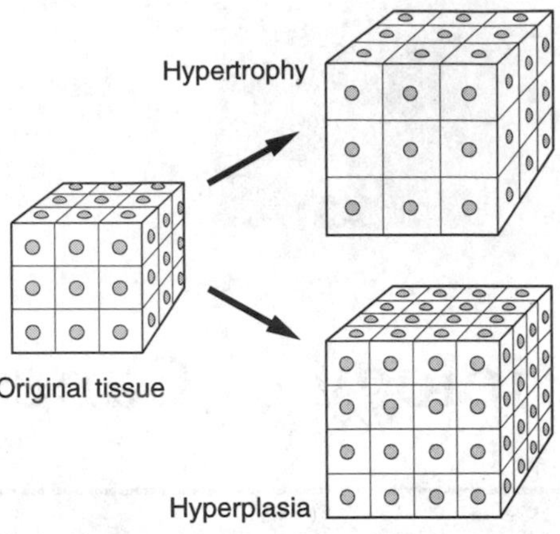

FIGURE 1–1 ■ Growth by Hyperplasia and Growth by Hypertrophy.

is termed *hypertrophy.* Growth by increasing the number of cells is termed *hyperplasia* (Figure 1–1).

A new cell growth that is not needed for normal development or replacement of damaged tissues that persists after removal of its initial stimulus is called *neoplasia.* Neoplasia, whether it results in benign tumors or cancer, is always considered abnormal. Neoplastic cells, whether they be benign or malignant, develop from normal cells (parent cells). Thus, cancer cells were once normal cells, but gene mutations occurred, resulting in the loss of the strict processes controlling normal growth and function. Any tissue can develop into cancer, but cancers more commonly develop among tissues that retain the ability to divide throughout the life span. Cancers are classified by the type of tissue from which they arise (e.g., glandular, connective). Terms that describe cancer by tissue origin are listed in Table 1–1.

■ Comparison of Normal Cells, Benign Tumor Cells, and Cancer Cells

Table 1–2 summarizes the characteristics of normal cells, benign tumor cells, and cancer cells.

Cell Appearance (Morphology)

Normal Cells Each normal mature cell type is differentiated, with a distinct and recognizable appearance, size, and shape. In addition, the

TABLE 1–1 ■ Nomenclature of Selected Neoplastic Tissues

Parent Tissues	Benign Tumors	Malignant Tumors
Epithelial (glandular)		
Breast (ductal)	Adenoma	Adenocarcinoma
Colon	Adenoma (polyps)	Adenocarcinoma
Liver	Hepatocellular adenoma	Hepatocellular carcinoma
Connective (mesenchymal)		
Adipose	Lipoma	Liposarcoma
Blood vessel	Hemangioma	Hemangiosarcoma
Bone	Osteoma	Osteosarcoma
Skeletal muscle	Rhabdomyoma	Rhabdomyosarcoma
Smooth muscle	Leiomyoma	Leiomyosarcoma

TABLE 1–2 ■ Comparison of Normal, Benign, and Cancer Cell Characteristics

Characteristic	Normal Cells	Benign Cells	Cancer Cells
Mitosis	Well regulated	Inappropriate	Nearly Continuous
Appearance	Defined size and shape	Defined size and shape	Anaplastic
Size of nucleus	Small	Small	Large
Specific functions	Maintains specific functions	Maintains specific functions	Loss of most or all specific functions
Adhesion	Tight	Tight	Nonadherent
Migration	Absent	Absent	Migrates/invades
Chromosomes	Euploid	Euploid	Aneuploid

size of the normal cell nucleus is usually small compared with the size of the rest of the cell, including the cytoplasm. Thus, normal cells generally have a small nuclear:cytoplasmic ratio.

Benign Tumor Cells Benign tumors look like the tissues they come from, retaining much of the specific morphology of parent cells. Just like completely normal cells, benign tumor cells also have a small nuclear:cytoplasmic ratio.

Cancer Cells Cancer cells lose the specific appearance of their parent cells. This loss of specific appearance makes many types of cancer cells look alike. The nucleus of a cancer cell is larger than that of a normal cell from the same tissue. Thus, cancer cells have a large nuclear:cytoplasmic ratio. Other common microscopic features of malignant cells include irregularly shaped nuclei and an increased proportion of cells undergoing mitosis.

■ Cell Functions

Normal Cells Every normal cell has at least one specific differentiated function that is important to optimal body function. For example, gastric cells secrete hydrochloric acid, nerve cells generate action potentials and conduct impulses, beta cells of the pancreas make insulin, and type II pulmonary epithelial cells make surfactant.

Benign Tumor Cells Benign tumor cells are normal differentiated cells growing in the wrong place or at the wrong time. Examples of common benign tumors are moles, colon polyps, and uterine fibroid tumors. Benign tumors retain both the appearance and the differentiated functions of their parent cells. For example, an adrenal adenoma secretes adrenal hormones, even when they are not needed.

Cancer Cells Along with losing the appearance of the parent cell, cancer cells lose some or all of the differentiated functions performed by the parent cells. Cancer cells have no useful function.

Cell Surface Properties

Normal Cells Normal cells make cell surface proteins (cell adhesion molecules) that allow cells of one type to bind closely and tightly together to one another and to the extracellular matrix (the glue-like molecules found in between cells). One such adhesion protein is fibronectin, which keeps most normal tissues bound tightly to each other. Cells that do not produce fibronectin, such as blood cells, do not adhere to each other. The tight adherence of normal cells makes them remain in a relatively fixed position in the body. With the exception of blood cells, they do not wander from one tissue into the next.

Benign Tumor Cells Benign tumor cells do make fibronectin and are tightly adherent. Many benign tumors are surrounded by fibrous connective tissue ("encapsulated"), which also limits cell movement. Thus, benign tissues do not invade other body tissues.

Cancer Cells Cancer cells make little, if any, fibronectin and adhere poorly to each other. Because cancer cells do not bind tightly together and have many enzymes on their cell surfaces that can digest the molecules of the extracellular matrix, they are able to break off from the main tumor, move through blood vessels and tissues, and spread to other body sites (metastasize).

Chromosomes/Genes

Normal Cells Most normal human cells have 23 pairs of chromosomes, the correct number for human beings, a state called *euploidy* or *diploidy*. All normal cells (except the sex cells and the mature red blood cells) have the entire human genome in every cell, although not all genes are expressed (i.e., are active or "turned on") in every cell. For example, the gene for insulin is expressed normally only in the beta cells of the pancreas, although this gene is present in the nucleus of all other cells. In cells other than the beta cells of the pancreas, the insulin gene is suppressed so that insulin is only produced by the pancreas.

Normal cells have about 35,000 genes. About 50 of these genes are very active during embryonic life, and their expression is critical to fetal development. These early development genes are called *proto-oncogenes,* and their activity is not needed after embryonic life. Other genes, called *tumor suppressor genes,* slow down cell division, repair DNA mistakes, and tell cells when to die (a process known as *apoptosis,* or programmed cell death). Tumor suppressor genes can also reduce expression of proto-oncogenes by negative-feedback mechanisms. Proto-oncogenes are not abnormal genes. They are part of every human's normal cellular DNA.

Benign Tumor Cells Just like totally normal cells, benign tumor cells generally have 23 pairs of chromosomes and, thus, are euploid. Most of the genes expressed in benign tumor cells are the same ones that are expressed in the normal tissue from which the benign tumor arose. All other genes are suppressed.

Cancer Cells As cancer cells become more malignant, they lose or gain whole chromosomes or parts of chromosomes, a state called *aneuploidy*. When cancer cells have more than the normal chromosome number, they are *hyperdiploid*. When they have less than the normal chromosome number, they are *hypodiploid*. Usually, the more malignant a cancer cell is, the more abnormal its chromosomes are.

The fact that cancer cells usually have abnormal chromosomes indicates that changes in these cells occur first at the gene level. The most important gene changes are those that allow cancer cells to revert to a less differentiated state that actually resembles embryonic cells much more than they resemble normal differentiated cells. These gene changes also increase the growth potential for cancer cells. Gene changes from normal are called *mutations*. In cancer cells, one or more suppressor genes have been mutated and are no longer able to control cell growth. Likewise, most cancers have one or more proto-oncogenes that have been activated by mutation. When proto-oncogenes are activated by mutation or by other mechanisms that cause their overexpression, they are called *oncogenes*. Overexpression of oncogenes and inactivation of tumor suppressor genes convert normal cells into cancer cells.

Cell Growth Characteristics

Normal Cells Normal cells undergo mitosis (cell division) either to develop normal tissue during embryonic development, childhood, and adolescence or to replace lost or damaged normal tissue. Not all differentiated tissues have cells that can undergo mitosis. Even when they are capable of mitosis, normal cells divide only when body conditions are optimal. These conditions include the need for more cells, adequate space, and sufficient nutrients. Cell division, occurring in a well-recognized pattern, is described by the cell cycle. Figure 1–2 explains the phases of the cell cycle.

Normal cells spend little time reproducing. Most are found at any one time in a reproductive resting state termed G_0. In this state, normal cells carry out their specific differentiated functions but do not divide.

Mitotic cell division makes one cell divide into two cells. The resulting two new cells are identical to each other and to the cell that started the mitotic cell division. The steps of entering and completing the cell cycle are tightly controlled. Much of this control is regulated by proteins produced by "suppressor genes."

Each normal cell divides only when it is not totally surrounded by other cells and when some of its membrane surface is not in direct contact with another cell. Once the normal cell is contacted on all surface areas with other cells, it no longer undergoes mitosis. Thus, normal cell division is *contact inhibited*. Contact inhibition is also called *density-dependent inhibition of cell growth*.

In addition to dividing only when needed, normal cells "know" when it is time to die. Each normal cell type has internal instructions to undergo programmed cell death, a process called *apoptosis*. Each differentiated cell type has a specific life span, measured in time, or a fixed number of cell divisions. Once a cell has reached the end of this normal life span, it essentially commits suicide, resulting in its own death. The process of apoptosis allows replacement (in mitotic tissues) with new cells to ensure continuing optimum organ or tissue function.

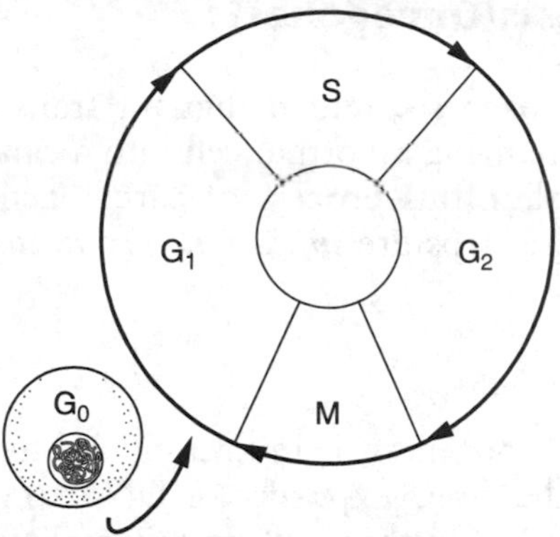

FIGURE 1–2 ■ The Phases of the Cell Cycle Are:

G_1 The cell takes up extra nutrients, synthesizes more energy, and produces extra membrane. The amount of cell fluid (cytoplasm) also increases.

S Because making one cell into two cells requires twice as much deoxyribonucleic acid (DNA), the cell doubles its DNA content through DNA synthesis in S phase.

G_2 This phase is characterized by the synthesis of proteins needed for both cell division and for normal physiologic function after cell division is complete.

M During the M phase, actual mitosis occurs, in which the single cell is separated into two cells.

(You really would not want all your bone marrow cells, for instance, to be geriatric citizens in your body.)

Benign Tumor Cells Benign tumor cells follow normal cell growth patterns even though their growth is not needed. Growth may continue beyond an appropriate time, but the rate of growth is normal. It is not clear whether benign tumor cells respond to apoptotic signals. Benign tumors grow by expansion and do not invade.

Cancer Cells Unlike normal cells or benign tumor cells, cancer cells divide nearly continuously. The gene changes that cause the cancer to form allow cancer cells to bypass the controls and restrictions on entering the cell cycle. Almost as soon as one round of mitosis is complete, the daughter cells begin a new round. In addition, cancer cells have an infinite life span that does not respond to apoptotic signals. This characteristic has been termed *immortality.* The persistence of cancer cell division makes cancer difficult to control.

■ Carcinogenesis/Oncogenesis

Carcinogenesis, oncogenesis, and malignant transformation are terms for the process of changing a normal cell into a cancer cell. As the term transformation implies, this process of carcinogenesis occurs through multiple steps. These steps are *initiation, promotion, progression,* and *metastasis* (Figure 1–3).

Initiation

The first step in carcinogenesis is initiation, and this occurs at the gene level. Initiation is the direct exposure of DNA to a carcinogen, resulting in irreversible changes that will permit malignant transformation. The initiated cell may appear somewhat abnormal, perhaps referred to as *dysplastic* or *premalignant,* but it is still able to function normally.

Several events are needed for carcinogenic exposure to result in initiation. The exposure must alter DNA structure—causing one or more breaks in the DNA chain (mutations), eliminating a genetic component, resulting in faulty DNA repair, or inserting new genetic information into the DNA strand. The change must be permanent and unrepairable.

Gene mutations (caused by exposure to carcinogens or by spontaneous DNA replication error) can activate proto-oncogenes and inactivate tumor suppressor genes. Any agent that can penetrate a cell, get into the nucleus, and damage the DNA can damage oncogenes and tumor suppressor genes. Substances that can irreversibly change the activity of

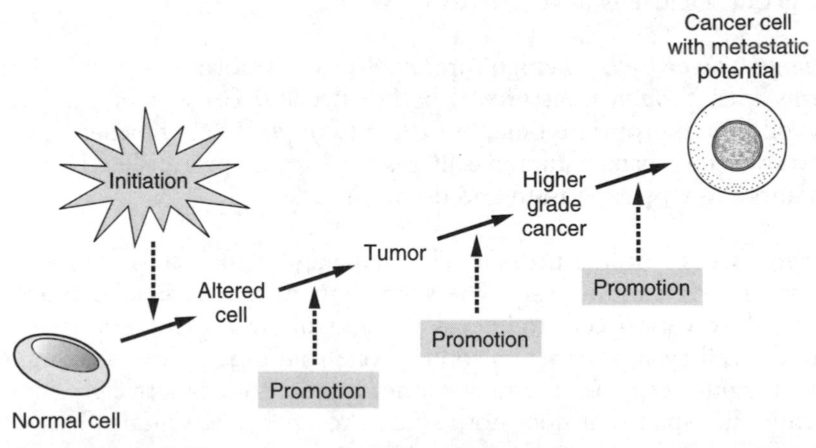

FIGURE 1–3 ■ The Steps of Carcinogenesis.

a cell's oncogenes and tumor suppressor genes are *carcinogens*. Carcinogens may be chemicals, physical agents, or viruses (see Chapter 2).

Once a cell has been initiated, it can become a cancer cell if it retains the ability to divide and if the cellular changes that occurred during initiation are enhanced by *promotion*. If the gene mutations prevent cell division, a tumor cannot form. However, it is possible for one mutated cell that has undergone malignant transformation to develop into widespread metastatic disease.

Promotion

Once a normal cell is initiated and becomes a cancer cell, growth enhancement can allow it to form a tumor. The time between a cell's initiation and development of an overt tumor may take months to years and is called the *latency period*. Substances that enhance growth of the initiated cancer cell are called *promoters*. Agents that promote tumor growth include chemicals, drugs, and hormones. In order for a tumor to form, initiation must be followed by promotion. If a person is first exposed to a promoter and then exposed to a pure carcinogen, the initiated cells do not form a tumor (Figure 1–4). Unlike those of initiators, the effects of promoters may be reversible if there are prolonged periods between exposures. Promoters have a definite threshold, that is, a specific minimum required dose or exposure, before their effect occurs (Figure 1–4).

Progression

After cancer cells have grown to the point that a detectable tumor is formed, other events are required for cancer to develop. At this point,

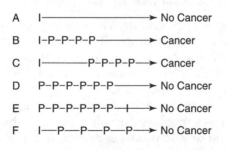

A I——————→ No Cancer

B I–P–P–P–P————→ Cancer

C I————P–P–P–P——→ Cancer

D P–P–P–P–P–P————→ No Cancer

E P–P–P–P–P–P——I——→ No Cancer

F I—P—P—P—P——→ No Cancer

FIGURE 1–4 ■ The Sequence of Initiation and Promotion Leading to Cancer Development.

Key: I = exposure to initiator; P = exposure to promoter.

the tumor must develop its own blood supply in order to survive. In early growth, the tumor receives nutrition only by diffusion. After the tumor reaches 1–2 mm in diameter, diffusion is not efficient. The tumor then makes *tumor angiogenesis factors,* which stimulate blood vessels in the area to grow new capillaries into the tumor.

Genetic instability within the colony of transformed cells results in the development of subpopulations that differ from each other in their growth properties, sensitivities to treatment modalities, and other such characteristics. Certain mutations eventually provide to one or more subpopulations a *selection advantage,* a mutation that enables survival despite environmental changes that are unfavorable to other tumor cell subpopulations. Changes that a tumor undergoes at this time can allow it to become even more malignant and less differentiated, expressing fewer and fewer normal cell features.

The original tumor or *primary tumor* is identified by the tissue from which it arose, such as in breast cancer or lung cancer. Primary tumors in vital organs can be lethal by severely damaging the vital organ or "crowding out" healthy organ tissue, reducing that organ's ability to perform vital functions. Primary tumors that develop in nonvital tissues can disrupt vital life processes by spreading into other areas.

Metastasis

Metastasis is the movement of cancer cells from the primary site location and the establishment of secondary tumors at remote sites. Although the metastasized tumor cells are now in a different organ, they are still known by the primary cancer type. Thus, when lung cancer metastasizes to the brain and the liver, the secondary tumors are still lung cancer cells in the brain and in the liver. Table 1–3 lists common sites of metastasis. Metastasis involves several distinct steps or processes known as the *metastatic cascade* (Figure 1–5).

1. *Vascularization or angiogenesis.* The tumor progresses in size and develops internal vascularization. Tumor angiogenesis factors stimulate growth and development of new blood vessels within the tumor; however, these newly formed vessels are often defective and are easily invaded by tumor cells.
2. *Invasion.* The malignancy extends into surrounding tissue by producing enzymes that dissolve substances that hold normal cells together. The tumor also produces agents that help move tumor cells into normal tissues.
3. *Intravasion.* The tumor penetrates into body cavities and blood vessels. Malignant cells produce enzymes that create holes in the capillary endothelium and allow cancer cells to escape.

TABLE 1–3 ■ Sites of Metastasis for Common Tumors

Cancer	Sites of Metastasis
Lung cancer	Lymph nodes, brain, bone, liver, pancreas
Colorectal cancer	Adjacent lymph nodes, liver
Breast cancer	Bone, brain, lung, liver
Leukemia	Visceral organs, central nervous system
Prostate cancer	Bone, adjacent lymph nodes, lung

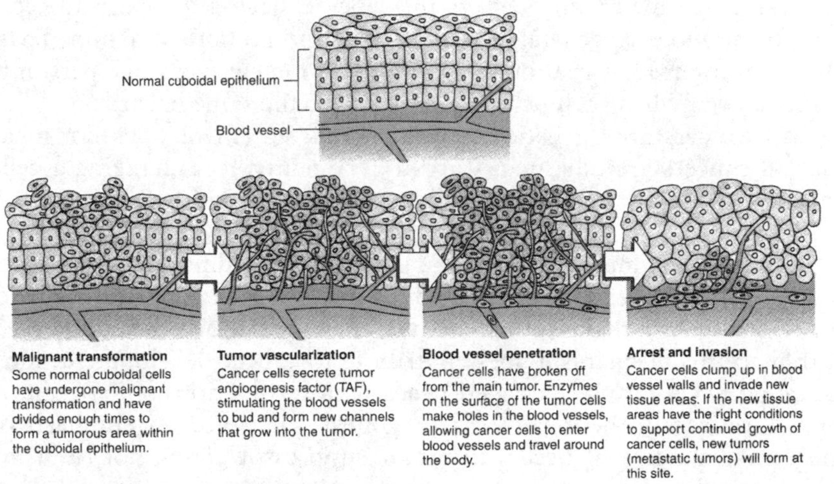

Normal cuboidal epithelium
Blood vessel
Malignant transformation
Some normal cuboidal cells have undergone malignant transformation and have divided enough times to form a tumorous area within the cuboidal epithelium.
Tumor vascularization
Cancer cells secrete tumor angiogenesis factor (TAF), stimulating the blood vessels to bud and form new channels that grow into the tumor.
Blood vessel penetration
Cancer cells have broken off from the main tumor. Enzymes on the surface of the tumor cells make holes in the blood vessels, allowing cancer cells to enter blood vessels and travel around the body.
Arrest and invasion
Cancer cells clump up in blood vessel walls and invade new tissue areas. If the new tissue areas have the right conditions to support continued growth of cancer cells, new tumors (metastatic tumors) will form at this site.

FIGURE 1–5 ■ The Metastatic Process.
Source: Ignatavicius, D. & Workman, M. L. (Eds.), *Medical-surgical nursing: Critical thinking for collaborative care* (4th ed.), Philadelphia: W. B. Saunders.

4. *Embolization and transport.* Tumor cells are carried to other body sites. En route, they interact with platelets, lymphocytes, fibrinogen, and other host-protective influences. It is estimated that only 1% of tumor cells reaching this stage survive for 24 hours, with less than 0.01% establishing metastatic colonies.
5. *Arrest.* Tumor cells are eventually trapped in the capillary bed of the target organ. The cell or cell cluster adheres to the blood vessel walls, stimulating the coagulation cascade. Development of a fibrin meshwork around the malignant cell or cell cluster protects it from detection by the host's immune system.

6. *Extravasation* The tumor cell releases enzymes that dissolve the blood vessel membranes and allow the cell to invade the surrounding tissues.
7. *Establishment.* The malignant cells manipulate the new environment to promote growth and development of the metastatic colony. If it is unable to establish its own vascular supply in this new location, the new colony will die.

■ Genetic Factors in Cancer Development

Carcinogenesis takes years and depends on several tumor and personal factors. Three interacting factors influence cancer development: exposure to carcinogens, genetic predisposition, and immune function. These factors account for variation in cancer development from one person to another, even when each person is exposed to the same hazards.

All cancers are "genetic"; however, this statement does not mean that all cancers are inherited. Carcinogenesis involves changing a cell's genes, allowing activation of oncogenes and inactivation of tumor suppressor genes.

Carcinogens mutate or damage genes. At one time, it was believed that exposure to carcinogens acted mainly by damaging the DNA of proto-oncogenes, making them active when they should be suppressed. Although this mechanism does contribute to cancer development, most mutating events cause damaged genes to lose function, not to gain it. Therefore, recent theories of carcinogenesis place greater emphasis on the gene damage that occurs to tumor suppressor genes, not to proto-oncogenes. Damaging cancer suppressor genes would result in the loss of suppressive function and remove negative-feedback mechanisms that normally control the proto-oncogenes, thereby causing their activation to oncogene status. This theory makes DNA damage or mutation a prerequisite that allows cancer development. Table 1–4 lists some specific cancer suppressor genes that when damaged, allow specific cancers to develop. Table 1–5 lists oncogenes that when expressed, result in the development of specific cancers.

Some cancer development is sporadic, that is, it appears randomly, probably as a result of multiple carcinogenic exposures. Other cancers may also have a predictable pattern of inheritance within a family. Cancers that have a known hereditary type as well as a sporadic type include breast cancer, prostate cancer, ovarian cancer, colorectal cancer, retinoblastoma, Wilms' tumor, and melanoma. In addition, many cancers occur more commonly within a family kinship but do not have any recognizable pattern of inheritance (*familial cancer*). It is possible for some families to have different members who have sporadic, hereditary, and familial forms of one type of cancer.

TABLE 1–4 ■ Selected Malignancies Associated with Altered Suppressor Gene Activity

Suppressor Gene	Malignancies
APC	Colorectal, stomach, and pancreatic
ATM	Leukemia, lymphoma, breast, ovarian
BRCA1	Breast, ovarian
BRCA2	Breast, ovarian
CDK4	Melanoma
CDKN1C	Wilms' tumor, rhabdomyosarcoma
CDKN2A	Mesothelioma, melanoma
DCC	Colorectal
DPC4	Pancreatic, colon
EXT1	Osteosarcoma
FUS1	Lung
Ink4a	Melanoma
MEN1	Parathyroid, pituitary, adrenal, carcinoid, pancreatic islet cell
MLH1	Colorectal
MSH2	Colorectal
MTS1	Melanoma, brain tumors, leukemia, sarcomas, breast, bladder, ovarian, lung, kidney
NF1	Neurofibroma, colon, astrocytoma
NF2	Neurofibroma, meningioma, schwannoma
NKX3.1	Prostate
PTEN	Breast, prostate, endometrial
RB1	Retinoblastoma, sarcomas, breast, bladder, esophageal, small-cell lung
SMAD3	Prostate
TP53	Breast, bladder, colorectal, esophageal, liver, lung, ovarian, brain tumors, sarcomas, leukemia, lymphoma
VHL	Renal cell carcinoma, pheochromocytoma, hemangioblastoma
WT1	Wilms' tumor (nephroblastoma)

Sporadic Cancers

To prevent problems caused by damaged genes, we have DNA repair mechanisms that can fix mutations that occur as a result of either spontaneous DNA replication errors or exposure to carcinogens. How active these mechanisms are for any one person and how well they perform the repair are genetically determined. Some people have very

TABLE 1–5 ■ Selected Malignancies Associated with Altered Oncogene Activity

Oncogene	Malignancies
ABL1	Chronic myelogenous leukemia, other leukemias
BRAF	Gastric
CCND1	Breast
ERBB-1	Glioblastomas, squamous cell carcinoma
ERBB-2 (HER-2/*neu*)	Breast, salivary gland, ovarian carcinomas
FES	Acute promyelocytic leukemia, lung, bladder
HRAS	Breast, melanoma, lung, kidney, bladder, colon
JUN	Lung
Ki-*RAS*	Colorectal
MYC	Burkitt's lymphoma, T-cell & B-cell neoplasms, breast, gastric, lung
MYCL	Lung
MYCN	Small cell lung cancer, neuroblastoma
NRAS	Ovarian, thyroid, melanoma, leukemia
PRAD-1	Breast, squamous cell cancers
RET	Thyroid, multiple endocrine neoplasias
TRK	Colorectal, thyroid

efficient DNA repair mechanisms. Such people tend to have longevity and a low rate of cancer development, even when exposed to multiple environmental carcinogens. Other people have faulty DNA repair mechanisms that either do not recognize DNA mutations or do not repair them properly. These people have a higher risk for cancer development, even when carcinogenic exposure is minimal.

Every cancer suppressor gene is located on a specific chromosome. For example, the TP53 cancer suppressor gene is located on chromosome 17. Because you have a pair of number 17 chromosomes, technically you have a pair of TP53 genes. Both genes of this pair need to be active to adequately suppress certain oncogenes. Therefore, the TP53 gene on both of the number 17 chromosomes must be damaged to allow a specific cancer to develop. This is known as the "two-hit" mechanism of carcinogenesis.

Sporadic cancers occur when carcinogenic exposures "knock out" the activity of both of the TP53 genes. The carcinogenic hits often occur separately, and the risk for acquiring these hits increases with age. Age is thought to be a risk factor for cancer development for two reasons: (a) the longer a person lives, the more exposure to carcinogens he or she experiences and the greater the accumulation of DNA mutations, and (b) the efficiency of DNA repair decreases with age. The vast majority of cancers that develop in the United States are sporadic, with no specific pattern of inheritance.

Hereditary Cancer

Some people have a genetic risk or inherited predisposition for cancer development. The most common reason for this increased genetic risk is the inheritance of a mutation in a cancer suppressor gene. If one of a pair of cancer suppressor genes is mutated, the function of the gene pair is reduced by about 50% and the person's risk for cancer development is increased. If both pairs of a cancer suppressor gene are mutated and nonfunctional, the tasks of regulating apoptosis, repairing DNA damage, and suppressing oncogene activity are disrupted, and the person's risk for cancer development is greatly increased.

Only about 5%–10% of all cancers appear to be hereditary. For a gene mutation to be inherited, the mutation must be present in the germline cells (ova or sperm). Then, the mutation would be present in all of the newly created person's cells. This means that the person's cells are already initiated (the first hit has occurred), and only promotion is needed for a cancer to develop. Inherited cancers have several characteristics. First, they tend to appear in family members in a recognizable pattern of mendelian inheritance. Often, they appear in both of paired organs (e.g., cancer in both breasts), and they tend to have an earlier age of onset. For example, the average age of onset for sporadic colon cancer is between 60 and 70 years. The average age of onset for inherited colon cancer-associated APC mutations is the mid- to late 30s.

Familial Cancer

In some families, the incidence of cancer development (usually of more than one type of cancer) is higher than could be expected by chance alone, but there is no recognizable mendelian pattern of inheritance. It is thought that there may be a true genetic predisposition that is influenced by other environmental factors. This type of problem is multifactorial or polygenic. There is an increased susceptibility (i.e., difficult to quantify), but exposure to the proper carcinogen (or carcinogens) is needed at a susceptible time in order for a cancer to develop.

■ Conclusion

Carcinogenesis is a multistep process by which a normal cell undergoes progressive changes and ultimately becomes malignant. Among the many differences between normal cells and their cancerous counterparts is cancer's lack of response to normal cell growth control mechanisms. Cancer cells continue to divide despite limited space and nutritional resources. They also have the ability to separate from the primary tumor and migrate to other body sites.

Recent cancer research findings have enhanced understanding about carcinogenesis, the metastatic cascade, and genetic factors that influence tumor growth and development. Although much still needs to be known before improvements can be made in cancer treatment, nurses can play important roles in cancer prevention by educating consumers about known carcinogens in the environment and emphasizing the importance of reducing exposure.

■ Resources

Publications

Websites

Fred Hutchinson Cancer Center, Molecular Biology of Cancer: *www.fhcrc.org/education/courses/cancer_course/basic/molecular/*

Cell Biology and Cancer: *science.education.nih.gov/supplements/nih1/cancer/guide/pdfs/NIH_cancer.pdf*

Bibliography

Hanahan, D., & Weinberg, R. (2000). The hallmarks of cancer. *Cell, 100,* 57–70.

Loescher, L. (2003). The biology of cancer. In A. Tranin, A. Masny, & J. Jenkins (Eds.), *Genetics in oncology practice: Cancer risk assessment.* Pittsburgh: Oncology Nursing Society. Pp 23–56.

Macleod, K. (2000). Tumor suppressor genes. *Current Opinion in Genetics and Development, 10,* 81–93.

Peters, J., Loud, J., Dimond, E., & Jenkins, J. (2001). Cancer genetics fundamentals. *Cancer Nursing, 24,* 446–461.

Ruoslahti, E. (1996). How cancer spreads. *Scientific American, 275,* 72–77.

Workman, M.L. (2002). Altered cell growth and cancer development. In D. Ignatavicius & M. L. Workman (Eds.), *Medical-surgical nursing: Critical thinking for collaborative care* (4th ed.), Philadelphia: W. B. Saunders. pp 407–422.

CHAPTER

2

Epidemiology of Cancer

Kimberly Rohan

Susan Budds

The American Cancer Society estimates that 1,368,030 people will be diagnosed with cancer in the United States in 2004. This number does not include the common skin cancers, basal cell and squamous cell, or noninvasive cancers (carcinoma in situ) except for bladder malignancies. Approximately 563,700 people will die of their disease this year, more than half of them from lung, colorectal, breast, or prostate cancer. Cancer continues to be the second leading cause of death in the United States. Although these numbers are dramatic and troubling, it is also important to recognize that the 5-year survival rates for cancer have steadily improved and that today, 62% of those diagnosed with cancer can expect to be alive in 5 years. In fact, both incidence and mortality rates for cancer have dropped approximately 1% per year since 1991, and there are nearly 9 million Americans living with a cancer diagnosis today. Cancer is disproportionately a disease of the elderly, and as the US population ages, we can expect an increasing number of people to be diagnosed with cancer. The total population is increasing, which also contributes to the increasing number of people diagnosed each year. One particularly encouraging trend is that increasingly, new cases are diagnosed at early stages, which should further increase survival rates.

Great strides in the prevention, early detection, and treatment of many types of cancer are reflected in overall declining incidence and mortality rates. The American Cancer Society has established the goal of a 25% reduction in the overall age-adjusted cancer incidence rate and a 50% reduction in the overall age-adjusted cancer mortality rate by 2015. Nurses should play a pivotal role in the attainment of these goals through active involvement in cancer prevention and early detection activities. In order to do this, nurses must understand basic concepts of epidemiology. This chapter acquaints the reader with basic concepts of epidemiology as they relate to cancer.

Epidemiology is the study of the incidence, prevalence, and mortality and identification of causes of disease in populations by the collection and analysis of statistical data. The analysis of prevalence, incidence, and mortality data help quantify the impact of cancer and cancer control efforts on the population.

■ Incidence and Mortality

Incidence refers to the number of new events or cases of a disease. *Incidence rate* is the number of people per 100,000 who are diagnosed with cancer within a specified period of time, usually 1 year. Incidence rates can be used to evaluate the changing patterns of disease occurrence within a population. *Mortality* refers to the number of deaths due to a disease. This may be expressed as a *mortality rate,* which is the number of deaths per 100,000 people; this statistic allows comparison between populations. Cancer mortality rates reflect the overall risk of dying of cancer in a specific population.

Currently, the American Cancer Society uses data that are age adjusted to the 2000 US standard population. This method allows more accurate contemporary comparisons among populations with different age distributions. This is important when cancer rates are examined because cancer is more often a disease of older people, and comparing elderly and younger populations as if they were the same would skew the analysis of data. For example, unless data were adjusted for age, Florida, which has a relatively large elderly population, would appear to have a higher incidence of, and death rate from, cancer than a state like Alaska, which has a younger population. Once that adjustment is made, the interpretation of data comparison is more accurate.

Prevalence is the number of existing cases of cancer in a given population at a specific time. *Survival rate* represents the percentage of persons alive 5 years after diagnosis, whether cured, in remission, or with evidence of disease. This rate is usually adjusted for normal life expectancy and is described as the *5-year relative survival rate*. These rates are useful in monitoring progress in cancer diagnosis and treatment, but they do not provide a complete picture. Differences between patients who are permanently cured and those who survive beyond 5 years but subsequently die of their cancer are not reflected in the 5-year relative survival rate data. For this reason, survival rates at other time points should also be considered.

Risk Factors

Epidemiologic features, when statistically associated with incidence of disease, identify a *risk factor.* Each of these factors becomes a part of the estimation of the likelihood of developing cancer. Many risk factors decrease or increase one's risk of developing the disease. This sometimes raises questions for further study, to define more clearly the significance of an identified risk factor. Risk can be expressed as *lifetime risk,* the probability of developing cancer over the course of one's life, or *relative risk,* the risk of developing cancer because of a biologic trait or exposure compared with the risk in someone who does not have that trait or exposure. Risk factors can be categorized as either endogenous or exogenous. Endogenous risk factors are risk factors that come from a genetic predisposition to a specific disease state, such as in a woman who carries the *BRCA1* gene mutation and would therefore be considered to have an endogenous risk factor. Typically, endogenous risk factors are beyond one's control to change in any way. Other examples include one's sex, age, race, or family history. Exogenous risk factors are environmental and are sometimes within one's control. Examples of exogenous risk factors include alcohol intake, diet, exercise, occupational exposure, cigarette smoking, and sexual activity. It is believed that 80% of all cancers may be associated with exogenous exposures that can be modified by personal behavior, thereby reducing cancer risk significantly. Table 2–1 lists known risk factors for common cancers.

Factors Influencing Cancer Risk and Mortality There are multiple factors that affect cancer risk, incidence, and mortality. Age, gender, race, ethnicity, and socioeconomic status are some of the most significant exogenous factors.

Age The incidence increases with age for nearly all cancers in adults. Approximately three fourths of all cancers occur in people over the age of 55. With the increasing age of the US population, the overall number of new cases of cancer diagnosed annually is expected to increase. Explanations for this increase include diminished DNA repair with age, decline in immune function and ability to recognize abnormal cells, and increased exposure to carcinogens over time.

TABLE 2–1 ■ Risk Factors and Signs and Symptoms of Common Cancers

Cancer Site	Risk Factors	Signs and Symptoms
Breast	• Female gender • Age >50 years • Family history • Personal history of breast cancer • 2 or more first-degree relatives • Known *BRCA1* or *BRCA2* mutation • Biopsy history • Atypical hyperplasia • DCIS or LCIS • Postmenopausal obesity • Early menarche/late menopause • Late first pregnancy/nulliparous • Oral contraceptives • Radiation to the chest wall • Alcohol • Obesity and high-fat diet • Hormone replacement therapy	• Lump or mass • Thickening in breast or axilla • Change in size or contour or texture • Skin dimpling or retraction • Peau d'orange skin • Nipple discharge, retraction, or scaliness • Erythema • Pain or tenderness
Prostate	• Male gender • Age > 50 years • African American ethnicity • Family history of first-degree relative (greater if first-degree relative diagnosed before age 40) • High-fat diet	• Weak urinary stream & urinary frequency • Difficulty in initiating stream or stopping urinary stream • Pain or burning on urination • Urinary retention • Hematuria

TABLE 2–1 ■ Risk Factors and Signs and Symptoms of Common Cancers—*Continued*

Cancer Site	Risk Factors	Signs and Symptoms
Colorectal	• Age > 60 years • Inflammatory bowel conditions • Sedentary lifestyle • Diet high in fat and low in fruits and vegetables • Heavy alcohol consumption • Family history of colorectal cancer especially if before the age of 40 • Familial genetic syndromes, e.g., familial adenomatous polyposis (FAP) and hereditary nonpolyposis colon cancer (HNPCC)	• Change in bowel habits • Rectal bleeding • Abdominal pain • Decreased diameter of stools • Anemia • Rectal pressure or pain • Weight loss • Anorexia
Lung	• Cigarette smoking • Occupational exposure to asbestos, arsenic, chromium, coal products, nickel refining, smelter workers, ionizing radiation, radon • Second-hand smoke	• Chronic cough and wheezing • Persistent respiratory infections • Dull chest pain • Hemoptysis • Dyspnea • Weight loss

Key: DCIS = ductal carcinoma in situ; LCIS = lobular carcinoma in situ.

Gender Overall cancer incidence in males has stabilized in recent years when compared with that in females. Men have a higher lifetime probability of developing and dying of cancer than women, but men have a greater recent decline in death rates. The three leading cancer types for men are prostate, lung, and colorectal. Lung cancer is the leading cause of death for males over the age of 40. For men aged 40–79 years, colorectal cancer is the second most common fatal cancer. For men aged 20–years, cancer is the fifth leading cause of death.

Overall cancer incidence has increased more in females than in males. Females have a higher probability of developing cancer when they are younger than 60 years. The three leading cancer types in order of occurrence are breast, lung, and colorectal cancer. The leading causes of cancer deaths in order of frequency for women are lung, breast and colorectal. Lung cancer mortality rates for women are expected to peak by the year 2010, largely because smoking causes damage over time. Although the prevalence of smoking may be decreasing overall, cancers related to smoking will continue to increase, and they are often diagnosed at later stages. Women have a slightly lower lifetime risk of developing cancer than men. Among women aged 20–59 years, breast cancer is the leading cause of death, and for women aged 60 years and older, lung cancer is the leading cause of cancer deaths. For males and females under the age of 20, leukemia is the most common fatal cancer.

Childhood Overall, cancer is the leading cause of death due to disease in children between 1 and 14 years of age. It is second only to accidents as the most common cause of death. Leukemia (acute lymphocytic leukemia), central and sympathetic nervous system tumors, lymphomas, soft-tissue sarcomas, and renal tumors are the most common cancers in children. The 5-year survival rates are encouraging. For the years 1992–1999, the 5-year survival for acute lymphocytic leukemia increased to 85%, compared with 69% in 1983–1985; for brain and other nervous system cancer, the 5-year survival was 71%, compared with 63% in 1983–1985. The mortality rate for all childhood cancers combined has declined by 47% since 1975. The progress seen in survival is due primarily to advances in treatment options for these tumors (see Table 2–2 for age-related cancer deaths).

Race and Ethnicity No scientifically accepted definition exists for race. There is an increase in multiethnicity in the US population, and differences among race and ethnicity should be interpreted with caution because these factors may not be classified uniformly among different sources. Socioeconomic factors may be more crucial than race in evaluating differences in incidence and mortality. Economics often limits access to care and influences personal health habits. Statistics related to race should be interpreted as descriptive. Some statistics stratified by race are noted in Table 2–3.

Hispanics Americans of Hispanic heritage is the fastest-growing minority group in the United States. Cancer incidence for Hispanic males decreased by 2.8% per year between 1992 and 1999. During that same time, cancer incidence decreased 0.6% in Hispanic females. Mortality decreased by 1.5 % per year in males and 1.1% in females during

TABLE 2–2 ▪ Cause of Cancer Death by Age

Age (yrs)	Males	Females
20–39	1. Brain/CNS 2. Leukemia 3. Lung	1. Breast 2. Uterine/cervix 3. Leukemia
40–59	1. Lung 2. Colorectal 3. Pancreas	1. Breast 2. Lung 4. Colorectal
60–79	1. Lung 2. Colorectal 3. Prostate	1. Lung 2. Breast 3. Colorectal
> 80	1. Lung 2. Prostate 3. Colorectal	1. Lung 2. Colorectal 3. Breast

Key: CNS = central nervous system.

those years. Although these statistics are encouraging for this population, Hispanic women with breast cancer have lower survival rates than their White counterparts, possibly because of later diagnosis and barriers in access to high-quality care. Current data suggest an increased use of mammography among Hispanic women, and rates are now similar to those of non-Hispanic whites. Breast cancer death rates could decline with this trend. The incidence and mortality of stomach, liver, gallbladder, and cervical cancers is higher among Hispanics than the general population and is especially high among first-generation immigrants to the United States. The incidence and mortality rates of all cancer types combined and for the most common cancers individually (breast, prostate, lung, and colorectal) are lower among Hispanics than in the general population. This is most likely related to cultural differences in health beliefs, dietary practices, language barriers, and socioeconomic status. As Hispanics adopt a more westernized culture, their cancer rates become similar to those of non-Hispanics. Obesity in Hispanic people, especially Hispanic women, is increasing and contributes to the increased incidence of cancer; obesity is a known risk factor for the development of cancers such as endometrial, breast, liver, gallbladder, and colon. Gallbladder cancer is more common in Hispanics than in any other studied ethnic group. This cancer is believed to be linked to chronic gallstones, a condition that is more common among Hispanics.

TABLE 2–3 ■ Incidence and Mortality Rates* by Site, Race and Ethnicity, United States, 1992–1999

Incidence	White	African American	Asian/ Pacific Islander	American Indian/ Alaskan Native	Hispanic
All Sites					
Males	568.2	703.6	408.9	277.7	393.1
Females	424.4	404.8	306.5	224.2	290.5
Total	480.4	526.6	348.6	244.6	329.6
Breast (female)	137.0	120.7	93.4	59.4	82.6
Colon and rectum					
Males	64.4	70.7	58.7	40.7	43.9
Females	46.1	55.8	39.5	30.8	29.7
Total	53.9	61.9	47.9	35.2	35.7
Lung and bronchus					
Males	82.9	124.1	63.8	51.4	44.1
Females	51.1	53.2	28.5	23.3	22.8
Total	64.3	82.6	44.0	35.4	31.5
Prostate	172.9	275.3	107.2	60.7	127.6
Mortality	**White**	**African American**	**Asian/ Pacific Islander**	**American Indian/ Alaskan Native**	**Hispanic**
All Sites					
Males	258.1	369.0	160.6	154.5	163.7
Females	171.2	204.5	104.4	110.4	105.7
Total	205.1	267.3	128.6	128.6	129.2
Breast (female)	29.3	37.3	13.1	14.8	17.5
Colon and rectum					
Males	26.7	34.8	16.5	14.6	16.6
Females	18.4	25.4	11.6	11.3	10.6
Total	21.9	29.1	13.7	12.8	13.2
Lung and bronchus					
Males	81.7	113.0	42.3	49.3	38.2
Females	41.1	39.6	19.3	24.9	13.8
Total	57.9	68.9	29.3	35.5	24.1
Prostate	32.9	75.1	15.1	18.8	22.6

*Per 100,000, age-adjusted to the 2000 US standard population. Incidence rates obtained from SEER registries covering 10%–15% of the US population. Mortality data are from all states.

Hispanics are not mutually exclusive from whites, African Americans, Asian/Pacific Islanders, and American Indian/Alaskan Natives.

Source: Surveillance, Epidemiology, and End Results Program, 1973–99, Division of Cancer Control and Population Sciences, National Cancer Institute, Bethesda, MD, 2002.

American Cancer Society, Surveillance Research, 2003

The three most common cancers for Hispanic men are prostate, colorectal, and lung, with the highest death rate being from lung cancer. For Hispanic women, the three most common cancers are breast, colorectal, and lung; breast cancer is the leading cause of cancer death.

African Americans African Americans continue to have the highest incidence and death rates, later stage at diagnosis, and reduced probability of survival than any racial or ethnic group. Incidence and mortality rates have dropped significantly since 1992 but are still higher than those for all other groups. This rate may be related to socioeconomic factors, unequal access to care, and higher prevalence of comorbidities. Cancer incidence for African Americans is 10% higher than whites, 50%–60% higher than Hispanics and Asians/Pacific islanders, and two times higher than American Indians. African Americans' death rate is 30% higher than whites and two times higher than Asian Pacific Islanders, American Indians, and Hispanics. The incidence of prostate cancer in African American males was 58% higher than in white men in 1999; the reason for this disparity is not certain. As conditions improve for this population, further improvements in cancer statistics should be seen. Lung cancer causes the highest number of cancer deaths in African American males; prostate cancer is the second and colorectal cancer the third leading cause of cancer deaths. Breast cancer is the most common cancer among African American women. The incidence is significantly lower than that of white women, but death rates for breast cancer are 28% higher than in white women. This difference may be due to several factors, including later diagnosis, less access to care, or greater incidence of more aggressive forms of breast cancer. Lung cancer is the second most common cancer in African American women, and it is the leading cause of cancer death.

American Indian/Alaskan Natives This population represents 560 federally recognized tribes and more than 100 state-recognized tribes, each of which has its own unique culture. Because of the differences among this group, it is difficult to reach conclusions from aggregate statistics. Overall, this population has the lowest incidence rates for breast, colorectal, and lung cancers, and for all cancer sites combined, of any U.S. racial or ethnic group. As a group, they showed a relatively stable incidence from 1992–1999, and mortality decreased by 1.2% annually during that same period. Among American Indian/Alaskan Native females, the most common cancer is breast cancer. For males, the most common cancer is prostate cancer. Mortality rates from the same analysis show that the most common cause of cancer death for females and males is lung cancer. This is probably due to smoking patterns and access to care. According to most recent Surveillance, Epidemiology, and End Results (SEER) data, this group has the lowest survival rates for cancer of the breast, lung, and prostate and for all cancer combined compared than any other ethnic group. This is most likely related to socioeconomic factors that limit access to care for screening, diagnosis, and treatment.

Asian American/Pacific Islanders Asians and Pacific Islanders make up one of the fastest-growing populations in the United States, increasing by more than 40% between 1990 and 2000. They showed a stable incidence of cancer during 1992–1999. Mortality decreased by 1.2 % annually from 1992–1999. Among females, breast cancer is the most common cancer, and prostate cancer has the highest incidence among males. Lung cancer is the most common cause of cancer death for both males and females. Liver cancer is common among this racial/ethnic group; it is the third leading cause of cancer death in Asian Americans because of high rates of exposure to, and infection with, the hepatitis B virus in immigrant Asian populations. Hepatitis B is a known cause of liver cancer. SEER data show that Asian Americans tended to be diagnosed as having cancer at older ages than other ethnic groups, most likely because of their longer life expectancy.

■ The Role of the Nurse

The interaction of nurses with patients in a wide array of settings provides them with multiple opportunities to educate individuals, families, and groups about cancer risks and risk-reduction strategies. For example, school nurses can educate children, parents, and teachers about the importance of diet, exercise, and physical activity in primary cancer prevention. These nurses can begin to educate young girls and boys about early cancer detection, and these discussions can be part of routine school physicals. Avoidance of tobacco products and overexposure to the sun should be part of the health education by nurses everywhere. Appropriate cancer screening can and should be encouraged by nurses practicing in any setting. Nurses working in many settings have the opportunity to develop long-term relationships with patients and their families, affording nurses multiple opportunities to provide patient education about cancer prevention and screening. As part of annual physicals, nurses can develop strategies for monitoring and teaching about cancer prevention and screening guidelines. Education about tobacco and nutrition affects not only the risk for developing cancer but also the risk for development of diabetes, heart disease, and nonneoplastic lung disease. It is essential for nurses in these settings to establish a mechanism for documenting these conversations but more importantly to assess the risk behaviors of individuals and to establish a dialogue. The American Cancer Society offers many excellent brochures and programs that can assist a nurse in teaching about cancer risks and risk reduction. Providing various pamphlets in the waiting and examination rooms for patients and families to read often stimulates questions and dialogue with the health care providers.

Nurses interacting with hospitalized patients may find that patients and families are particularly anxious to understand cancer risks and risk-reduction strategies when someone close to them has been hospitalized with a diagnosis of cancer or for testing to rule out a malignancy. They also have other health care providers available to assist in that teaching.

Making a health behavior change is difficult for most people. Nurses play an important role in helping people recognize the risks, identify possible behavior changes, and consistently reinforce their attempts at making those changes. Helping people make small changes that will positively affect their health in a cumulative way is rewarding for both the nurse and the individual. Being a positive role model can have perhaps the most significant impact in promoting health among those with whom a nurse comes in contact. Nurses who eat a well-balanced diet, exercise, avoid tobacco, and follow cancer screening guidelines give positive behavioral messages about health.

It is essential that nurses in any setting understand trends in cancer incidence, mortality, and survival rates; be knowledgeable about cancer risk factors; and use every opportunity to assist those in our care to reduce their cancer risk. We can have a positive impact on the health of our patients and our community when our knowledge is up to date and our messages accurate and positive.

■ Resources

The American Cancer Society's Cancer Facts and Figures series is available online at *www.cancer.org*.

Bibliography

American Cancer Society. (2003). *Cancer facts & figures for African Americans 2003–2004.*

American Cancer Society. (2003). *Cancer facts & figures for Hispanics/Latinos 2003–2005.* Retrieved July 2003, cancer.org

Brittain, A. (Ed.). (2003) *Cancer: What causes it, what doesn't.* Atlanta: American Cancer Society.

Jemal, A., Murray, T., Samuels, A., Ghafoor, A., Ward, E., Thun, M. (2003). Cancer statistics, 2003. *CA: A Cancer Journal for Clinicians, 53,* 5–26.

CHAPTER

3

Cancer Screening, Early Detection, Risk Reduction, and Genetic Counseling

Marilyn Frank-Stromborg

This chapter addresses the issues surrounding cancer screening and early detection, risk-reduction behaviors, and genetic counseling. Cancer screening and early detection are part of secondary cancer prevention (the early detection and diagnosis of cancer), and they have become an essential part of cancer care in the United States. By detecting cancer at the earliest stage possible, curing it or slowing its progression, preventing complications, and limiting disability, both length and quality of life can be maximized.

Cancer screening, that is, the search for disease in persons without symptoms, is an organized effort to find cancer in its early stages in a defined population. Screening is conducted at intermittent time intervals and is usually site specific. Nurses frequently play an important role in educating the public about screening programs and in conducting screening tests. Once a person has had a positive screening test result, or once signs or symptoms have been identified, further tests are considered diagnostic.

Early detection is the identification of disease in an individual—when it is still localized, curable, or manageable—or the identification of a precancerous lesion. The individual may or may not be asymptomatic, and identification is made through tests, examinations, and observations. In an era of health care cost containment and limited funding, existing resources must be focused on screening and early-detection of cancers that have a high incidence and in which early diagnosis contributes to increased survival.

In the secondary prevention of cancer, nurses' responsibilities may include assessment, counseling, teaching, screening and detection, and planning, as well as being an advocate and role model. An emerging role for nurses is providing information to the public about available resources in their community and on the Internet to assist them in making decisions related to cancer prevention and early detection. Nurses in advanced-practice roles conduct screening and detection tests, such as Papanicolaou smears, clinical breast examinations, and physical examinations. In addition to fulfilling these roles, nurses provide support and guidance while performing these functions.

■ Screening Issues

Many issues are involved in screening specific populations, in particular, cost containment, limited state and federal funding, and managed care. Questions raised about screening include the following: Can screening recommendations by the American Cancer Society or the National Cancer Institute decrease deaths from cancer? Are they cost effective? How can their performance be optimized?

An implicit assumption underlying any screening program is that early detection will lead to a more favorable prognosis because treatment begun early in the disease course will be more effective than later treatment. This assumption holds true for some cancers, such as cervical and colorectal cancer, but it is not true for others, such as lung cancer. Research has shown that using routine cytology and x-ray studies on people who smoke heavily has no effect in reducing lung cancer mortality. Thus, the American Cancer Society and other groups do not recommend that smokers be screened yearly for lung cancer with the use of these methods. However, using spiral computed tomography to screen high-risk asymptomatic individuals for lung cancer has been encouraging. Several large randomized clinical trials of lung cancer screening are taking place in the United States and Europe and may provide evidence that early detection with spiral computed tomography lowers mortality from lung cancer. Table 3–1 summarizes The American Cancer Society's recommendations for the early detection of cancer in asymptomatic individuals. These should be incorporated into the regular physical examination as appropriate. Federal legislation in the early 1990s mandated Medicare coverage for cervical and breast cancer screening; this has enhanced compliance with the American Cancer

TABLE 3-1 ■ Guidelines for the Early Detection of Cancer in Asymptomatic People

Site	Recommendation
Breast	Women age 40 and older should have a mammogram every year, and should continue to do so for as long as they are in good health. Women in their 20s and 30s should have a clinical breast examination (CBE) as part of a periodic (regular) health exam by a health professional preferably every 3 years. Starting at age 40, women should have a breast exam by a health professional every year. Women should report any breast changes to their health professional right away. BSE is an option for women starting in their 20s. Women should be told about the benefits and limitations of BSE. Women at increased risk (e.g., family history, genetic tendency, past breast cancer) should talk with their doctor about the benefits and limitations of starting mammograms when they are younger or having additional tests (e.g., breast ultrasound or MRI).
Colon & rectum	Beginning at age 50, men and women should follow one of the examination schedules below: • A fecal occult blood test (FOBT) every year • A flexible sigmoidoscopy (FSIG) every 5 years • Annual fecal occult blood test and flexible sigmoidoscopy every 5 years • Annual double-contrast barium enema every 5 years • A colonoscopy every 10 years • Combined testing is performed over either annual FOBT, or FSIG every 5 years, alone. People who are at moderate or high risk for colorectal cancer should talk with a doctor about a different testing schedule.
Prostate	The PSA test and the digital rectal examination should be offered annually, beginning at age 50, to men who have a life expectancy of at least 10 years. Men at high risk (African American men and men with a strong family history of one or more first-degree relatives diagnosed with prostate cancer at an early age) should begin testing at age 45. For both men at average risk and high risk, information should be provided about what is known and what is uncertain about the benefits and limitations of early detection and treatment of prostate cancer so that they can make an informed decision about testing.
Uterus	Cervix: Screening should begin approximately 3 years after a woman begins having vaginal intercourse, but no later than 21 years of age. Screening should be done every year with regular Pap tests or every 2 years using liquid-based tests. At or after age 30, women who have had three normal test results in a row may get screening every 2–3 years. However, doctors may suggest a woman get screening more often if she has certain risk factors, such as HIV infection or a

(continued)

TABLE 3-1 ■ Guidelines for the Early Detection of Cancer in Asymptomatic People—*Continued*

Site	Recommendation
	weak immune system. Women 70 years and older who have had three or more consecutive normal Pap tests in the last 10 years may choose to stop cervical cancer screening. Screening after total hysterectomy (with removal of the cervix) is not necessary unless the surgery was done as treatment for cervical cancer.
	Endometrium: The American Cancer Society recommends that all women should be informed about the risks and symptoms of endometrial cancer, and strongly encouraged to report any unexpected bleeding or spotting to their physicians. Annual screening for endometrial cancer with endometrial biopsy beginning at age 35 should be offered to women with or at risk for hereditary nonpolyposis colon cancer (HNPCC).
Cancer-related checkup	For individuals undergoing periodic health examinations, a cancer-related checkup should include health counseling, and depending on a person's age, might include examinations for cancers of the thyroid, oral cavity, skin, lymph nodes, testes, and ovaries, as well as for some nonmalignant diseases.

Source: The American Cancer Society. (2004). Cancer facts and figures—2004 (no. 5008.04). Atlanta: Author.

Society recommendations. For women over the age of 65, Medicare Part B currently covers a Papanicolaou smear and a mammogram every 2 years. Since 2000, Medicare has also allowed average-risk beneficiaries to have a screening colonoscopy once every 10 years. As a result of this coverage, many men and women are able to take advantage of national screening recommendations.

Certain inherent characteristics must be present in a cancer for screening to be cost effective and efficient:

- The cancer must have a poor prognosis when symptoms appear.
- There must be a high prevalence of the cancer in the population being screened.
- The cancer must be detectable in the presymptomatic stage.
- There must be an improved prognosis when the cancer is found by screening.
- There must be consensus on the efficacy of treatment for the early stages of this disease.
- The test to detect the cancer must be available.

It is important for nurses to be aware of cancer screening recommendations so that they can promote those tests that have been shown to reduce cancer deaths, increase the percentage of cases that are detected in the early stages, reduce cancer complications, prevent or reduce cancer recurrences or metastases, and improve the quality of life of screened individuals.

Another issue that arises with cancer screening concerns the sensitivity, specificity, and predictive value of the screening test itself. The screening test should be able to detect cancer before the onset of signs and symptoms. *Specificity* is defined as the probability that a screening test will correctly classify an individual as negative for cancer when the individual does not have the disease. In contrast, *sensitivity* is defined as the probability that a screening test will correctly classify an individual as positive for cancer when that person actually does have the disease. The *predictive value* of a test refers to the percentage of persons with positive screening test results who actually have cancer. Presently, there is no perfect test. Generally, the more sensitive a test is, the less specific it will be, and a balance must be struck between the two indices of sensitivity and specificity.

In tests with less than 100% sensitivity, a proportion of preclinical cancers are not diagnosed at screening. A major problem with tests with low sensitivity is that they lead individuals to believe that they do not have cancer. In contrast, in tests with less than 100% specificity, false-positive results are expected. Tests with low specificity not only overwhelm diagnostic services and result in prohibitive follow-up costs, but they also expose individuals to the risks of unnecessary diagnostic work-ups, resulting in potentially substantial physical and psychological morbidity and possible mortality. This is one of the issues with the use of prostate-specific antigen to detect prostate cancer because the argument is that the test detects and consequently leads to the treatment of some clinically insignificant tumors. Another concern with the prostate-specific antigen test is that many men with benign conditions, such as benign prostatic hypertrophy, have elevated prostate-specific antigen levels, and thus the test yields numerous false-positive results. The consequences are that many men may be subjected to unnecessary prostate needle biopsies to rule out the possibility of prostate cancer. Therefore, the current recommendation to test for prostate cancer is to offer the test, and then discuss the benefits and limitations of further testing so that men can make an informed decision about testing.

The cost-benefit ratios are favorable for screening for cervical and colorectal cancers. Less is known about the cost-benefit ratios for screening for cancers of the stomach, esophagus, bladder, or liver.

It is known that sensitivity and specificity can vary from setting to setting. Factors that can influence these two indices include optimal laboratory practice and clinical expertise. Nurses can have a substantial impact on the accuracy of such screening techniques as the Papanicolaou smear, digital rectal examination for prostate cancer, colonoscopy or sigmoidoscopy for colorectal cancer, and physical breast examination. For instance, nurses assisting with either sigmoidoscopy or colonoscopy can make sure that the patient (a) has been given all bowel and diet instructions to ensure the success of the test, (b) understands the preparation necessary to ensure that the bowel is thoroughly emptied before the procedure, (c) is contacted the day before the test to review the preparation procedure and answer any questions, and (d) is given information after the test about the specific recommended interval frequency for screening based on the results of the screening test.

Effective screening practices should begin with a health history and physical examination. The accuracy and completeness of history taking and physical examination are essential to a differential diagnosis. Information gathered during history taking includes medical, family, social, occupation, and sexual background. When obtaining the health history, the nurse should make sure that every individual is asked about known risk factors and early symptoms of cancer. This is an excellent opportunity for the nurse to educate the individual about behaviors that can reduce risks, what specific symptoms merit medical attention, and the recommended early-detection tests that have been proved to assist in lowering death rates from cancer. The nurse may also gather information about exposure to cancer-causing agents, high-risk personal habits (e.g., tobacco use, excessive alcohol use, infection with human papillomavirus, obesity, and lack of exercise), and membership in a particular racial or ethnic group (e.g., Hispanic, African American, Native American, Asian), all of which may influence the individual's risks for cancer. It is essential that the nurse devote time to securing a thorough family history and, if necessary, assist the patient by drawing a pedigree chart. A pedigree chart frequently helps the patient visually see relationships and avoid including "kin" that are not blood relatives. The history may lead to the detection of vague symptoms that the patient may be unaware of or be denying. A comprehensive history enables the nurse to more effectively counsel the patient about their cancer risks and what specific prevention/detection strategies are recommended. This thorough history taking is followed by the physical examination of body systems, which includes inspection, palpation, percussion, and auscultation.

The screening process is more than a set of examinations and tests. It is an excellent opportunity for nurses to educate patients about self-examination techniques, stop-smoking programs, the importance of nutrition and physical activity in reducing cancer risk, weight reduction programs, and personal and occupational health hazards. Table 3–2 lists the nursing interventions that can be implemented to assist in

TABLE 3-2 ■ Nursing Interventions to Promote Risk Reduction Behaviors

Risk Factor	Nursing Interventions
Tobacco use	• Advocate politically for decreasing access to tobacco for minors and smoke-free environments. • Provide smokers with specific information on effective methods for stopping smoking and community resources to assist them, including counseling. • Provide young people with specific information on the short- and long-term health consequences of smoking.
Nutrition and diet	• Provide individuals with material that details what constitutes healthy eating and the community resources to support their efforts to adopt health diets. • Provide young people with information on healthy diets that will ensure them healthy bodies, lifestyles, and optimal weight. • Advocate for healthy food in settings focused on young people (e.g., schools, camps, recreational parks, day care centers).
Physical Activity	• Explain that physical activity is one of the most easy cancer risk factors to modify and thus decrease the risk of cancer. • Assist individuals to increase their physical activity level by supplying information on community resources that will help them adopt a healthier lifestyle. • Advocate for more opportunities in the work setting for employees to have physical activity.
Ultraviolet Radiation	• Provide information on how to safely enjoy the sun: use SPF of at least 15, use wide-brimmed hats and protective clothing. • Provide information on the known long-term dangers of using tanning salons and healthy alternatives to using tanning salons. • Educate high-risk individuals on how to do skin self-assessments.
Environment factors	• Provide individuals with the information necessary for them to make the appropriate lifestyle changes to limit or decrease their exposure to known carcinogens. • Advocate politically for changes to decrease environmental carcinogens (e.g., clean air, clean water).
Occupational	• Assist individuals in identifying unhealthy exposure in their workplace and the most effective means of reducing or eliminating these exposures. • Explore the occupational hazards the individual is exposed to, workplace recommendations for decreasing these exposures, and compliance with these recommendations. Explore ways to increase compliance if necessary.

(continued)

TABLE 3-2 ■ Nursing Interventions to Promote Risk Reduction Behaviors—*Continued*

Risk Factor	Nursing Interventions
Alcohol	• Provide information on what defines moderately using alcohol.
Estrogen	• Counsel about the risks vs benefits of using hormone replacement • Provide resources for obtaining scientifically sound information as new research emerges on use of hormone replacement.
Increasing age	• Provide materials that explain the relationship between increasing age and rising incidence of cancer. • Provide materials and community resources that will help the elderly obtain appropriate cancer screening tests.

Note: All information supplied should be age, educationally, and culturally appropriate for the individual the nurse is counseling. It is essential that nurses know their community resources and Internet sites that are easy to access and that will supply valid, reliable, and scientifically sound information to help the individual make informed decisions.

reducing high-risk factors. Because there is controversy about some of the high-risk factors, nurses can support individuals in making decisions by providing them with resources and reliable Internet sites for obtaining more information. The public is inundated with conflicting information about the prevention of cancer, and an essential nursing role is to help guide individuals to sources of information that provide factual, unbiased, scientifically sound information. Existing scientific evidence suggests that one third of cancer deaths occur each year because of smoking. Another one third of cancer deaths are caused by dietary factors. It is believed that more than two thirds of cancer-related deaths could be prevented by not smoking, making appropriate nutrition and dietary choices, and engaging in regular physical activity.

Patients can perform self-examination of breasts, testes, skin, and the oral cavity. The American Cancer Society has excellent materials to teach self-examination techniques that are available via the Internet.

Nurses can receive specialized training in screening techniques, such as oral examinations, pelvic examinations, rectal examinations, and breast examinations from organization-sponsored programs. Counseling, especially for high-risk individuals, is an integral part of care. Nurses who provide screening services can also make an important contribution by educating employers and third-party payers about the benefits of screening.

■ Counseling About Genetic Predisposition

The identification of genetic mutations associated with increased risk for certain cancers has created the demand for cancer predisposition testing and genetic counseling and education. About 5%–10% of cancers are thought to be related to hereditary factors. Nurses can play multiple roles in genetic counseling, depending on their educational preparation, interest level, and specialty training. The basic role for every nurse is to be able to provide information to patients about genetic testing, Internet sites to obtain more information, and appropriate referrals.

Some of the most important tasks for the nurse in the area of genetic counseling are to (a) identify those factors in the patient's history that warrant genetic services; (b) provide patients and families with genetic resources for informed decision making; (c) to obtain a patient and family medical history, including a three-generational pedigree chart to assist individuals in understanding family relationships and generational risks; (d) to assist patients in the identification of cancer risk factors related to their life and family history; and (e) to provide educational materials and community resources to assist in risk-reduction behavior and developing a healthy lifestyle. Nurses do not have to be experts in the genetics field to provide help to families in making the decision to seek genetic counseling. Rather, the nursing role that is most useful is to provide educational materials and resources that assist patients and their families in making decisions about seeking genetic counseling.

A difficult question to answer is when is it appropriate to refer a patient to a cancer genetics program? The following questions illustrate the clinical histories that merit making a referral. Remember that testing is a patient decision, and a referral to a genetic program does not imply that the patient must be tested.

- My mother's sisters and aunts have all been diagnosed with breast cancer. Should I have a genetic work-up?
  Yes, when there is cancer in two or more close relatives on the same side of the family, a referral for a work-up is merited.
- My aunt was found to have a mutation for cancer. Should I have a work-up?
  Yes, a referral is warranted when a blood relative has been tested and found to carry a mutation known to be associated with increased cancer risk.

- We were told that my father had prostate and colorectal cancer and that they were primary cancers, not metastatic spread. Should I have a genetic work-up?
  Yes, when there is a family history of a relative having multiple primary cancers, a genetic referral is appropriate. Also, if the family history includes bilateral cancer in paired organs, such as cancer of the ovary and breast, a referral should be made to a genetics clinic.
- I have multiple relatives with ovarian and breast cancer and a cousin with both of these cancers. Should I have a work-up?
  Yes, there are specific patterns of cancers known to comprise a cancer syndrome, and when these are present, the individual needs a referral to a genetics clinic. Another common hereditary cancer syndrome is hereditary nonpolyposis colon cancer, which is evidenced by early-onset colorectal cancer and other tumors, such as uterine and ovarian.
- I have a couple of relatives who have cancer at an earlier age than you would expect. For instance, my brother had colorectal cancer at age 35, and an aunt had breast cancer at age 29. Do I need to have a genetic work-up?
  Yes, a diagnosis of cancer at an earlier age than is seen in the general population is a common characteristic seen in families with a hereditary cancer syndrome.

Although genetic testing has many benefits, it also has significant risks and problems. The risks and benefits associated with genetic testing relate to whether the results were positive or negative, or whether there was a mutation of unknown clinical significance. In general, when the test results are positive, there is a removal of uncertainty and reduced anxiety because individuals know their genetic status and can make medical decisions about surveillance, chemoprevention, or prophylactic surgery. It may be the stimulus for increasing the individual's motivation to engage in positive health behaviors. However, there may also be feelings of depression, fear, or hopelessness and guilt that genetic mutations have been passed on to children. Individuals with positive results may fear discrimination by insurance companies/employers and concerns about the increased costs associated with cancer surveillance tests or risk-reduction interventions, such as prophylactic surgery, necessitated by the genetic mutations.

On the other hand, negative results may result in relief that (a) children cannot inherit the altered gene, (b) they do not have to worry about having an increased risk for the cancer, and, (c) they will not have to spend money on surveillance tests or surgery. These feelings may be tempered by survivor guilt, strained relationships within the family because they do not have the mutated gene, and the potential for the individual to think they are "home free" and do not have to adopt a healthy lifestyle or adhere to any cancer surveillance plan. Nurses need to be aware of the multiplicity of responses that can occur and follow up on patients referred for genetic counseling and testing to determine the type of responses they have. There may be a need for continuing psychological support of the patient and/or family, information to answer questions/concerns, or additional referrals based on the issues raised by the genetic testing.

■ Early Detection and Diagnosis Issues

As defined earlier, early detection refers to the application of screening tests that allow presumptive diagnoses of various cancers in asymptomatic persons. The process of cancer diagnosis involves the recognition of a complaint by the individual, its evaluation by a health care professional, and confirmation by laboratory tests or procedures (e.g., endoscopy).

One of the biggest issues concerning early detection and diagnosis of cancer is that the individual with the physical complaint or positive test result from a screening program is responsible for bringing himself or herself to the health care professional. It is not uncommon, once symptoms appear or the individual is told of the positive screening result, to delay seeking medical attention for months. Nurses can have an important role in decreasing this delay by (a) contacting people who have been through a screening program and have positive test results, and (b) discussing the importance of follow-up. Follow-up phone calls allow individuals to discuss the fears, apprehensions, and misconceptions they have about follow-up for a positive screening result. Nurses can reduce the misconceptions about cancer by providing accurate information about procedures and providing an opportunity for individuals to verbalize their fears. Many factors influence whether or not individuals access screening programs or follow-up once they experience symptoms or have a positive screening result. These factors are listed in Table 3–3, along with suggested nursing activities to decrease the barriers to accessing screening and early-detection programs.

Compliance, a significant issue in any discussion of cancer self-examination practices and early detection, is another area that merits further attention. Nurses can increase compliance by addressing the issue in a forthright manner. To teach self-examination techniques (e.g., breast self-examination, oral self-examination) effectively, the nurse

TABLE 3–3 ■ Factors Influencing Participation in Screening and Early Detection

Factor	Manifestation	Nursing Role
Delay	Individual may delay reporting symptom or follow-up on a positive test result for months.	1. Phone follow-up on positive test results found during a screening program. 2. Educate the public about national recommendations for cancer screening. 3. Include questioning about cancer risk factors in every health history.
Lack of knowledge of the early symptoms of cancer	Research documents that both the public and health care professionals are not knowledgeable about cancer screening national recommendations and early symptoms of the leading cancers. Ignorance results in lack of recognition that the symptom merits immediate attention.	1. Nurses must be familiar with the national symptoms of cancer as well as the early signs and symptoms of the most common cancers. 2. Educate the public about the national cancer screening recommendations as well as the early signs and symptoms of the most common cancers. 3. Encourage other health professionals to become familiar with the national cancer screening recommendations and early signs and symptoms of the most common cancers. 4. Post national cancer screening recommendations in areas that the public would see. 5. Computerized office reminder systems have been shown to be effective in improving cancer screening with medical settings.
Individual personality	Barriers to accessing screening programs or early detection: • low self-esteem • denial • fear • embarrassment	Discuss the personality characteristics that are barriers to both screening and early detection. Open discussion enables the nurse to present accurate information about the disease, tests, and value of early detection.
Confidence	Lack of confidence in the value of early detection. For instance, the	1. Provide the individual with information and literature that documents the value of early detection.

TABLE 3-3 ■ Factors Influencing Participation in Screening and Early Detection—*Continued*

Factor	Manifestation	Nursing Role
	public believes that detecting colorectal cancer early makes no difference in terms of survival.	2. Address misconceptions held about the value of early detection with the public.
Attitudes	Research has shown that individuals who participate in screening programs have positive attitudes about the value of preventive health practices, are better informed about serious illnesses, and are more optimistic and less frightened about cancer.	1. Provide patients with accurate information on the disease and the value of early detection. 2. Have an individual who exemplifies the value of early detection of cancer talk to individuals or make presentations at education programs designed for the public.
Age	The elderly are less likely to participate in screening programs or report suspicious symptoms.	1. Provide information, literature, and programs on the normal symptoms of aging and differentiate these from the warning signs of cancer. 2. Provide information affirming that age doesn't necessarily mean poor health. 3. When designing screening programs, keep in mind that the elderly are less likely to participate, and make special accommodations to encourage this group to participate.
Access to care	Lower socioeconomic status frequently results in lack of access to care and poorer survival.	1. Literature and community educational programs for individuals and groups from low socioeconomic backgrounds must reflect the reality of lack of access and specific suggestions for gaining access to health care services. 2. Special efforts must be made to reach lower socioeconomic groups

(continued)

TABLE 3-3 ■ Factors Influencing Participation in Screening and Early Detection—*Continued*

Factor	Manifestation	Nursing Role
		in the community and bring screening and early detection programs to them only when follow-up health care is assured. 3. Increased use of advanced practice nurses in screening programs may assist in increasing access for the poor.
Socioeconomic status	Higher income affects access to care and participation in screening programs and lessens delay with suspicious symptoms.	1. See Access to Care above.
Race/ethnicity	1. African Americans tend to know less about cancer than whites and delay longer than whites when confronted with suspicious symptoms. 2. Hispanics tend to be pessimistic about cancer, and may have	1. Nurses need to be knowledgeable about the health beliefs and practices of the racial/ethnic group they work with and address these beliefs. 2. If language barriers exist, literature and all written information needs to be in the language the community members can read.

needs to spend time understanding how people feel about each technique, what barriers prevent them from practicing it, what is needed to help them practice it, and what benefits they feel are inherent in the procedure. These areas need to be discussed with the person learning the techniques, and consumer-generated (rather than health professional-generated) solutions should be encouraged.

TABLE 3–3 ■ Factors Influencing Participation in Screening and Early Detection—*Continued*

Factor	Manifestation	Nursing Role
	language barriers and have knowledge deficits. 3. Native Americans tend to view cancer as a white man's disease or as a punishment for something they did (Burhans-stipanov & Olsen, 2001). 4. Asian/Pacific Islanders may tend to view cancer as caused by personal life-style choices or external forces. They may believe illness represents an imbalance or disorder or that illness is caused by an imbalance in morals and spirit (Phillips & Price, 2002).	

■ Conclusion

Secondary preventive efforts, such as screening and early detection, provide a very real and potent weapon against some cancers that only 20 years ago were considered incurable. Nurses need to understand the technical, psychological, and financial aspects of screening and early detection procedures in order to create an atmosphere of openness and trust that will encourage patients' participation in secondary prevention activities. The nurse's primary responsibilities in cancer screening and early detection are to

- Be knowledgeable about the barriers to participation in screening and early-detection programs.
- Provide accurate information about cancer screening and early detection to individuals and the public.
- Encourage individuals to discuss their perceptions and fears about cancer screening/early detection tests and clarify misconceptions.
- Collect accurate information during the health history that includes questions about the seven warning signs of cancer and site-specific questions designed to identify the early signs and symptoms of cancer.
- Assist in the collection of specimens during screening and early detection activities in a way that will ensure that they are as accurate as possible.
- Perform screening examinations commensurate with the nurse's educational background.

■ Resources

- American Cancer Society Resources
  - American Cancer Society Guidelines on Nutrition and Physical Activity for Cancer Prevention
    www.cancer.org/docroot/COM/content/div_Midwest/COM_11_2x_American_Cancer_Society_Guidelines_on_Nutrition_and_Physical_Activity_for_Cancer_Prevention.asp?sitearea=COM
  - American Cancer Society Cancer Facts & Figures 2003: reports the Society's annual estimates of expected numbers of new cancer cases and deaths.
    www.cancer.org/docroot/STT/stt_0.asp
  - American Cancer Society Prevention & Detection Programs: provides information about cancer prevention and detection programs by the American Cancer Society in different areas of country.
    www.cancer.org/docroot/PED/ped_2.asp?sitearea=PED
  - Cancer Prevention & Early Detection. Facts & Figures 2003: provides a wonderful overview and discussion of all aspects of cancer prevention and detection.
    www.cancer.org/docroot/STT/stt_0.asp

- CancerNet (National Cancer Institute): download pamphlets and articles related to genetics.
  cancernet.nci.nih.gov/prevention/genertics.shtml
- Gene Clinics (University of Washington School of Medicine and Children's Hospital Regional Medical Center, Seattle, Washington): an overview of the diagnosis, management, and genetic counseling of people with specific genetic disorders.
  www.geneclinics.org
- Genetics Alliance Support Groups: a nationwide list of genetics support groups.
  www.geneticalliance.org/

Bibliography

American Cancer Society. (2003). *Cancer facts & figures 2003.* (no. 5008.03) Atlanta: author.

Burhansstipanov, L., & Olsen, S. J. (2001). Cancer prevention and early detection in American Indian and Alaska native populations. In M. Frank-Stromborg, & S. J. Olsen (Eds.), *Cancer prevention in diverse populations: Cultural implications for the multidisciplinary team.* (pp. 5–52). Pittsburgh: Oncology Nursing Society Publishing.

Fletcher, S.W. (2002). Screening for breast cancer. *UpToDate, 10,* 1–12.

Greco, K.E. (2002). Genetic counseling and screening. In K. Jennings-Dozier, & S. M. Mahon (Eds.), *Cancer prevention, detection, and control: A nursing perspective* (pp. 727–766). Pittsburgh: Oncology Nursing Society Publishing.

Jennings-Dozier, K., & Foltz, A. (2002). An epidemiological approach to cancer prevention and control. In K. Jennings-Dozier, & S. M. Mahon (Eds.), *Cancer prevention, detection, and control: A nursing perspective* (pp. 33–78). Pittsburgh: Oncology Nursing Society Publishing.

Phillips, J. M., & Price, M. M. (2002). Breast cancer prevention and detection: Past progress and future directions. In K. Jennings-Dozier, & S. M. Mahon (Eds.), *Cancer prevention, detection, and control: A nursing perspective* (pp. 389–444). Pittsburgh: Oncology Nursing Society Publishing.

Rieger, R.T. (2000). Counseling on genetic risk for cancer. In C. H. Yarbro, M. Goodman, M. H. Frogge, & S. L. Groenwald (Eds.), *Cancer nursing: Principles and practice* (5th ed., pp. 189–213). Boston: Jones & Bartlett.

Smith, R.A., Cokkinides, V., & Eyre, H. (2003). American Cancer Society guidelines for the early detection of cancer, 2003. *CA: A Cancer Journal for Clinicians, 53,* 27–43.

CHAPTER

4

Culturally Competent Care

Janice Phillips

Shanita Williams-Brown

Anne E. Belcher

Cancer is a complex, multistage disease process. The factors that contribute to cancer initiation and progression are interwoven and complex as well. There are numerous opportunities and challenges related to providing quality cancer care, and the changing diversity of the US population presents one of these challenges. The purposes of this chapter are to highlight some of the cancer-related issues among racial and ethnic minority populations and the aged and to identify implications for providing quality cancer care for these two groups, the fastest-growing segments of our society. Special emphasis is placed on providing culturally competent care for these populations.

■ The Cancer Profile of Racial and Ethnic Minority Populations

The need for quality cancer care will become increasingly important as the growth in racial/ethnic diverse populations continues. Race is a sociopolitical concept that theoretically defines discrete and separable population groups based on common inherited physical characteristics, such as skin and hair color, facial features, and other superficial external criteria. By contrast, an ethnic group is a population within the larger society that shares a common ancestry, history, or culture, such as language, values, cultural norms, religious traditions, and dietary preferences. Racial and ethnic classification schemes are social, political, and cultural constructs that do not reflect genetic homogeneity or discrete biologic categories. Currently, there are five categories of race and ethnicity: White, Black or African American, American Indian or Alaska Native, Asian or Pacific Islander, and Hispanic or Latino. These federal classifications are frequently used to monitor federal programs. However, there are other race and ethnicity categories. Demographic trends reveal that in 2000, America's population was 71.4% White, 11.8% Hispanic/Latino, 12.2% African American, 3.9% Asian and Pacific Islander, and 0.7% Native American. The 2020 projections are 67.3% White, non-Hispanic; 14.6% Hispanic, 12.5% Black, non-Hispanic; 0.8% Asian, non-Hispanic; and 4.8% Asian-Pacific Islander (US Census Bureau, 2003). When working with minority populations, one must take into account the diversity that exists within and among the various groups. For example, when addressing Hispanics, one must be careful not to assume that Hispanics and their various subgroups (e.g., Mexicans, Cubans, and Puerto Ricans) are alike. Although racially and ethnically diverse populations share common beliefs, values, and practices, there may be substantial variations with regard to culture, social norms, and level of acculturation or assimilation. As such, health care interventions must be assessed and designed in collaboration with the targeted population. Nurses working with diverse populations must avoid the "one size fits all" approach.

Racially and ethnically diverse populations show marked variations with regard to cancer incidence, mortality, and survival. Table 4–1 depicts the cancer incidence and mortality for males and females by race and ethnicity between 1996 and 2000.

Despite the advances in cancer diagnosis and state-of-the-art-treatment, many racially and ethnically diverse populations still lag behind in survival when compared with their white counterparts. For example, from 1992–1998, the 5-year survival rate for all cancers combined was 62% overall but was 64% for whites and 53% for African Americans. Clegg et al (2002) found that the risk of cancer death was significantly higher among all minority groups (except Asian/Pacific Islanders) when compared with whites.

The disparities in cancer survival are even more striking among the economically disadvantaged. Statistics reveal that economically disadvantaged populations have overall 5-year survival rates that are 10%–15% lower than those of the general population. This is particularly important, given that racial and ethnic minority populations are more likely to be disproportionately represented among the economically disadvantaged. Poverty remains a major risk for high cancer incidence and high cancer mortality, regardless of race or ethnicity.

TABLE 4–1 ■ Selected Cancer Incidence[a] and Mortality,[b] Male and Female, by Race/Ethnicity, 1996–2000

Incidence

Rank	African American, Non-Hispanic	Hispanic[c]	Asian/ Pacific Islander	American Indian/ Alaska Native	White, Non-Hispanic
1	Prostate (272.1)	Prostate (137.2)	Prostate (100.0)	Breast (female) (58.0)	Prostate (163.3)
2	Breast (female) (121.7)	Breast (female) (89.8)	Breast (female) (97.2)	Prostate (53.6)	Breast (female) (148.3)
3	Lung (81.2)	Colorectal (40.0)	Colorectal (46.9)	Colorectal (34.7)	Lung (64.9)
4	Colorectal (62.6)	Lung (33.2)	Lung (43.2)	Lung (33.1)	Colorectal (54.8)
5	Pancreas (15.9)	Pancreas (9.8)	Liver/hepatic (13.8)	Pancreas (8.5)	Pancreas (10.8)

Mortality

Rank	African American, Non-Hispanic	Hispanic[b]	Asian/ Pacific Islander	American Indian/ Alaska Native	White, Non-Hispanic
1	Prostate (73.0)	Lung (25.8)	Lung (28.5)	Lung (37.2)	Lung (58.8)
2	Lung (66.4)	Prostate (24.1)	Prostate (13.9)	Prostate (21.9)	Prostate (30.5)
3	Breast (female) (35.9)	Breast (female) (17.9)	Colorectal (13.1)	Breast (female) (14.9)	Breast (female) (27.4)
4	Colorectal (28.5)	Colorectal (14.3)	Breast (female) (12.5)	Colorectal (14.7)	Colorectal (20.8)
5	Pancreas (14.4)	Pancreas (8.3)	Liver/hepatic (10.9)	Pancreas (6.6)	Pancreas (10.2)

[a]Incidence data are from the 12 SEER areas (San Francisco, Connecticut, Detroit, Hawaii, Iowa, New Mexico, Seattle, Utah, Atlanta, San Jose-Monterey, Los Angeles, and Alaska Native).

[b]Mortality data are from the National Center for Health Statistics (NCHS).

[c]Hispanic is not mutually exclusive from White, African American, Asian/Pacific Islander, and American Indian/Alaska Native.

■ Cancer and Racial and Ethnic Minorities across the Cancer Continuum

Quality cancer care should occur along the cancer continuum, with targeted prevention strategies, early diagnosis, state-of-the-art treatment regimens, intensive palliation, and the resources necessary to promote survival. Because minority populations may not receive the same level of care as majority populations do at various points along the cancer care continuum, nurses have multiple opportunities to serve as advocates for these groups.

Prevention

Leading health officials predict that approximately 60,000 deaths and 1,000,000 new cases of cancer could be prevented by the year 2015. Epidemiologists estimate that approximately one third of all of the 556,500 projected new cancers for 2003 will be related to a number of lifestyle factors, including smoking, poor diet, sedentary lifestyle, and obesity, all of which are amenable to preventive intervention. These lifestyle behaviors show variation across minority populations as well as their subpopulations. A few facts include the following factors.

Tobacco Use

- American Indians and Alaska Natives were more likely to smoke than other racial and ethnic groups.
- Between 1978 and 1995, decreases in smoking were noted for all groups except American Indian/Alaska Native populations.

Physical Activity

- African Americans and Hispanics have the highest percentage of no-leisure activity.
- Individuals with lower levels of education are also at risk for inactivity.

Overweight/Obesity

- High rates of obesity are noted among African American women and Mexican American men and women.
- Overweightness and obesity are higher among those with limited education and income.

Nutrition A diet high in vegetables and fruits is considered important in preventing cancer. Recent data show that 24.5% of Blacks and 23.3% of Hispanics reported consuming five or more fruits or vegetables a day. This compares with 20.2% among Whites.

Early Detection The early detection of cancer via screening has the potential to reduce significantly the burden of cancer. For the eight accessible screening sites (e.g., breast, cervical, colon, rectum, oral, skin, prostate, testes), the American Cancer Society estimates that the 5-year relative survival rates would increase from 82% to more than 95% if these cancers were to be diagnosed at a localized stage. Figure 4-1 depicts the most commonly reported screening rates among racially and ethnically diverse populations. As shown, screening rates are suboptimal for all populations; however, rates are particularly low among minority populations.

Decreased utilization of cancer screening services among racial and ethnic minorities has been attributed to lack of education; lack of access to care and state of the art cancer treatment; lack of awareness of

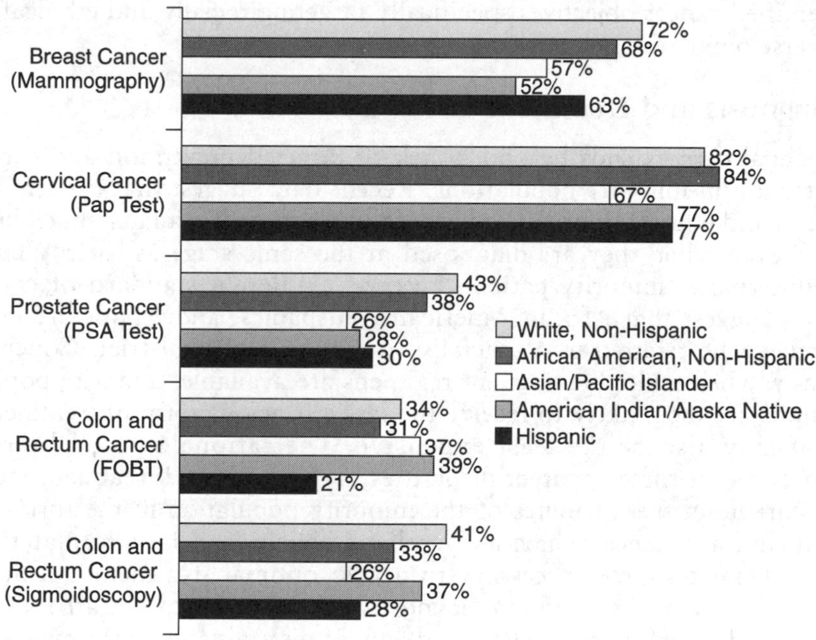

FIGURE 4–1 ■ Cancer Screening by race/ethnicity, 2000. NOTE: Age-adjusted to the 2000 US standard population. Percentages of women 40+ who reported mammography use within past 2 years; women 18+ who reported Pap test in past 3 years; men 50+ who reported PSA test within past year; men & women 50+ who reported fecal occult blood test and within past 2 years; and men and women who ever received a sigmoidoscopy.
Source: National Center for Health Statistics, National Health Interview Survey, 2000.

screening recommendations and related benefits; misconceptions about cancer screening; cultural and language barriers for both provider and patient; life priorities, which take precedence over cancer screening; fear of treatment, especially radiation therapy and chemotherapy; fear of contagion; and a fatalistic perspective regarding cancer outcomes among others. Table 4–2 (beginning on pages 66–67) summarizes reported health beliefs and practices thought to influence the cancer care—seeking behaviors of racial and ethnic minorities and whites. Health beliefs and practices may vary by subpopulations or according to degree of acculturation, assimilation, socioeconomic status, and other sociocultural factors. Because of these potential variations, nurses should conduct careful assessments to identify the specific barriers for the target population. In an effort to improve cancer screening and early detection, the landmark document Healthy People2010 (*www.healthypeople.gov/document/pdf/Volume1/03Cancer.pdf*) has identified cancer objectives specifically targeting racially and ethnically diverse populations.

Diagnosis and Treatment

Unequal care extends beyond a lack of targeted prevention and early detection in minority populations. Recent data suggest that cancers in racial and ethnic minorities are generally diagnosed at a later stage, but that even when they are diagnosed at the same stage as their White counterparts, minority patients receive a different standard of care. Data suggest that African Americans, Hispanics, and Asians are less likely to be referred to a specialist and/or to a clinical trial. Concurrently, when multiple treatment regimens are available, minority populations are most likely to receive the less efficacious form of treatment that may also be the least expensive. The rationale posed by researchers for these apparent disparities in diagnosis and treatment may in part lie in the attributes of the minority population in the form of fear and avoidance behaviors, fatalistic beliefs, and lack of material and social resources necessary to access optimal treatment options. However, many disparities in diagnosis and treatment can be attributed to provider preferences, biases, and lack of dissemination of knowledge and information regarding available options. The Institute of Medicine's report documented that provider decision making and interventions were frequently not based on evidence.

Survivorship

Quality treatment translates into increased survival. Racial and ethnic minorities experience increased mortality and decreased survival after a cancer diagnosis. Some of the disparity in mortality and survival may be attributed to issues of biology; however, the data clearly suggest that biology alone cannot account for much of the observed disparity. The time has come to move from creating laundry lists of racial and ethnic minority population attributes to strategic efforts to ensure quality cancer care for all. This requires health care providers, especially nurses, to be alert to the potential for unequal treatment. It is the provider's responsibility to be constantly aware of systematic biases, both subtle and overt, and to commit themselves to decreasing the cancer burden among minority populations by delivering consistent, quality cancer care.

Cancer in the Elderly

More than 12% of Americans are over the age of 65. By 2030, approximately 70 million people will be "young old" (65–74 years), "middle-old" (75–84 years), or "oldest-old" (85+ years). The oldest-old are the fastest growing group in the United States. Many older adults are, and increasingly will be, from ethnically diverse cultures. By 2040, almost 160 million people will be living with chronic conditions, such as cancer. Age is the most important factor in determining cancer risk because more than 50% of all cancers occur in persons over the age of 65.

Myths and misconceptions held by both the elderly and the public in general are obstacles to prevention, early detection, diagnosis, and treatment of cancer in this group. Health care providers may practice ageism, the stigmatizing effect of societal prejudices toward older persons. The presence of elder bias prevents the application of new scientific knowledge and new ways of thinking to clinical practice in caring for older adults. The following beliefs may present barriers to cancer care in the elderly: older people are senile or demented and cannot give a reliable health history; many elders are unhealthy and cannot care for themselves without assistance; the aging process is inevitable and results in general physical deterioration. In reality, most elderly persons are not mentally disturbed, are able to carry on their preferred lifestyle, and have widely varying rates of declining organ and system function. There are, however, other barriers to early detection, diagnosis, and treatment of cancer in the elderly, some of which are based on their beliefs and behaviors:

- Taking their aches and pains for granted
- Viewing ill health and disability as inevitable
- Experiencing the gradual loss of friends and relatives who are used as a support and referral system
- Not having or using access to accurate health information

TABLE 4–2 ■ Summary of Reported Health Beliefs/Practices Among Racial/Ethnic Minority and White Populations

Race/Ethnicity	Spiritual/Natural Supernatural	Fate/Punishment
African American/Black	Health is related to harmony in nature Faith and prayer may eliminate disease	Illness may represent God's punishment Illness/suffering may be unavoidable
Asian/Pacific Islander	Health is a state of harmony in mind, body, & spirit Achieving harmony with nature is essential to healing Balance between hot and cold is needed for health	Suffering is a part of life Defer care at beginning of year (lunar New Year)
American Indian/Alaska Native	Wellness is harmony with nature in mind, body, and spirit Illness may be caused by witchcraft, violation of sacred or tribal taboo	Cancer is punishment for personal or family actions Cancer is a white man's disease
Hispanic	Hot and cold imbalances may lead to illness Faith and prayer may alleviate/cure disease	Health is a result of good luck Disease is God's will Illness may be caused by evil eye (*mal ojo*), spirits, or past sins
White	Faith and prayer may alleviate/cure disease	No

Sources: Andrews, M. M. (2003). The influence of cultural and health beliefs systems on health care. In M. M. Andrews, & J. S. Boyle (Eds.). *Transcultural concepts in nursing care practices* (pp. 73–92). Philadelphia: Lippincott Williams & Wilkins; Frank-Stromborg, M., & Olsen, S. J. (Eds.) (2001). *Cancer prevention in diverse populations: Cultural implications for the multidisciplinary teams* (2nd ed.). Huff, R. M., & Kline, M. (1999). *Promoting health in multicultural populations: A handbook for practitioners.* Thousand Oaks, CA: Sage Publications; Phillips, J., Cohen, M., & Moses, G. (1999). Breast cancer screening and African American women: Fear, fatalism, and silence. *Oncology Nursing Forum, 26,* 561–571; Taoka, K. N., &

Fatalism/Fear	**Holistic/Alternative Medicine**	**Western Medicine**
Fatalistic views	Traditional folk healers, herbal remedies	Combine holistic/alternative medicine with Western medicine May be the primary and/or only treatment choice[a]
Fear of intrusive procedures	Traditional medicine and faith healers	Combine holistic/alternative medicine with Western medicine May be the primary and/or only treatment choice[b]
Cancer is contagious	Use of traditional healers, medicine men, and herbal remedies Traditional healing ceremonies used to promote mental, physical, and spiritual balance and well-being	Combine native traditional medicine with Western medicine
Fatalistic views	Folk healers are frequently sought out as the primary treatment of choice	Western medicine sought after/preferred in advanced illnesses[c]
No	Complimentary and alternative medicine (e.g., acupuncture, massage therapy) herbal remedies	Primary treatment of choice

Itano, J. K. (2000). Cultural Diversity among individuals with cancer. In C. H. Yarbro, M. Goodman, M. H. Frogge, & S. L. Groenwald (Eds.), *Cancer nursing: Principles and practice* (pp. 100–134). Boston: Jones & Bartlett Publishers.

[a]Younger, middle-class, and wealthy African-Americans seek treatment sooner and utilize the health-care system more readily.

[b]Frequently the case in young, middle-class, and wealthy Asian/Pacific Islanders.

[c]Younger, middle-class, and wealthy Hispanics seek Westernized medical treatment sooner and utilize the health care system more readily.

- Possessing negative and often fatalistic attitudes about cancer and about the value of early detection, diagnosis, and treatment
- Experiencing the constraints of a fixed income and inadequate funds for health care

Cancer mortality is especially high in the elderly, particularly among the socioeconomically disadvantaged, because of a delay in diagnosis but also because of patients' comorbidities, such as cardiovascular disorders, pulmonary alterations, renal and neurologic changes, diabetes mellitus, and hypertension. These comorbidities, rather than chronological age, should be used by health care providers as guides to early detection and treatment decisions. For example, such factors as obesity, inadequate nutritional status, lung disease, complications of vascular and cardiac status, and impaired immunity may place older persons at additional risk when undergoing surgery, radiation therapy, and chemotherapy. In addition, the use of polypharmacy (multiple drug use) among the elderly may create individual problems and drug interactions and enhanced side effects in persons receiving cancer treatment. Elderly persons' experience with cancer may also be complicated by their increasing likelihood of living alone and losing supportive resources as they grow older. Poverty may intensify these changes in lifestyle. Out-of-pocket expenses associated with cancer and its treatment impact most severely on those with a fixed income. However, in spite of these potential constraints, many older persons can tolerate and benefit from standard or experimental treatment protocols.

■ Other Factors Affecting Cancer Care

In addition to the impact of racial and ethnic diversity and age on cancer care, there are other factors that health care providers should identify and incorporate into prevention, detection, diagnosis, and treatment strategies. These include gender, sexual orientation, language, physical limitations, and geographic location. As seen in Table 4–1, there are gender differences with regard to cancer site, incidence, and mortality.

Sexual orientation also affects cancer care, particularly in lesbians. Numerous studies have suggested that lesbians are at increased risk for breast and other cancers because of such behavioral and lifestyle factors as smoking and alcohol consumption, poor diet, higher body mass index, and null parity. Perceived barriers to adequate cancer care for both lesbians and gay men include physician ignorance regarding homosexual health issues, discrimination in health care settings, decreased access to care, and mistrust of the medical establishment. Language can serve as a barrier to understanding messages regarding the value of cancer prevention and detection as well as affecting the person's ability to question the health care provider and to make informed decisions. Physical limitations may affect the individual's ability to access care and to tolerate the side effects; for example, the mobility-challenged person may not be able to use exercise as a strategy for coping with the fatigue induced by chemotherapy and/or radiation therapy.

Geographic location is another factor that affects access to cancer care all along the cancer care continuum; when combined with poverty, it negatively affects individuals' and groups' ability to receive preventive education, early detection and diagnosis, and state-of-the art treatment.

Culturally Appropriate Care

Numerous authors have provided definitions and guidelines related to achieving cultural competence in nursing practice, research, and education. In 1994, the Oncology Nursing Society Multicultural Advisory Council developed the *ONS Multicultural Outcomes: Guidelines for Cultural Competence* (2000) to assist nurses when providing care to and/or conducting research with racially and ethnically diverse populations. The Multicultural Advisory Council defined cultural competence as "being sensitive and responsive to issues related to culture, race, ethnicity, gender, age, socioeconomic status, and sexual orientation. Cultural competence indicates a translation of cultural sensitivity and awareness into credible behaviors and actions." This document provides a comprehensive discussion on culture, cultural assessments and implications for oncology nursing practice, education, and research and is available on line at *www.ons.org*. Although there are many models that address cultural competence, the Cultural Competency Model by Campinha-Bacote (1999) is one of the most popular. This author emphasizes that becoming culturally competent is an ongoing and continuous process that consists of four components: cultural self-awareness, cultural knowledge, cultural skill, and cultural encounters.

Purnell and Paulinka (1998) provide an organizing framework that can be used when conducting cultural assessments in any culture, across any setting and disease state. In this model, the authors examine the culture of an individual or group by collecting data from 12 domains: (1) overview, inhabited localities, and topography; (2) communication; (3) family roles and organization; (4) work force issues; (5) biocultural ecology; (6) high-risk behaviors; (7) nutrition; (8) pregnancy and childbearing practices; (9) death rituals; (10) spirituality; (11) health care practices; and (12) health care practitioners. These data can be used when in the development of cancer-related education and services targeting racially and ethnically diverse populations. A detailed discussion of this framework and other implications for providing culturally relevant care is located within the Oncology Nursing Society guidelines previously mentioned.

■ Conclusions and Future Recommendations

The authors have provided a beginning discussion on cancer and two of the fastest growing segments of our society: racially and ethnically diverse populations and the aged. Although there is a growing body of knowledge regarding cancer-related issues for minorities, much remains unknown with regard to their various subpopulations. Nurses working with these populations are encouraged to develop a working knowledge of culture and its influence on the cancer care—seeking behaviors of culturally diverse populations. The cultural values, beliefs, and practices of minority populations should be assessed and incorporated into the entire cancer continuum. When working with racially and ethnically diverse populations and the aged, the authors offer the following recommendations for action:

- Expand outreach activities to enhance cancer awareness, cancer prevention/early detection, and prompt treatment.
- Continue to advocate for access to state-of-the-art treatment for all patients.
- Increase awareness of resources for supportive care once a diagnosis of cancer is made.
- Collaborate to expand the number of supportive care resources.
- Develop interventions to enhance compliance with recommended screening guidelines for asymptomatic culturally diverse and aged populations.
- Strive toward learning and respecting the world views of those from different cultural backgrounds and walks of life.
- Include the target population when planning and delivering cancer-related services.
- Tailor health education and other activities to address the customs and language needs of diverse individuals.
- Incorporate sociocultural factors into educational and outreach programs targeting diverse populations.

■ Resources

- Intercultural Cancer Council
  iccnetwork.org
  713-798-4617
- National Center for Chronic Disease Prevention and Health Promotion, Centers for Disease Control and Prevention
  www.cdc.gov/health/cancer.htm
- Office of Minority Health Resource Center
  www.omhrc.gov/omhrc
  800-444-6472

Bibliography

American Cancer Society. (2003). *Cancer facts and figure series.* Atlanta: Author.

Campinha-Bacote, J. (1999). A model and instrument for addressing cultural competence in healthcare. *Journal of Nursing Education, 38,* 203–207.

Clarke-Tasker, V. (2003). Socioeconomic status and African Americans' perceptions of cancer. *Journal of National Black Nurses Association, 14,* 13–19.

Clegg, L., Li, F., Hankey, B., Chu, K. & Edwards, B. (2002). Cancer survival among US whites and minorities: A SEER (Surveillance, Epidemiology, and End Results) program population-based study. *Archives of Internal Medicine, 162,* 1985–1993.

Edwards, B., Howe, H., Ries, L., Thun, M., Rosenberg, H., Yancik, R., Wingo, P., Jemal, A., Feigal, E. (2002). Annual report to the nation on the status of cancer, 1973-1999, featuring implications of age and aging on US cancer burden. *Cancer, 94,* 2766–2792.

Institute of Medicine (2003). *Fulfilling the potential of cancer prevention and early detection.* Washington, DC: The National Academies Press.

Oncology Nursing Society (2000). Oncology nursing society multicultural outcomes: guidelines for cultural competence. *Oncology Nursing Press.* Pittsburgh: Author.

Purnell, L. D., & Paulanka, B. J. (1998). *Transcultural health care: A culturally competent approach.* Philadelphia: F. A. Davis.

Rankow, E. (1995). Breast and cervical cancer among lesbians. *Women's Health Issues, 5,* 123–129.

Shavers, V. & Brown, M. (2002). Racial and ethnic disparities in the receipt of cancer treatment. *Journal of the National Cancer Institute, 94,* 334-357.

United States Department of Health and Human Services. *Healthy People 2010 Cancer. www.healthypeople.gov/document/pdf/Volume1/03Cancer.pdf.* Retrieved July 14, 2003.

CHAPTER

5

Complementary and Alternative Medical Approaches to Management of Cancer and Symptoms

Janice Post-White

Susan Bauer-Wu

Adults and children with cancer use complementary and alternative medicine (CAM) to help fight cancer, reduce symptoms and side effects, and promote healing and recovery. Most therapies are used as adjuncts (complementary) to conventional medical therapy, as opposed to those that replace standard care (alternative). Cancer patients are actively seeking and using CAM, but they do not necessarily tell their health care team about their CAM use, frequently because they are never asked. It is important to know what therapies patients are using or considering to ensure that informed decisions are made and to help determine interactions with medical treatment. Side effects are specific to the type of CAM used, with few adverse responses to mind-body interventions, touch therapies, or energy therapies. Biologic therapies can interfere with chemotherapy or radiation therapy and cause liver, cardiac, or renal toxicities, or they may have hormonal and anticoagulant effects. Despite patients' use of CAM, few studies document its safety and effectiveness or whether CAM improves quality of life and other positive clinical outcomes. Despite that, it is clinically imperative that nurses be aware of the types of CAM patients use and their potential risks and benefits.

■ What Is CAM?

According to the National Center for Complementary and Alternative Medicine of the National Institutes of Health, CAM is defined as a group of diverse medical and health care systems, practices, and products that are not presently considered to be part of conventional medicine. CAM can be grouped into five major domains: alternative medical systems, mind-body interventions, biologically based treatments, manipulative and body-based methods, and energy therapies.

■ CAM Use in Cancer: Prevalence and Reasons

The use of CAM among cancer patients is higher than in the general population. Recent surveys indicate that 50%–84% of adults and children with cancer use CAM, and CAM use increases at times of disease recurrence or progression. Interestingly, educated women undergoing chemotherapy who have sufficient income to self-pay for CAM are the patients who are most likely to use CAM. Children are more likely to use CAM if their parents use CAM. Despite widespread use, most patients and families do not divulge their use of CAM to a health care professional unless they are specifically asked.

Reasons patients give for using CAM include palliation of side effects from the disease or treatment, attempt to slow down cancer growth with the goal to live longer and have a better quality of life, obtainment of a sense of control, and hope for a cure. Many CAM therapies are considered holistic, which is attractive to patients and families who are also looking for care of the whole person, beyond the conventional high-technology oncology treatments.

Most of the National Cancer Institute's designated cancer centers have staff with CAM expertise, and many offer CAM therapies that have some scientific evidence of safety and effectiveness. Integrative medicine, offered at these cancer centers, combines CAM therapies with conventional cancer treatment to improve quality of life, enhance coping, and encourage active participation in care.

■ Types of CAM

Alternative Medical Systems

Alternative medical systems have long histories of practice that have been passed down from generation to generation. These practices differ from the conventional medical practices in the United States because they evolved apart from and preceded modern Western medicine. Homeopathy and naturopathy developed from Western cultures and Ayurveda and traditional Oriental/Chinese medicine from non-Western cultures. Examples of alternative medical systems are listed in Table 5–1. Acupuncture is one aspect of traditional Oriental/Chinese medicine that has become increasingly popular in the United States because of scientific evidence supporting its benefits to cancer patients for pain and for chemotherapy-related nausea and vomiting.

TABLE 5–1 ■ Alternative Medical Systems

Homeopathy	Naturopathy	Ayurveda	Traditional Oriental/Chinese Medicine
• Based on principle that "like cures like" • Minute doses of plant extracts stimulate body's defenses to specific conditions	• Views disease as alterations in the natural healing process • Recognizes integration of the whole person • Includes a combination of clinical nutrition, botanical medicine, hydro(water) therapy, and physical medicine (e.g., massage, manipulation)	• Views disease as natural end result of living out of harmony with environment • Recognizes uniqueness of the person and the manifesting disease • Treatment based on understanding own body constitution within the elements of nature	• Emphasizes proper balance of *qi* (chi), as life force or energy, to connect body, mind, spirit, and environment • Recognizes value of person's constitution and symptoms • Includes acupuncture, diet and herbal medicine, meditation, and body movement

Mind-Body Interventions Cancer patients use mind-body interventions to reduce stress, increase their sense of control, and to enhance their quality of life. Mind-body techniques (Table 5–2) are generally quite safe and without adverse effects, and many can be easily taught by nurses and incorporated into the day-to-day care of cancer patients.

Biologically Based Therapies Biologically based therapies encompass ingestible or injectable agents and include herbal therapies, dietary supplements, special diets, and other "natural" but unproven therapies (Table 5–3). Vitamins and herbs have the potential to interact with cancer medical treatment. Because radiation and some chemotherapy agents kill tumors through oxidative damage, antioxidants can interfere with medical treatment and should not be taken during anthracycline therapies or radiation therapy. Herbs that stimulate the immune system may also interfere with treatments for leukemia and lymphoma. Other concerns about biologic therapies are the lack of standards for recommended adult or pediatric dosages and little oversight of the herbal and nutritional industries, resulting in inconsistent products and uneven quality and purity.

TABLE 5–2 ■ Categories and Examples of Mind-Body Interventions

Sensory	Cognitive	Expressive	Physical
Smell: Aromatherapy	Meditation	Expressive writing, poetry, and journaling	Physical exercise
Hearing: listening to music, sounds of nature, calming or uplifting voice	Guided imagery/ visualization	Creative therapies—art therapy, drama, arts and crafts	Dance and movement
Sight: colors/visual images	Humor	Music therapy/singing, playing an instrument, composition	Yoga, T'ai chi , Qi gong
Touch: massage; back, foot, hand, or scalp rubs	Cognitive restructuring and reframing; affirmations	Group support and psychotherapy	Progressive muscle relaxation
Taste: eating pleasurable and flavorful foods	Hypnotherapy, biofeedback, and autogenic training Prayer and spiritual healing		

TABLE 5-3 ■ Biologic Approaches to Cancer Treatment and Care

Biologic Agent	Possible Effects	Precautions
Antineoplastons Burzynski Clinic, TX	Cell differentiation and apoptosis.	Phase I/II trials in adults. No RCT. High cost. Mild side effects.
Antioxidants Vitamins A, C, E, B6, melatonin, coenzyme Q10, grape seed extract, carotenoids	Enhanced immune function. Repair or prevention of cellular damage from toxins.	Vitamins A and E may progress lung and prostate tumors or cause liver damage (vitamin A). Anticoagulants (vitamins C, E). May interfere with chemotherapy and radiation therapy.
Astragalus Traditional Chinese medicine herb	T lymphocyte function, interferon production, macrophage activity.	Nontoxic. No studies in children. Caution if hypoglycemic or on anticoagulants. Avoid in transplant patients.
Essiac Herbal Tea (Flor-Essence). 7 herbs	Supports immune system, decreases tumor size, improves appetite.	No efficacy. Not for young children. No adverse events in adults. Avoid if renal stones or intestinal obstruction.
Green Tea Flavenol polyphenols	Antitumor, prevents tumor angiogenesis.	Safe in moderate amounts without side effects. Includes caffeine.
Milk thistle *Silybum marianum* Herbal tea	Reduces liver dysfunction. Inhibits TNF alpha.	Prostate cancer effect. Strong antioxidant may interfere with chemotherapy and radiation therapy.
Mistletoe (ISCAR, iscador) *Viscum Album L.*	Stimulates NK cells, TNF alpha, IFN gamma, IL-1, IL-6.	No efficacy in head and neck cancer and melanoma, but some efficacy in patients with various tumors.
St. John's Wort *Hypericum perforatum*	Mild antidepressant.	Interferes with irinotecan, indinavir, cyclosporin.
Shark cartilage	Antiangiogenic proteins.	No effect in advanced cancer. Caution in pregnancy/children.
Soy products Isoflavenoid Phytoestrogens	Antioxidants. Weak estrogenic effects compete with estradiol.	Avoid soy if on tamoxifen. Prostate cancer effect. Inhibits platelet aggregation.

Key: NK = natural killer; TNF = tumor necrosis factor; IFN = interferon; IL = interleukin; RCT = random controlled trial.

Manipulative and Body-Based Methods Touch therapies can reduce fatigue and restore structure and function of the musculoskeletal and nervous systems. Massage increases circulation, muscle tone, and relaxation and reduces blood pressure, heart rate, and cortisol. In cancer, massage has reduced anxiety, pain, fatigue, lymphedema, and nausea, and it has improved quality of life. Although side effects are rare, bleeding and tissue swelling can occur, and common advice is to avoid massage when platelet counts are less than 20,000 m^3, as well as to avoid massage directly over solid tumor sites, central or peripheral venous catheters, and surgical or radiation sites. Children may be distrustful of strangers touching them, and parents can be taught to do gentle massage strokes. Licensure is required in many states, but not all. Certification for massage therapists is provided by The American Massage Therapy Association.

Chiropractic involves skeletal manipulation of the spine and joints and can reduce low back pain. Although chiropractic is reportedly one of the most common forms of CAM used by children, little evidence supports its effectiveness. Chiropractic is not recommended for patients with spinal lesions (e.g., myeloma or bone metastases) or for those at risk for vascular events, such as strokes.

Energy Therapies Energy healing therapies are based on the belief that all matter is energy and that disease or illness represents an imbalance in the person's energy flow. Healing occurs when the person's energy system is removed of blockages and is "balanced." Practitioners of energy therapies channel spiritual or healing energy to manipulate or interrupt energy fields within the body (biofields) or external to the body (electromagnetic fields). External qi gong, reiki, therapeutic touch, and healing touch involve identifying and correcting energy imbalances and promoting energy flow by applying pressure or placing the hands in or through the energy fields. These therapies are used in cancer for pain and symptom management and for general relaxation and well-being. Nurses can incorporate energy therapies such as therapeutic touch, healing touch, and Reiki into their care of patients with cancer. Training and certification for therapeutic touch and healing touch are provided through Healing Touch International and the American Holistic Nurses Association.

■ The Role of the Nurse

Nurses need to have a general understanding of CAM and to know how to access information on CAM to inform their own practice and

TABLE 5–4 ■ Complementary and Alternative Medical (CAM) Guidelines for Nursing Practice

- Ask patients if they are using or are considering using CAM therapies.
- Listen in nonjudgmental, objective way regarding therapies using or considering using.
- Explore the patient's expectations and goals for using the CAM therapy.
- Ask questions to ensure the family has considered risks, benefits, and cost.
- Document what is being used and why, including dosages and frequency.
- Ascertain all potential side effects and interactions with treatment.
- Monitor and assess for positive and negative responses, including symptoms and side effects, mood, allergic reactions, and interactions with medical treatment.
- Encourage patients/families to evaluate the need and value of each therapy.
- Provide reliable resources for information on specific CAM therapies.
- Provide a list of local resources, including credentialed practitioners.
- Make referrals and/or provide CAM therapies that can be safely integrated with care.
- Receive proper training and credentialing, and check state regulations before incorporating CAM therapies into nursing practice.
- Assess for financial hardship and discuss options for insurance reimbursement.

educate patients (Table 5–4 and Resources). The Oncology Nursing Society's position on the use of CAM requires that nurses assess for CAM use; rely on credible sources and providers when giving information to patients; evaluate CAM for safety, efficacy, cost, third-party payer coverage, ethics, and liability; and evaluate their own beliefs regarding CAM (Oncology Nursing Society, 2000). Use of CAM and potential interactions with treatment should be assessed at diagnosis, during each hospitalization, and at every phase of medical treatment.

■ Conclusion

CAM can be safe and effective if it is used in combination with standard cancer care. Because some herbal, dietary, and biologic therapies interfere with cancer treatment, it is important to know what CAM is being used. The position of the American Cancer Society on CAM is to encourage health care professionals to ask their patients about their use of alternative and complementary methods. Health care professionals should listen and know how to communicate with their patients with an open, trusting, noncritical dialogue.

■ Resources

American Botanical Association, *www.herbalgram.org*
American Cancer Society: Complementary and Alternative Therapies: *www.cancer. org/docroot/eto/eto_5.asp?sitearea=eto*
American Holistic Nurses Association, *www.ahna.org*
The Longwood Herbal Task Force, *www.mcp.edu/herbal*
Memorial Sloan-Kettering Cancer Center Information Resource: About Herbs, Botanicals & Other Products: *www.mskcc.org/mskcc/ html/11570.cfm*
National Cancer Institute (NCI) Physicians Data Query (PDQ): *cancer-net.nci.nih. gov/cam*
NIH Medline Plus (for CAM literature searches): *www.nlm. nih.gov/medlineplus/alternativemedicine.html*
NIH National Center of Complementary and Alternative Medicine: *www.nccam.nih.gov/*
NIH Office of Cancer Complementary and Alternative Medicine: *www3.cancer. gov/occam*
NIH Office of Dietary Supplements: *ods.od.nih.gov/index.aspx*

Bibliography

American Cancer Society. (2000). *American Cancer Society's guide to complementary and alternative cancer methods.* Atlanta: American Cancer Society.

Bauer-Wu, S. (2002). Psychoneuroimmunology part II: Mind-body interventions. *Clinical Journal of Oncology Nursing, 6,* 243–246.

Oncology Nursing Society (2000). Oncology Nursing Society position on the use of complementary and alternative therapies in cancer care. *Oncology Nursing Forum, 27,* 749.

Post-White, J., Sencer, S., & Fitzgerald, M. (2002). Complementary and alternative treatments in children with cancer. In K. Kelly, C. Baggott, G. Foley (Eds.). *Nursing care of the child with cancer* (2nd ed., pp. 256–263). Philadelphia: W. B. Saunders.

Weiger, W. A., Smith, M., Boon, H. Richardson, M. A., Kaptchuk, T. J., & Eisenberg, D. M. (2002). Advising patients who seek complementary and alternative medical therapies for cancer. *Annals of Internal Medicine, 137,* 889–905.

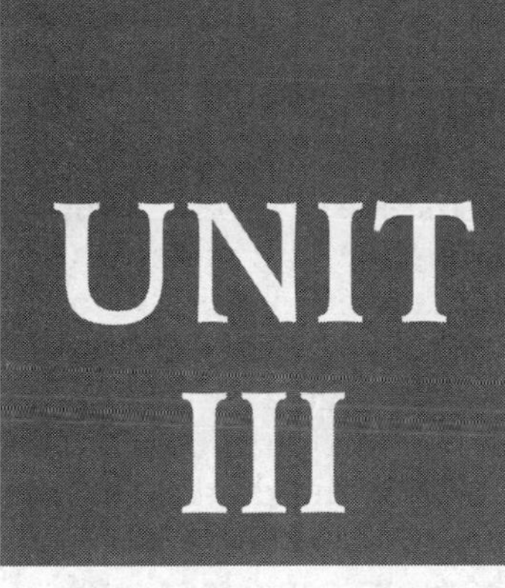

Treatment Approaches

Kathi Mooney

There are a variety of approaches to treating cancer. The three main treatments include surgery, radiation therapy, and chemotherapy. These treatments remove or kill cancer cells but are nonspecific to cancer and therefore may also affect normal tissue, causing side effects. Surgery and radiation therapy provide focused or localized treatment of cancer, whereas chemotherapy is systemic treatment. A fourth approach, biotherapy, has played a secondary role in cancer treatment for many years.

As more has been learned about the biology of cancer, new approaches called *targeted therapies* are now under development. These novel approaches target tumor-specific molecules that regulate tumor growth and progression. Because they have a precise tumor target, there is less impact on normal tissue, producing fewer side effects and toxicities.

■ Diagnostic Evaluation

Before a cancer treatment plan is chosen, a comprehensive diagnostic evaluation is performed to determine whether a malignancy is present and if so, to determine the tissue type, the primary site of the malignancy, the extent of the disease throughout the body, and the biologic, molecular, and genetic characteristics of the malignancy. A key component of this evaluation is a histologic examination of the suspected cancer, usually accomplished through a surgical biopsy. Various techniques can be used, including aspiration biopsy, needle biopsy, excisional biopsy, and incisional biopsy. In addition, presenting signs and symptoms, individual and family health histories, physical examination, and extensive imaging, laboratory, and biochemical analyses make up a comprehensive evaluation.

What Kind of Cancer?

Once the relevant tests and examinations have been performed, the malignancy can be named and staged. Naming is generally descriptive of the type of tissue involved. For example, a sarcoma is a malignant tumor of connective tissue, and an osteosarcoma is a malignant tumor of the bone. A carcinoma is a malignant tumor of epithelial tissue, and a breast adenocarcinoma is cancer that arises from glandular epithelial tissue in the breast. The naming of cancer is based on the tissue of origin. It is possible that a biopsy may be taken from a metastatic site rather than the originating organ. For example, a woman may be diagnosed with metastatic breast cancer from a lung biopsy, because the malignant tissue taken from the lung reflects the histology of the original epithelial breast tissue.

Staging Systems

Staging provides additional information about the extent and special characteristics of the cancer. Although a variety of staging systems exist, the most broadly recognized and used is the TNM system that was developed by the International Union Against Cancer and the American Joint Committee on Cancer. In this system, three areas are quantified and together provide specific yet concise information about the extent of the cancer.

The *T* of TNM indicates the size of the primary tumor, so that a T_0 means no evidence of a primary tumor and T_1–T_4 represent increasing size or levels of local invasion by the primary tumor. The *N* identifies the amount of regional lymph node involvement, with N_0 representing no involvement and N_1–N_4 representing increasing involvement of regional lymph nodes. The *M* indicates the presence (M_1) or absence (M_0) of distant metastases.

Because staging systems are meant to provide useful information for treatment planning, they will continue to evolve to include new indicators of malignant and metastatic potential based on emerging molecular and biologic information.

Treatment Choices

Treatment of cancer is focused on achieving one of three goals: cure, tumor control, or palliation of symptoms. Whenever possible, the desired outcome of treatment is cure of the disease. For some cancers in which curative treatments have yet to be identified or once the disease has recurred after initial treatment, treatment goals may instead focus on disease control. If treatment is no longer effective in controlling disease and prolonging life, the focus of treatment then shifts to comfort and palliation of symptoms. This may include, for example, treatment of a collapsing vertebral body or a painful bone metastasis or relief of a bowel obstruction.

Treatment options depend on the tumor type and the stage of disease. Other factors that may affect treatment choices include previous treatment, comorbidities, health status, and personal preferences of the individual. Often, multidisciplinary tumor boards that bring together the health care providers involved in a patient's care are used to review all pertinent information and discuss treatment options.

Treatment may involve a single therapy, such as surgery alone, or it may be multimodal, such as a combination of surgery, chemotherapy, and biotherapy. Similarly, when chemotherapy is given, it may involve a single agent or a combination of several agents.

Clinical Trials

Treatments for cancer are developed through research and systematic comparisons called *clinical trials*. Once a treatment approach has been shown to be the most effective for a particular cancer, it is considered standard treatment. New approaches are tested in clinical trials against current standard treatment. Many clinical trials are conducted through a multi-institutional system of academic institutions and cancer treatment centers known as *cooperative groups*. Pharmaceutical companies also conduct clinical trials with drugs they are developing.

Clinical trials are divided into four phases (see Table 7–1 in Chapter 7, Chemotherapy), depending on the purpose of the trial. Phase I studies establish the maximum dose that can safely be given and the associated toxicities. Phase II studies test the effectiveness of the treatment for specific cancers, using the dose established in the phase I trial. Phase III clinical trials compare the effectiveness of the new treatment with that of standard treatment. Patients are randomly assigned to receive either the new treatment or the standard treatment. Phase IV clinical trials may be conducted after treatment approval and are sometimes called postmarketing studies. Although not required, they provide additional information about the use of the treatment over time.

Although clinical trials are the primary method of improving treatment outcomes, few cancer patients actually participate in a clinical trial. However, when offered a clinical trial, most patients agree to participate. Increasing the opportunities for patients to participate in clinical trials is important so that treatment advances can be identified more quickly and so that there is greater diversity among patients who participate.

■ Patient Involvement in Decision Making

The diagnostic and treatment planning period can be extremely stressful to patients and their families. While they attempt to adapt to an unwelcome and life-threatening diagnosis, they must complete many diagnostic tests and scans, interact with a variety of new health care providers, and make decisions about a treatment plan.

There is variability in how involved patients want to be in making a treatment decision. Historically, many cancer patients have taken a passive role in treatment planning, and even today, some physicians offer patients only one approach to treatment. However, increasingly, patients express a desire to be an active partner in choosing treatment.

Degner and colleagues (1997) have identified five preferred roles that range from active to collaborative to passive. Patients who prefer to make the final treatment decision themselves or prefer to make the final decision after considering their physician's advice want an active role. Patients who prefer a joint decision between themselves and their physician want a collaborative role. Patients who prefer that their physician consider their input but make the treatment decision or prefer that the physician take all responsibility for the decision want a passive role.

No matter the decision role preference chosen, most patients want detailed information about their disease, treatment options, what is involved with treatment, and potential side effects of treatment. The nurse plays a very important role in reinforcing and clarifying disease and treatment information both before and after a treatment decision is made.

It is important to ask patients about their preferred treatment decision role and their values and preferences about treatment so that they can be coached in how to get their questions answered and their needs met when the treatment decision is made. If, for example, the nurse learns that a patient would be interested in learning about available clinical trials for their disease, the patient can be coached to ask his or her physician if a clinical trial is available, rather than waiting for the physician to bring it up.

Occasionally, a patient wants minimal information. This may be due to the anxiety that is created by thinking about their situation. The nurse may need to assist the patient in coping with the negative emotions associated with the diagnosis and the need for treatment before providing treatment information.

Nurses are in the best position to help patients understand the process of treatment. Preparatory information that identifies exactly what the patient will hear, see, feel, and smell has been shown to decrease treatment-related anxiety and negative mood.

Because treatment is associated with a variety of toxicities and side effects, detailed systematic symptom assessment is a cornerstone of nursing care during the active treatment period. Patients and their families must be well educated to anticipate and respond to toxicities and side effects because these generally occur while the patient is at home.

The chapters that follow in this unit provide an overview of the most common treatment approaches to cancer. The rationale and principles for each treatment approach are described, as are common toxicities and side effects, issues of administration, and nursing considerations. All of this information provides readers with an appreciation for the complexity of cancer treatment.

■ Resources

The American Cancer Society web site at *www.cancer.org* has a wealth of information for patients and their families during diagnostic, treatment decision-making, and active treatment periods. This includes a specific section entitled "Making Treatment Decisions," which provides information such as descriptions of types of treatment, a detailed discussion about considering clinical trials, hints on how to talk about cancer to others, support group resources, and suggestions on how to stay active during treatment. A treatment decision tool is available at the site that allows patients to input their specific diagnostic information and then generate a guide to treatments that might be appropriate for their situation.

Bibliography

Degner, L.F., Sloan, J.A., & Venkatesh, P. (1997). The control preferences scale. *Canadian Journal of Nursing Research, 29,* 21–43.

Surgical Oncology

Robin Gemmill

Surgery is the oldest method used in the treatment of cancer, dating as far back as early 1600 B.C. Throughout history, surgical procedures for the removal of cancer have correlated with our knowledge of tumor biology. During the time of Hippocrates (460–375 BC), cancer was believed to be caused by black bile, one of the body's four humors (phlegm, yellow bile, blood, and black bile). Surgery at that time used a form of lancing or bloodletting to release the collection of cancer-causing humor.

The 19th century proved to be a milestone in our understanding of human anatomy and physiology when a more sophisticated view of the cellular nature of cancer led to the concept of cancer as a local disease, thus replacing the humoral theory.

This was the basis, for example, for the Halstead radical mastectomy procedure, which is the surgical removal of the breast, chest wall muscles, and local lymph nodes that often left patients with drastic disfigurement and loss of function. This procedure remained the treatment of choice up until the 1960s. Scientific advances and discoveries during the last decades of the 20th century increased our understanding of the genetic and molecular basis of cancer and the mechanisms of metastasis, leading to more conservative surgery, sparing lymph nodes and tissue whenever possible.

Although surgery continues to be the primary treatment for localized disease, it is more common for cancer patients to receive a combination of treatment modalities. For example, the patient with early-stage breast cancer may have a lumpectomy followed by radiation therapy and/or chemotherapy. Combining treatment modalities has led to a decreased length of stay in the hospital, an increase in outpatient services, and minimizing the risk of decreased function in the adjacent arm. All together, these new treatment options, along with more sophisticated diagnostic technology, improved anesthesia, improved operative techniques, and infection control measures, have led to better patient outcomes, an improved quality of life, and a reduction in cost.

■ Principles/Rationale

There are several basic principles used to guide decision making in the surgical treatment of cancer. These include the following:

- Slow-growing and locally confined tumors are most suitable to surgical intervention.
- A border (margin) of normal tissue is removed with the tumor while functional and physical outcomes are preserved as much as possible.
- Before surgery, adequate staging should be performed to determine the best therapeutic approach.
- Operative techniques used during surgery should minimize the local and systemic spread of cancer.
- Any possible dysfunction related to the surgery must be explained beforehand and be acceptable to the patient.

The initial surgery for the removal of a primary cancer has a better chance for success than subsequent surgery for recurrent disease.

■ Role of Surgical Oncology

Surgical intervention for the treatment of cancer serves many purposes, including diagnosis, staging, prevention, treatment, palliative treatment, reconstruction, insertion of vascular access devices and ambulatory pumps, and treatment of oncologic emergencies.

Diagnosis

Advances in diagnostic technology, such as magnetic resonance imaging, positron emission technology scan, computerized tomography scan, and tissue sampling (biopsy), have facilitated interdisciplinary diagnosis and treatment planning. The diagnosis of cancer largely depends on pathological examination of a sample of tissue taken from the lesion in question, including both the affected area and adjacent tissue, to confirm diagnosis and determine the specific type of cancer present.

The choice of biopsy technique is based on the type, size, location, and growth characteristics of the suspected tumor. General guidelines for performing a biopsy are as follows:

- The biopsy site should be in an area that will be removed at the time of surgery, or the specimen obtained at biopsy should contain the entire tumor with clean margins, to reduce the possibility of seeding cancer cells along the incision site.
- The incision line, when possible, should be cosmetically acceptable and in skin folds.
- The tissue sample must be intact and contain normal tissue for comparison. For an overview of the various biopsy procedures, see Table 6–1.

TABLE 6–1 ■ Surgical Techniques for the Diagnosis of Cancer

Technique	Method	Benefits/Risks
Needle aspiration/ biopsy Use: diagnosis	Needle inserted into tumor Percutaneous or during surgery Sample may be fluid or tissue Fine needle (21–22 gauge) or core needle (cutting needle)	Simple to perform Less tissue trauma Needle may miss the tumor or malignant cells May not get enough specimen for definitive diagnosis Possible to seed (spread) tumor cells along the needle tract, causing recurrence
Excisional biopsy Use: diagnosis, treatment	Removal of the whole tumor with an effort to obtain clean margins Most commonly used biopsy method Tumor usually £ 3cm and accessible	Can be definitive therapy Outcome should be cosmetically acceptable Possible to seed tumor cells into tissue and incision, causing recurrence
Incisional biopsy Use: diagnosis	Removal of a piece of the tumor Tumors usually > 3cm	Additional surgery required to remove tumor Risk of profuse bleeding Specimen may be too small to make a diagnosis Margins not defined

(continued)

TABLE 6–1 ■ Surgical Techniques for the Diagnosis of Cancer—*Continued*

Technique	Method	Benefits/Risks
Needle localization biopsy Use: diagnosis, treatment	Needle placed by stereotactic guidance to mark the tumor, then tumor excised Tumor usually nonpalpable, but seen as radiographic abnormality Commonly used for breast cancer	Radiograph of specimen is necessary to ensure correct tissue was excised Done in outpatient radiology clinic
Sentinel node biopsy Use: diagnosis	Injection of blue dye and/or radioactive substance into area of tumor to identify lymph node closest to the tumor site, which is then removed and examined	Prevents removal of unaffected nodes Done during primary surgery Shorter recovery time Less pain Risk of false-negative result
Endoscopy Use: diagnosis, treatment	Tumor visualized through endoscope and a piece of tumor removed with forceps Commonly used for tumors of GI, GU, and respiratory tracts Can be incisional or excisional	Risk of perforation, hemorrhage Increases accessibility to tumors Avoids surgical trauma
Laparoscopy Use: diagnosis, staging, treatment	Tumor visualized through laparoscope and a specimen can be taken using one or more techniques (incisional, excisional, scraping, or peritoneal washing)	Can detect metastatic disease not seen on imaging scans Risk of perforation, hemorrhage Increase accessibility to tumors Requires small incisions but avoids surgical trauma
Laparotomy Use: diagnosis, staging, treatment	Exploratory surgery used to rule out metastases to other organs All types of biopsies can be performed (needle biosy, incisional, excisional, scraping, or peritoneal washing)	Useful when tumors are incorrectly staged by other techniques (e.g., computed tomographic scan), inaccessible, or difficult to evaluate

Source: Stahl, C.(1997). Surgical oncology. In *A cancer source book for nurses* (pp. 80–90). Sudbury, MA: Jones & Bartlett Publishers.

Needle biopsies are usually performed in an outpatient setting with the use of a local or topical anesthetic. The procedure is generally well tolerated by the patient. Hematoma and infection are potential complications.

A new surgical strategy for biopsy is the sentinel node biopsy. Because cancer cells may migrate to the sentinel node (the lymph node closest to the tumor) before spreading to other lymph nodes in the area, this node can be located by injecting blue dye and/or a radioactive substance into or around the tumor. Once the dye or radioactive substance is injected, it travels to the sentinel node, where the surgeon uses a scanner to find it. The sentinel node is then removed and sent for pathological review to identify the presence of cancer. If the sentinel node is determined to have no cancer, then no other nodes are removed. This prevents the removal of unaffected nodes and facilitates faster recovery with less pain. Common side effects of sentinel node biopsy include minor pain or bruising at the site and the rare possibility of an allergic reaction to the blue dye.

Nurses can help ease patient anxiety by educating patients and their families about the procedure and the time required to obtain results. It is not unusual to have a 2-week waiting period between the time of biopsy and surgery. Patient/family education should include caring for the biopsy site, identifying and reporting signs of infections or continued bleeding, and accessing the health care system to ask questions and report untoward symptoms during and after office hours.

Staging

Staging of disease using laparoscopic and endoscopic technology allows the physician to determine whether the disease has spread from the original site of tumor to other parts of the body. Laparoscopic procedures are usually performed as an outpatient or same-day procedure, thus avoiding a lengthy hospital stay and recovery time. Once the physician knows the stage of the disease, the most appropriate treatment plan for the patient can be created. In general, the lower the stage of disease (i.e., the more localized it is), the more amenable it is to surgical intervention. The higher the stage of disease, the more problematic surgical intervention becomes.

Prevention

Certain conditions, diseases, and genetic or congenital traits are associated with a higher risk for developing cancer. These include familial adenomatous polyposis, benign polyps of the colon, and ulcerative colitis. Preventive or prophylactic surgery to remove a portion of the affected bowel can lower the incidence of disease and possibly prevent occurrence of cancer. The following factors are taken into consideration when the need for preventive surgery is suggested:

- The presence or absence of symptoms
- Potential risks related to the age of the patient
- Risk for cancer based on medical and family history
- The ability to detect cancer at an early stage if prophylactic surgery is not performed
- Postoperative outcome (is it acceptable to the patient?)

Surgery for precancerous or in situ lesions (e.g., skin, cervix) is considered preventive. In situ tumors are at an early stage of growth, when the cancer cells are still confined to one layer of tissue. Because in situ cancers tend to have a high cure rate, preventive surgery is the treatment of choice and is usually curative.

Treatment

Surgical treatment for cancer varies depending on the goal. Surgical resection of the primary tumor is the treatment of choice for tumors that are localized or regionally contained and do not invade major organs or vascular structures. An example is breast conservation surgery, including lumpectomy (removal of the lump), quadrantectomy (removal of one quarter, or quadrant, of the breast), and segmental mastectomy (removal of the cancer as well as some of the breast tissue around the tumor and the lining over the chest muscles below the tumor). Eradicating all visible tumor cells, maintaining tissue and organ function, and minimizing alteration in appearance are the goals of treatment.

Radiofrequency ablation, commonly used for the treatment of hepatic tumors, is a relatively new laparoscopic treatment approach designed to produce complete coagulative necrosis of the tumor and surrounding nonmalignant tissue. A needle electrode that emits radio waves is placed through the skin directly into the liver tumor. The radio wave energy creates heat in the electrode inside the tumor, which spreads out to destroy the entire affected area. This procedure is usually performed on an outpatient basis and can take about 2 hours. After the procedure, patients are watched closely for about 4 hours before discharge to make sure that there are no problems. There is a small risk of bleeding and a very small possibility of infection or damage to the liver or lung near the tumor. Minor aches and pains or tiredness are common for a few days after procedure. This procedure, although effective, does not prevent cancer from returning or destroy micrometastases. For patients who cannot be treated by conventional surgery or chemotherapy, radiofrequency ablation is a good option.

Surgery as an adjuvant treatment is aimed at removing the bulk of tumor cells (cytoreduction), thus reducing tumor size so that other therapies (e.g., chemotherapy, radiation therapy, biotherapy) can be used to kill the remaining tumor cells.

Removal of recurrent tumor after a more conservative initial treatment has failed is known as salvage treatment. This type of surgery is usually more radical because more tissue is removed in an attempt to excise all of the cancer. The goal is still to cure, but as was stated before, secondary surgery for recurrence has less chance of success.

Palliative Treatment The goal of palliative surgery is to minimize symptoms of disease, enhance patient comfort, and optimize overall quality of life. It is not intended to be curative. The decision to have surgery for palliation depends on the patient's life expectancy, tumor growth rate, expected outcome, and expected benefit to the patient. Examples of palliative surgery include surgical relief of ascites with shunt procedures, neurosurgical intervention for chronic pain, fixation of pathological fractures, placement of feeding tubes to deliver food and medications, and relief of gastrointestinal, urinary, or respiratory obstruction.

Reconstruction

Cancer surgery may result in anatomic defects and loss of function. Reconstructive surgery to improve function or cosmetic appearance is often offered to patients who have had extensive cancer surgery. Some reconstructive surgeries, such as postmastectomy breast reconstruction, can take place during the primary surgery. Other reconstructive surgeries may be delayed and may necessitate multiple surgeries, such as for patients with head and neck cancer.

Vascular Access Devices and Ambulatory Pumps Many cancer patients require surgically implanted, long-term vascular access devices (VADs) and ambulatory pumps to facilitate the delivery of treatment and increase patient comfort. Although care for the various VADs is similar (e.g., need for patient education and aseptic technique), the differences in flushing techniques, catheter clamping, blood withdrawal, and complication management require close attention. There are three major types of long-term VADs: tunneled catheters, peripherally inserted central catheters (PICCs), and implantable venous ports. Each VAD offers distinct advantages and disadvantages (Table 6–2).

Tunneled catheters were originally designed for the long-term administration of parenteral nutrition. The catheter is tunneled under the skin from the insertion site to the superior vena cava. A Dacron cuff is located on the catheter to secure the device within the subcutaneous tissue approximately 2 inches from the exit site and to minimize the risk of ascending bacteria within the tunnel. These catheters can be used for months to years as long as they are cared for adequately.

TABLE 6–2 ■ Overview of Available Vascular Access Devices

Type	Description	Longevity	Comments
Peripheral catheter Intima	• Catheter over needle • Teflon or polyurethane • Single and double lumen • 26 to 14 gauge	Hours to days	• Excellent for multiday infusional therapy • Provides greater patient mobility and less likely to infiltrate
Nontunneled central venous catheter	• Polyurethane or silicone catheter • Single, double, and triple lumen	Hours to months	• Excellenht for emergency need for CVC • Can augment existing VAD for acute care needs or longer-term use • Inserted by physician at bedside or in procedure room
Peripherally inserted central catheters (PICCs)	• Silicone elastomer or other polymers • Single and double lumen • 24 to 16 gauge	Weeks to months	• Excellent for continuous infusion over several weeks or months • Can be inserted at bedside by specially trained nurse • Quick, easy central access without surgical procedure • Requries external site care and routine flushing
Tunneled central venous catheter	• Silicone catheter with Dacron cuff • Single, double, and triple lumen • 4.2–19.2 Fr; 40- to 90-cm length • Groshong has slit valve, requiring less flushing	Months to years	• Excllent for long-term, continuous, or intermittent therapy • Preferred for long-term TPN administration • Preferred by many for vesicant infusional therapy • Requires surgical placement • Requires external site care and routine flushing
Implantable port	• Titanium, stainless steel, Silastic, or plastic portal attached to catheter • Single and double lumen • Access with noncoring needle • Low profile ports available	Months to years	• Excellent for long-term, intermittent infusional therapy • No site care required when not in use so excellent for patients unable to perform site care • Surgical procedure required for placement and removal

TABLE 6-2 ■ Overview of Available Vascular Access Devices—*Continued*

Type	Description	Longevity	Comments
Peripheral port	• Titanium portal attached to Silastic catheter • Single lumen • Access with noncoring 22-gauge needle	Months to years	• Ideal for intermittent access, particularly for those patients with active lifestyles or body image concerns • No external site care when not in use • Not ideal for blood draw due to small volume

Key: CVC = central venous catheter; VAD = venous access device; TPN = total parenteral nutrition.

Reprinted with permission of Jones & Bartlett. Adapted from © 2003 CancerSource—All rights reserved

Insertion of this device is a surgical procedure, but it can be safely removed at the bedside. Tunneled catheters are an appropriate choice for patients undergoing intensive intravenous therapies, such as high-dose chemotherapy and bone marrow transplantation.

PICCs can be inserted at the bedside by specially trained registered nurses, without the need for a surgical procedure. Most PICCs placed are not sutured to the skin after insertion; therefore, care of the catheter must be meticulous. The insertion site is in the antecubital area, which may limit the patient's activity and pose problems in caring for the catheter (e.g., flushing and dressing change). Patients who have undergone a radical neck dissection, mastectomy, or radiation therapy to the chest; have neck veins that cannot be cannulated; or require short-term intravenous therapy are appropriate candidates for PICC lines.

Implantable ports are the only devices that are designed to access the peritoneal, arterial, venous or epidural body systems through a portal septum. Surgery is required for each implantable port placement. The port is a hollow housing of stainless steel, titanium, or plastic; it contains a latex septum over a portal chamber connected by a small tube to a silicone or polyurethane catheter inserted into a blood vessel. Venous ports commonly used for intravenous fluid or medication are placed in the upper chest area. The major advantage of an internal venous port is the infrequent need for flushing (every 3–4 months with sterile heparinized saline) when not in use. It is an ideal choice for a person who is unwilling to care properly for an external device, is receiving intermittent therapies, is concerned about body image, or is physically active. The major disadvantage is that it requires a needle to pass through the skin into the port for access.

The nurse is in a perfect position to continually assess the need for a VAD based on the frequency of access and the condition of the patient's veins. Ideally, VAD selection is a collaborative multidisciplinary decision, with the various types of VADs, the condition of the patient's peripheral veins, the anticipated frequency of access, the patient's ability to care for the device, the availability of support systems, and the cost being taken into consideration.

Occlusion of the VAD is commonly the result of a blood clot within the catheter. Other causes might be associated with incompatible drugs or lipids that have crystallized or precipitated. Although blood clots occur over time, drug precipitates tend to be directly related to a recent infusion. Key principles for prevention of occlusion include:

- Maintain positive pressure within the catheter and vigorously flush the catheter if there is no resistance. Intermittent resistance may mean that the catheter is being pinched off at the level of the clavicle and the first rib. Flushing forcefully in this case can cause an aneurysm in the catheter.
- Avoid excessive manipulation of external catheters.
- Vigorously flush with at least 20 ml of sterile saline to prevent sludge build-up within the port.
- Assess patient and family activities related to catheter care and maintenance, and provide supplemental education as needed.
- Flush in between each drug administration with at least 10 ml of solution to prevent precipitation.
- When administering total parenteral nutrition or lipids, vigorously flush catheter every 8–12 hours.

Principles for management of sluggish or partial occlusion and infection include the following:

- Catheter position can affect flow, so a partial occlusion in the absence of pain or discomfort should be managed first by teaching the patient to change position, raise the arms, deep breathe, and/or cough.
- Fibrin sheaths can form at the catheter insertion site and float, like a sleeve, around the outside of the catheter. If the sheath extends beyond the end of the lumen, it can cause withdrawal occlusion. Declot the fibrin sheath by instilling alteplase, 2 mg/2 ml, into the catheter with a dwell time of 30–120 minutes. If catheter function

is not restored after 120 minutes a second dose may be instilled to restore function.

- Infections in the catheter tunnel or port usually present with redness, edema, tenderness or discomfort, exudates, skin warmth, and/or fever.

Oncologic Emergencies

Surgery for an oncologic emergency is aimed at relieving symptoms and improving the patient's quality of life. Emergency surgery is most frequently used for gastrointestinal hemorrhage, spinal cord compression, or pericardial effusion. It is important for nurses to be familiar with the patient's advanced directives or wishes so that prompt interventions can be instituted quickly if needed.

■ The Role of the Nurse

Surgical care for the cancer patient poses many challenges for the nurse. Nurses need to be familiar with general surgical nursing principles, the disease process, the effects of radiation therapy and chemotherapy treatment, and the potential physical and psychosocial effects of cancer surgery. Preoperative assessment should include the following: diagnosis, patient age, developmental stage, goals of the surgery proposed, patient and family understanding of the diagnosis and proposed surgery, self-concept, coping skills/styles, expected outcomes, caregiver needs after surgery, and possibility of adjuvant therapies (e.g., chemotherapy, radiation therapy). Nurses play a crucial role in answering patient questions related to the cancer diagnosis and the proposed surgery. Addressing patient and family misconceptions and fears about the surgery helps reduce anxiety, thereby improving the patient's ability to learn about what to expect, self-care activities, and what symptoms to watch for and report to the physician. In addition, nurses can help the patient explore the meaning of cancer and surgery by validating concerns, providing emotional support through education, and identifying potential resource needs, such as support groups or preoperative counseling (e.g., Reach to Recovery, Wellness Community).

Nutritional Support for the Surgical Oncology Patient

For the surgical oncology patient, disease process, surgical stress, anorexia, prior chemotherapy, and radiation therapy increase catabolic requirements and contribute to protein-calorie malnutrition. In addition, many surgical procedures can alter the body's ability to maintain adequate nutrition. The most common nutrition-related alterations occur with surgery for gastrointestinal tract or head and neck cancer. These patients usually experience severe postoperative complications unless their nutritional status is fully assessed and an aggressive multidisciplinary treatment plan of support is developed and initiated before surgery.

Nutritional support, including oral diets, enteral tube feedings, and parenteral nutrition, provides the needed protein and calories. Pneumonia, ileus, sepsis, wound infection, wound dehiscence, and diminished tolerance of subsequent antineoplastic therapies are common complications associated with malnutrition resulting from surgery. It is standard practice to plan for postoperative enteral or parenteral nutrition for the patient for whom oral intake is not possible for more than 7–10 days after surgery. Preoperative nutritional support for the surgical oncology patient has significantly reduced postoperative morbidity and mortality.

■ Other Issues to Consider

Smoking

For patients undergoing surgery, smoking can pose numerous problems during recovery. Nicotine and carbon monoxide alter wound healing by causing vasoconstriction and tissue hypoxia that can lead to an increased risk of wound infection, delayed healing, and wound dehiscence. Numerous studies have shown that the relative risk for recurrence of cancer is doubled in patients who have quit smoking and quadrupled in those who continue to smoke, regardless of the amount they smoke.

Bleeding

The cancer patient is at risk for multiple hematologic alterations due to tumor burden and/or treatment. It is imperative for the nurse to assess the patient's hematologic status before surgery by looking for anemia, thrombocytopenia, neutropenia, and hypercoagulation in order to avoid intraoperative and postoperative bleeding or infection. Hypercoagulability is of particular concern for the cancer patient as clotting factors become elevated and the partial thromboplastin time becomes shortened, putting the patient at risk for deep vein thrombosis.

■ Late Effects

As the number of cancer survivors increases, nurses need to become more focused on late treatment effects in relation to quality of life. Ideally, all patients and families should be informed about possible late treatment effects in order to make informed decisions about treatment before surgery. The degree and the likelihood of late effects from cancer surgery depend on the type of surgery performed, the amount of tissue and/or organ removed, the age of the patient, and the significance the patient places on the treatment outcome. Possible late effects from oncologic surgery include the following: physical asymmetry, renal effects, lymphedema, and sexual dysfunction.

■ Physical Asymmetry

Surgery to remove a portion of bone (e.g., long bone) usually results in a shortening of the affected limb, resulting in physical asymmetry. Nursing can provide the patient with anticipatory guidance and counseling to address questions or concerns, making referrals to support groups to ease the emotionally stressful preoperative period.

Renal Effects

Surgery for gynecologic, prostate, or bladder cancer can result in recurrent urinary tract infections, hydronephrosis, renal stones, stress incontinence, and urgency, all of which, over time, can lead to renal impairment.

Lymphedema

Patients who have undergone a lymph node dissection of the groin, pelvis, or axilla are at risk for development of lymphedema. Damage to the lymph nodes or vessels during surgery impairs the body's ability to transport lymph fluid, causing an accumulation of fluid in the affected extremity. Numerous factors can contribute to development of lymphedema, including infection, inflammation, obesity, thrombophlebitis, arm dominance, and habitual dependent position of the arm. An example, commonly seen today, is the patient who has undergone radical mastectomy. The greatest incidence of lymphedema occurs in women who have had high-dose radiation therapy before surgery. The woman's self-image and emotional well-being may be adversely affected.

Sexual Dysfunction

Often, patients who have undergone a radical prostatectomy for prostate cancer, radical cystectomy for bladder cancer, and abdominoperineal resection for removal of the lower colon and rectum for colon cancer report sexual dysfunction and urinary incontinence related to surgery.

■ Conclusion

Advances in technology, both diagnostic and procedural, as well as our increased understanding of cancer biology, are changing the landscape of surgical oncology nursing. The increased use of laparoscopic procedures is resulting in shorter hospital stays and more care being provided in outpatient ambulatory care settings. Nurses play a vital role in helping patients and families navigate the health care system through coordination of care among the medical oncologist, surgeon, and radiologist while continuing to assess, teach, and provide quality patient care. Having a basic understanding of the foundational principles of surgical oncology, the dimensions of surgical treatment options, and an appreciation for some of the late effects cancer survivors might face are all pivotal aspects of care for the nurse caring for the surgical oncology patient.

■ Resources

- The American Cancer Society (ACS): *http://www.cancer.org/*
  - ACS Reach to Recovery program offers support and education for women with breast cancer.
  - ACS Man to Man—for men diagnosed with prostate cancer
- National Cancer Institute (NCI): *http://www.cancer.gov/*
- *www.cancersourcern.com*—provides information to nurses caring for cancer patients

Bibliography

Curley, S. (2001). Radiofrequency ablation of malignant liver tumors. *The Oncologist,* 6, 14–23.

Frogge, M. H., Cunning, S. M., (2000) Surgical Therapy. In C. H. Yarbro, M. H. Frogge, & M. Goodman. (Eds.), *Cancer nursing: Principles and practice* (pp. 272–283 & 408–421). Boston: Jones & Bartlett Publishers.

Goodman, M. (2002). Principles of chemotherapy administration: Vascular access devices. In C. H. Yarbro, M. H. Frogge, & M. Goodman. (Eds.), *Cancer nursing: Principles and practice* (5th ed.). Boston: Jones & Bartlett Publishers. See also: *http://www.cancersourcern.com/Nursing/CE/CECourse.cfm?courseid=146&contentid=22883*

Knobf, M.T. (1998). Surgical oncology. In S. B. Baird, R. McCorkle, & M. Grant (Eds.), *Cancer nursing: A comprehensive textbook* (pp. 22—33). Philadelphia: W. B. Saunders.

Weintraub, F., Neumark, D., (2001). Surgical oncology. In B. L. Johnson, & J. Gross (Eds.), *Handbook of oncology nursing.* (pp. 315—329). Boston: Jones & Bartlett Publishers.

CHAPTER

7

Chemotherapy

Mary Magee Gullatte

Janese Gaddis

With continued emphasis on cancer prevention and early detection coupled with advances in treatment, the overall cancer mortality continues to show a steady decrease. The American Cancer Society has published a goal of 50% reduction in cancer mortality rates by the year 2015. A major factor in this reduction in cancer mortality will be successful treatment outcomes. Chemotherapy plays a key role in the treatment plan for most cancers. For the estimated 1,368,050 new cases of invasive cancers in 2004, most will have been treated with a regimen including chemotherapy to effect cure, control, or palliation. Chemotherapy is a systemic treatment that can reach metastatic and sanctuary sites not always amenable to other treatment modalities, such as surgery and radiation therapy.

The development and evaluation of new cancer treatment agents includes a process spanning preclinical research through phase III clinical trials. This cancer agent development process takes an average of 100 months from bench research to approval. The US Food and Drug Administration statutes related to new agent development came into effect as early as 1906. It was not until 1962, with the Kefauver-Harris Drug amendments, that a manufacturer was required to prove that an agent was both safe and effective for its intended use before the manufacturer obtained marketing approval. From bench to bedside, cancer drug development is a four-phase process that ends with a new treatment in the armamentarium against cancer. Therapeutic clinical trials are essential to determine the effectiveness of the drug for the intended

TABLE 7–1 ■ Clinical Trials in Cancer

Phase I	Phase II	Phase III
• Define tolerable dose • Describe side effects • Administration • Safety profile	• Determine drug activity • Determine response rate and efficacy to specific cancer type	• Determine survival and quality of life • Compare to standard therapy

Source: Gullatte, M. M. (Ed.) (2001). *Clinical guide to antineoplastic therapy: A chemotherapy handbook.* Pittsburgh: Oncology Nursing Society.

treatment goal. The three primary types of clinical trials are listed in Table 7–1. In Phase IV, postmarketing studies are conducted to define new uses and dosing schedules and to gather additional information about the agent.

Principles/Rationale for Chemotherapy Use

To understand the rationale for using chemotherapy as treatment, one must have a working knowledge of the normal cell cycle kinetics, the changes occurring during malignant transformation and apoptosis (programmed cell death), the goals of chemotherapy treatment, and the mechanisms of action of these agents.

The normal cell cycle is an orderly sequence of steps through which cells divide and replicate. Malignant cells also undergo cellular division and replication. The process of cell replication and growth involves five phases designated by the letters and subscripts G_0, G_1, S, G_2, and M (see Figure 1–2 and Chapter 1 for more on the cell cycle).

Most antineoplastic agents are classified according to both where they affect cell cycle activity and how they affect cellular function. If classified by cellular activity, the agents are considered either cell cycle (phase) specific or cell cycle (phase) nonspecific. Functional classifications specify the antineoplastic agents as alkylators, antimetabolites, anthracyclines or antitumor antibiotics, plant alkaloids, hormonal agents, heavy metals, biotherapeutics, and miscellaneous agents (Table 7–2; which begins on page 106) .

The goals of chemotherapy are cure, control, or palliation. Additionally, when there is a large propensity for a cancer to have microscopic disease and with increased risk for systemic recurrence, agents may be given as neoadjuvant therapy or as adjuvant therapy; that is, as a treatment before either surgery or radiation therapy or biotherapy or in addition to these treatment modalities. Combining local and systemic modalities causes a greater tumor cell kill and hence a greater host response to treatment.

Having an understanding of the mechanisms of action and the purpose of treatment is paramount to understanding the logic behind the use of combination therapy.

In combination therapy, agents that differ in both cell-cycle specificity and toxicity are combined to achieve maximum cell kill with minimum side effects to the patient. Examples of standard combination therapy include AC (doxorubicin [Adriamycin], cyclophosphamide), one of several regimens for breast cancer, and MOPP (mechlorethamine), vincristine (Oncovin), prednisone, procarbazine), a standard combination therapy regimen for Hodgkin's disease.

■ Chemotherapeutic Agents

Alkylating agents are drugs that work by interacting chemically with the cellular DNA to prevent replication of the cell. As a class, these chemotherapy agents are considered cell cycle (phase) nonspecific. Alkylating agents have been proved to be cytotoxically active against chronic leukemias, lymphomas, Hodgkin's disease, and certain carcinomas of the breast, lung, prostate, and ovary. Nitrosoureas act similarly to alkylating agents by inhibiting enzymatic changes necessary for DNA repair. These agents cross the blood-brain barrier and are used to treat brain tumors, lymphomas, multiple myeloma, and malignant melanoma.

Antimetabolites are a group of agents that interfere with DNA and RNA synthesis by mimicking the chemical structure of essential metabolites. They prohibit cell replication in one of two ways: (a) by deceiving cells into incorporating the agent into metabolic pathways essential for the synthesis of RNA or DNA so that a false genetic message is transmitted, or (b) by blocking the enzymes necessary for the synthesis of essential compounds. The end result is that DNA synthesis is prevented. These drugs are cell cycle (phase) specific and are used in the treatment of leukemias and tumors of the gastrointestinal tract, breast, and ovary.

Anthracyclines, which are antitumor antibiotics, are cytotoxic agents synthesized from microorganisms and have both antimicrobial and cytotoxic activity. Anthracyclines are some of the most potent and widely used chemotherapeutic agents. However, large cumulative doses damage the heart muscle, an effect that limits the amounts that can be

TABLE 7–2 ■ Antineoplastic Drug Classification

Drug Class	Common Agents	Method of Action
Alkylating agents	Mechlorethamine Mitomycin Chlorambucil Melphalan Thiotepa Carmustine Lomustine Dacarbazine Procarbazine	Cell cycle nonspecific. Inhibit protein synthesis as RNA, DNA, function. Forms DNA cross-links.
Antimetabolic	Methotrexate Thioguanine Mercaptopurine 5-Fluorouracil	Cell cycle dependent, effects DNA, RNA, and protein synthesis. Greatest effect on rapidly dividing cells. Inhibit purine and pyrimidine nucleotide synthesis. Folic acid antagonist. Excreted unchanged in urine.
Anthracyclines and antitumor antibiotics	Mitomycin Doxorubicin Bleomycin Epirubicin Dactinomycin Daunorubicin Idarubicin Liposomal carriers: • Doxil® • Lipodox®	Bind with DNA to inhibit DNA and RNA synthesis.

Key: IV = intravenous; IM = intramuscular; MD = physician; NP = nurse practitioner; FSH = follicle-stimulating hormone; LH = luteinizing hormone; BUN = blood urea nitrogen; CNS = central nervous system; GI = gastrointestinal.

TABLE 7–2 ■ Antineoplastic Drug Classification—*Continued*

Side Effects/Toxicity	Administration	Patient Education
Dose dependent and cumulative Myelosuppression Anorexia Nausea, vomiting Diarrhea Alopecia Stomatitis Skin rashes Hemolytic uremic syndrome (HUS) Interstitial pneumonitis and/or fibrosis Cardiac failure CNS toxicities Mutagenic, Teratogenic, Carcinogenic effects	Do not extravasate Routes of administration may include: oral, IV, topical, depending on the agent and treatment plan	Educate patient about expected side effects based on agent, dose intensity, and route of administration.
Gastrointestinal mucosa Myelosuppression Stomatitis Diarrhea	Routes of administration based on agent and protocol: Topical Oral IV Intrathecal IM	Educate patient about sun exposure, skin color changes, hands, and nail beds. Education patient about sore mouth and some swallowing difficulties. Teach oral care.
Cardiotoxicity in nonliposomal products Myelosuppression Pulmonary toxicity Alopecia Fever and chills Pain at peripheral administration site Mucositis GI toxicity Hepatic and renal dysfunction Blood clotting disorders	IV Intra-arterial Intravesical (bladder instillation)	Monitor fever. Notify MD/NP for chills and fever or bleeding. Monitor for arrhythmias. Body image with hair loss.

(continued)

Key: IV = intravenous; IM = intramuscular; MD = physician; NP = nurse practitioner; FSH = follicle-stimulating hormone; LH = luteinizing hormone; BUN = blood urea nitrogen; CNS = central nervous system; GI = gastrointestinal.

TABLE 7–2 ■ Antineoplastic Drug Classification—*Continued*

Drug Class	Common Agents	Method of Action
Plant alkaloids	Vinca alkaloids • Vinblastine • Vincristine Taxanes • Paclitaxel • Docetaxel Epipodophyllotoxins • Etoposide • Teniposide	Cell cycle phase specific.
Hormonal agents (agonists and antagonists)	Androgens • Testosterone • Methyl testosterone Estrogens • Diethylstilbestrol • Conjugated estrogens Progestin • Megestrol Antiestsrogens • Tamoxifen • Toremifene • Raloxifene GnRH agonists • Goserelin • Leuprolide • Flutamide	Androgens: Inhibit gonadotropin-releasing hormone release and estrogen production. Estrogens decrease FSH and LH from the pituitary gland. Progestins effect serum estrogen. Antiestrogens bind to estrogens.
Biotherapy	Hematopoietic growth factors • Sargramostim • Filgrastin • Erythropoietin • Oprelvekin Interferons • Interferon—alpha 2a Interleukins • IL-2 Monoclonal antibodies • Gemtuzumab • Rituximab • Transtuzumab	Increase production of specific hematologic cell line Interferons: Induce antiproliferative and immunomodulatory responses Interleukins: Promotes proliferation of T and B cells and natural killer cells Monoclonal Antibodies: Selective binding to receptor proteins

Key: IV = intravenous; IM = intramuscular; MD = physician; NP = nurse practitioner; FSH = follicle-stimulating hormone; LH = luteinizing hormone; BUN = blood urea nitrogen; CNS = central nervous system; GI = gastrointestinal.

TABLE 7-2 ■ Antineoplastic Drug Classification—*Continued*

Side Effects/Toxicity	Administration	Patient Education
Myelosuppression Neuropathy Allergic reactions Hypotension Alopecia Cardiac arrhythmias Myalgia Mucositis Nausea Vomiting	Based on agent and protocol: Oral IV Intrathecal	Notify provider for fever, chills, dizziness from sitting or lying to standing position, numbness in fingers and toes. Unusual heart beats.
Changes in weight, mood Skin changes Cardiac changes Nausea and vomiting Hirsutism Male pattern baldness Hot flashes Gynecomastia Fluid retention Liver toxicity	Oral Depot Topical	Educate about relevant gender-specific side effects: hot flashes, gynecomastia, hirsutism.
Intensity of side effects directly related to dose intensity and duration of therapy Refer to specific information on each agent	Based on agent: Subcutaneous, IM, IV	Educate patient about side effects based on specific agent administered

(continued)

Key: IV = intravenous; IM = intramuscular; MD = physician; NP = nurse practitioner; FSH = follicle-stimulating hormone; LH = luteinizing hormone; BUN = blood urea nitrogen; CNS = central nervous system; GI = gastrointestinal.

TABLE 7–2 ■ Antineoplastic Drug Classification—*Continued*

Drug Class	Common Agents	Method of Action
Platinum compounds	Cisplatin Carboplatin Oxaliplatin	Cell cycle phase non specific. Inhibit RNA and DNA and protein synthesis by forming DNA cross-links.

Key: IV = intravenous; IM = intramuscular; MD = physician; NP = nurse practitioner; FSH = follicle-stimulating hormone; LH = luteinizing hormone; BUN = blood urea nitrogen; CNS = central nervous system; GI = gastrointestinal.

given. This has led, in recent years, to the development of cardioprotective agents, and more recently, liposomal (phospholipids membrane) formulations, which increase drug selectivity either by targeting the drug to the tumor or by diverting the drug from highly sensitive organs, such as the heart.

Plant alkaloids and natural products fall into three categories: mitotic inhibitors, enzymes, and enzyme inhibitors. Plants form the foundation of many of our modern pharmaceuticals. Mitotic inhibitors have two primary mechanisms of action: (a) crystallization of the microtubules during mitosis, causing mitotic arrest and apoptosis, and (b) enhanced microtubule formation, resulting in a stable, albeit nonfunctional, microtubules capable of causing cellular death. Enzymes act by inhibiting protein synthesis, thereby depriving tumor cells of the amino acids necessary for cell replication. Enzyme inhibitors, such as topoisomerase inhibitors (e.g., etoposide, topotecan, irinotecan), inhibit enzymes that break and reseal DNA strands. These drugs form a stable complex by binding to DNA and topoisomerase enzymes, resulting in DNA damage that interferes with replication and transcription. Vinca alkaloids used as antineoplastic agents include vinblastine and

TABLE 7–2 ■ Antineoplastic Drug Classification—*Continued*

Side Effects/Toxicity	Administration	Patient Education
Peripheral neuropathy Renal tubular damage Elevations in BUN and Bilirubin Hearing loss Myelosuppression Tinnitus Raynaud's phenomenon Nausea Vomiting Thrombocytopenia Abdominal pain Hypokalemia Liver abnormalities	IV	Educate patient regarding associated side effects and what and when to report to the physician or nurse.

Source: Data from Gullatte, M. M. (Ed.) (2001). *Clinical guide to antineoplastic therapy: A chemotherapy handbook.* Pittsburgh: Oncology Nursing Society; Adams, V. R., & Bence, A. K. (2003). Guide for the administration and use of cancer chemotherapeutic agents 2003. *Oncology special edition: The annual clinical reference.* New Jersey: Novartis Oncology; Brown, K. A., Esper, P., Kelleher, L. O., et al. (2001). *Chemotherapy and biotherapy: Guidelines and recommendations for practice.* Pittsburgh: Oncology Nursing Society.

vincristine. Another class of plant alkaloids are the taxanes paclitaxel and docetaxel, which have become important agents in treating breast, lung, and ovarian cancers.

A platinum compound, Cisplatin is the first established member of one of the most active classes of anti-cancer agents in clinical use (Calvert, H., Judson, I., and van Der Vijgh, W. 1993). Subsequent analogues developed include Carboplatin and Oxaliplatin compounds. The mechanism of action for the platinum compounds effect their action by inhibiting DNA replication and transcription, and in this way likely produce the cytotoxicity characteristic of the drug (Canal 1998).

Hormones and *hormone antagonists* are useful in treating some types of tumors by changing the environment in which the tumor originates and grows. Once the environment is changed, tumor growth is impaired or arrested. However, the specific mechanism of action is not clear. This group of agents is effective against hormone-dependent tumors, such as breast, ovary, prostate, and testicular cancers.

Biotherapy is defined as the use of agents derived from biologic sources, or agents that affect biologic responses and stimulate an immune response (see Chapter 10). The use of growth factors in the oncology treatment plan has made a significant positive impact on patient tolerance and outcomes of chemotherapy.

■ Administration Issues

The administration of cancer chemotherapeutic agents requires a knowledgeable, skilled, and competent oncology professional. Competency programs should minimally include information about cancer biology, treatment goals, drug information (vesicant or irritant), preparation, admixture, and safe handling and disposal guidelines. Chemotherapy doses are usually given based on body surface area per meters squared and are calculated from an individual's height and weight. The sequence of drug administration may be crucial to effectiveness; therefore, familiarity with the chemotherapy protocol is critical. Careful adherence to written chemotherapy orders prevents errors in scheduling, method of administration, or dose.

Based on the drugs and protocol, chemotherapeutic agents may be administered by the following routes: oral, intravenous, intramuscular, intracavitary, intraperitoneal, intrathecal, intrapleural, intravesicular, topical, and intra-arterial. Several chemotherapeutic agents are considered irritants and vesicants. When given intravenously, they can cause either irritation to the vein or, if improper technique is used, extravasation and subsequent tissue damage. Such damage might include hyperpigmentation, burning, erythema, inflammation, ulceration, necrosis, prolonged pain, tissue sloughing, infection, and loss of mobility (Table 7–3). Ensuring competent intravenous access before administration of intravenous agents is essential to preventing extravasation.

A comprehensive chemotherapy administration checklist may be found in Table 7–4; which begins on page 000. Some chemotherapeutic agents cause allergic or hypersensitivity reactions that vary from mild to life threatening. Although it is impossible for a nurse to recall all the side effects for every drug, it is the nurse's responsibility to be aware of potential allergic or hypersensitivity reactions to specific drugs. These drugs must be given with caution, and emergency medications should be readily available in case of anaphylactic reaction.

■ Nursing Care

The effects of antineoplastic agents are systemic and nondiscriminatory to human tissue. These agents damage proliferating and resting cells, healthy and cancerous cells alike. The most vulnerable cells are those

TABLE 7–3 ■ Vesicant and Irritant Chemotherapy Agents

Vesicants	**Irritants**
Anthracyclines/antitumor antibiotics • Dactinomycin • Daunorubicin • Doxorubicin • Idarubicin	Anthracyclines and antitumor antibiotics • Bleomycin • Carmustine • Daunorubicin (liposomal) • Doxorubicin (liposomal)
Alkylating agents • Mechlorethamine • Mitomycin C • Menogaril • Mitoxantrone	Alkylating agents • Dacarbazine • Streptozocin
Plant (vinca) alkaloids • Vinblastine • Vincristine • Vinorelbine • Teniposide	Plant alkaloids • Docetaxel • Paclitaxel • Etoposide
Miscellaneous • Plicamycin	Antimetabolite • Fluorouracil
	Platinum compounds • Cisplatin • Carboplatin
	Miscellaneous • Irinotecan

Source: Data from Gullatte, M. M. (Ed.) (2001). *Clinical guide to antineoplastic therapy: A chemotherapy handbook.* Pittsburgh: Oncology Nursing Society; Wilkes, et al., 1999; Peters, 1998; Brown, K. A., Esper, P., Kelleher, L. O., et al. (2001). *Chemotherapy and biotherapy: Guidelines and recommendations for practice.* Pittsburgh: Oncology Nursing Society.

with rapid doubling times in the hematopoietic, integumentary, gastrointestinal, respiratory, cardiovascular, genitourinary, nervous, and reproductive systems.

A prechemotherapy nursing assessment guide is presented in Table 7–5, which begins on page 116. This table includes assessment parameters as well as the drug- and dose-limiting side effects for chemotherapeutic agents. This information forms the foundation for care of patients receiving chemotherapy as treatment for their cancer.

Safe Handling of Hazardous Drugs

Recommended guidelines for safe handling of hazardous drugs have been in place since 1986. The Occupational Safety and Health Administration (OSHA) established these guidelines to protect workers in the

TABLE 7–4 ■ Chemotherapy Administration Check List

1. Verify informed consent before chemotherapy administration.
2. Know the drug pharmacology: mechanism of action, usual dosage, route of administration, acute and long-term side effects, and route of excretion.
3. Review laboratory data, keeping in mind acceptable parameters. Report abnormalities to the physician or oncology NP/PA.
4. Complete prechemotherapy assessment of patient, medical history, vascular access, height, and weight before chemotherapy.
5. Check physician order for name of drug(s), dosage, route, rate, and timing of drug(s) administration. (Question anything that seems out of the ordinary.)
6. Recalculate dosage, based on body surface area (BSA). Check height and weight; calculate body surface area.
7. Verify physician orders and dosage calculations with another clinician or pharmacist.
8. Premedication: administer most premedications at least 20–30 minutes before chemotherapy starts. In some cases, you may want to start the patient on an antiemetic or antianxiolytic therapy the night before or the morning of the therapy.
9. Patient education: teach and review with the patient and family details of the chemotherapy schedule, expected side effects, and self-care/preventive management suggestions to minimize untoward side effects. Provide written explanations the patient can refer to later because this information may be overwhelming. Refer questions to physician, nurse practitioner, or physician assistant as necessary.
10. Provide patient with telephone numbers for medical follow-up as appropriate.
11. Reconstitute drug(s) according to manufacturer suggestions, Occupational Safety and Health Administration (OSHA) guidelines, and intuition procedures. This may be the responsibility of the nursing or the pharmacy department depending on the institution's policy.
12. Gather appropriate equipment. Use the correct intravenous solution, based on compatibility and volume. Protect from direct sunlight if applicable.
13. To ensure patient safety, administer chemotherapy agents according to written policies and procedures using proficient intravenous therapy skills and techniques.
    a. Administer all medications using the five rights:
        i. Right patient
        ii. Right drug
        iii. Right dose
        iv. Right route (antineoplastic agents may be administered IV, IM, PO, IT, IP, IA, SQ, or topical).
        v. Right time
    b. If no information is available, proceed as if a vesicant and administer it with caution, according to institutional policy and procedure.

TABLE 7-4 ■ Chemotherapy Administration Check List—*Continued*

c. Avoid drug infiltration. If unsure whether the IV is infiltrated, discontinue it and restart IV rather than risk extravasation. *When in doubt, pull it out.*
d. Do not mix drugs together when administering multi drug regimen. Use syringe or intravenous of normal saline to flush before first drug, in between drugs, and on completion of all drugs.
e. It is not optimal to administer vesicant drugs through an indwelling peripheral IV (one that has been in place 4–6 hours or more). It is important to preserve veins, but it is more important to prevent potential extravasation.
f. Nonvesicant chemotherapy drugs may be administered through an existing IV, once the site has been fully assessed for patency and lack of infiltration.
g. If you are unable to start an IV after two attempts, consult a colleague for assistance.

14. Do not allow anyone to distract you during the preparation or administration of chemotherapy.
15. Do not foster a patient's dependency on one nurse.
16. Always have emergency drugs and an extravasation kit readily available should an adverse reaction occur.
17. Always listen to the patient. The patient's knowledge and preference should be used as frequently as possible. As the patient becomes more knowledgeable regarding IV techniques, his or her personal experience with successful IV sites, methods, and sensations can be a great aid to the nurse. There are times when the patient's preference may not be the best choice, but his or her participation should always be encouraged.
18. Dispose of intravenous supplies according to OSHA guidelines and institution policy and procedure.
19. Document drug administration according to institution policy and procedures. Use time savers in documentation. For example, instead of writing step-by-step how a vesicant was given, document "(Name of drug) administered according to institution policy and procedure for vesicants."
20. Observe for adverse reactions.
21. Use the opportunity to teach and counsel the patient and the family while administering the chemotherapy.

Key: IV = intravenous; IM = intramuscular; PO = oral; IT = intrathecal; IP = intraperitoneal; IA = intra-arterial; SQ = subcutaneous.

Sources: Data from Barton Burke, M., Wilkes, G., & Ingwersen, K. (1996). *Cancer chemotherapy: A nursing process approach* (2nd ed.). Sudbury, MA: Jones & Bartlett Publisher; Gullatte, M. M. (Ed.) (2001). *Clinical guide to antineoplastic therapy: A chemotherapy handbook.* Pittsburgh: Oncology Nursing Society; Polovich, M. (2003). *Safe handling of hazardous drugs.* Pittsburgh: Oncology Nursing Society; Brown, K. A., Esper, P., Kelleher, L. O., et al. (2001). *Chemotherapy and biotherapy: Guidelines and recommendations for practice.* Pittsburgh: Oncology Nursing Society.

TABLE 7–5 ■ Prechemotherapy Nursing Assessment Guidelines*

Potential Problems/ Nursing Diagnosis	Physical Status Assessment Parameters/ Signs and Symptoms	Drug- and Dose-Limiting Factors
Hematopoietic system A. Impaired tissue perfusion related to chemotherapy-induced anemia	• Hgb Norm, men 13.5–18g/dl, women 12–16g/dl • Hct Norm, men 40–54%, women 38–47% • Vital signs (BP, pulse, respiration) • Pallor (face, palms, conjunctiva) • Fatigue or weakness • Vertigo	Critical value: Hgb < 6.0g/dl Critical value: Hct < 14% Initiate blood transfusions or RBC growth factor.
B. Impaired immune competence and potential for infection related to chemotherapy-induced leukopenia	• WBC Norm, 5,000–10,000/mm^3; no gender differences • Pyrexia/rigor, erythema, swelling, pain any site • Abnormal discharges, draining wounds, skin/mucous membrane lesions	Critical value WBC< 1,00–1,500/mm^3 • Notify oncologist for possible hold of myelosuppressive agents (exceptions may include leukemia, lymphoma, and/or situations in which there is neoplastic marrow infiltration) Fever > 101° F:
C. Potential for injury (bleeding) related to chemotherapy-induced thrombocytopenia	• Productive cough, SOB, rectal pain, urinary frequency • Platelet count (150,000–450,000/mm^3) • Spontaneous gingival bleeding or epistaxis • Presence of petechiae or easy bruisability on skin (legs and arms) • Melena, hematemesis, hemoptysis • Hypermenorrhea	Critical value platelet count < 210,000/mm^3: • Notify oncologist to dose reduce or hold myelosuppressive agents (exceptions may include leukemia, lymphoma, and/or situations in which there is neoplastic marrow infiltration)

*All decisions to hold therapy should be in collaboration with oncologist and/or oncology nurse practitioner.

TABLE 7–5 ■ Prechemotherapy Nursing Assessment Guidelines—*Continued*

Potential Problems/ Nursing Diagnosis	Physical Status Assessment Parameters/ Signs and Symptoms	Drug- and Dose-Limiting Factors
	• S/s of intracranial bleeding (irritability, sensory loss, unequal pupils, headache, ataxia, acute change in level of consciousness)	
Integumentary system Alteration in mucous membrane of mouth, nasopharynx, esophagus, rectum, anus, or ostomy stoma related to chemotherapy-induced tissue changes	• Administer rescue agent as prescribed (e.g., leucovorin, mesna) Mucositis Scale 0 = pink, moist intact mucosa; absence of pain or burning +1 = generalized erythema with or without pain or burning +2 = isolated small ulcerations and/or white patches +3 = confluent ulcerations with white patches on 25% mucosa +4 = hemorrhagic ulcerations	+2 mucositis: • Notify oncologist for hold of antimetabolites (esp. methotrexate, 5-FU) • Notify oncologist for hold of antitumor antibiotics (esp. doxorubicin, dactinomycin)
Gastrointestinal system Discomfort, nutritional deficiency, and/or fluid and electrolyte disturbances related to chemotherapy-induced: A. Anorexia	• Lab values: albumin and total protein • Normal weight/present weight and % of body weight loss • Normal diet patterns/changes in diet pattern • Alterations in taste sensation • Early satiety	

TABLE 7–5 ■ Prechemotherapy Nursing Assessment Guidelines—*Continued*

Potential Problems/ Nursing Diagnosis	Physical Status Assessment Parameters/ Signs and Symptoms	Drug- and Dose-Limiting Factors
B. Nausea and vomiting	• Lab values: electrolytes • Pattern of nausea/vomiting (incidence, duration, severity) • Antiemetic plan: Drug(s), dosage(s), schedule, efficacy • Other (dietary adjustments, relaxation techniques, Diversion activities and environmental manipulation)	Intractable nausea/vomiting > 24 hours Initiate IV hydration
C. Bowel disturbances 1. Diarrhea	• Normal pattern of bowel elimination • Consistency (loose, watery/bloody stools) • Frequency and duration (no./day and no. of days) • Antidiarrheal drug(s), dosage(s), efficacy	Diarrheal stools × 3 per 24 hours: • Notify oncologist and hold antimetabolites (esp. methotrexate, 5-FU) • Evaluate antimicrobial therapy
2. Constipation	• Normal pattern of bowel elimination • Consistency (hard, dry, small stools) • Frequency (hours or days beyond normal pattern) • Stool softener(s), laxative(s), efficacy • Lab values: LDH, SGOT, alk phos, bilirubin • Pain/tenderness over liver, feeling of fullness	No BM × 48 hours past normal bowel patterns: • Hold vinca alkaloids (vinblastine, vincristine) Evidence of chemical hepatitis: • Notify MD and hold hepatotoxic agents (esp. methotrexate, 6-MP) until differential diagnosis established

TABLE 7–5 ■ Prechemotherapy Nursing Assessment Guidelines—*Continued*

Potential Problems/ Nursing Diagnosis	Physical Status Assessment Parameters/ Signs and Symptoms	Drug- and Dose-Limiting Factors
	• Increase in nausea/vomiting or anorexia • Changes in mental status • Jaundice • High-risk factors Hepatic metastasis Viral hepatitis Abdominal radiation therapy Concurrent hepatotoxic drugs Graft vs host disease Blood transfusions	
Respiratory system Impaired gas exchange or ineffective breathing pattern related to chemotherapy-induced pulmonary fibrosis	• Lab values, PFTs, CXR • Respiration (rate, rhythm, depth) • Chest pain • Nonproductive cough • Progressive dyspnea • Wheezing/stridor • High-risk factors: Total cumulative dose of bleomycin Preexisting lung disease Prior/concomitant XRT Age > 60 years Concomitant use of other pulmonary toxic drugs Smoking hx	Acute unexplained-onset respiratory symptoms: • Notify oncologist and hold all antineoplastic agents until differential dx established

TABLE 7–5 ■ Prechemotherapy Nursing Assessment Guidelines—*Continued*

Potential Problems/ Nursing Diagnosis	Physical Status Assessment Parameters/ Signs and Symptoms	Drug- and Dose-Limiting Factors
Cardiovascular system Decreased cardiac output related to chemotherapy-induced:	• Lab values: cardiac enzymes, electrolytes, EKG, ECHO, MUGA	Acute S/s CHF and/or cardiac arrhythmia: • Notify oncologist and hold all antineoplastic agents, especially anthrocycline, until differential dx established
A. Cardiac arrhythmias B. Cardiomyopathy	• Vital signs • Presence of arrhythmia (irregular radial/apical) • S/s of CHF (dyspnea, ankle edema, nonproductive coughs, rales, cyanosis) • High-risk factors: Total cumulative dose anthracyclines Preexisting cardiac disease Prior/concurrent mediastinal XRT	If total dose of doxorubicin or daunorubicin has exceeded > 550 mg
Genitourinary system A. Alteration in fluid volume (excess) related to chemotherapy-induced: 1. Glomerular or renal tubule damage 2. Hyperuricemic nephropathy	Lab values: BUN, creatinine clearance, serum creatinine, uric acid, electrolytes, urinalysis Serum creatinine Norm, men 0.6–1.3 mg/dl, women 0.5–1.0 mg/dl • Color, odor, clarity of urine • 24-hour fluid I&O(estimate/actual)	Assess S/s hematuria: • Vigorous hydration • Monitor BUN and creatinine • Notify oncologist and hold cyclophosphamide Serum creatinine > 2.0 and/or creatinine clearance: men 85–125 mL/min, women 75–115 mL/min

TABLE 7–5 ■ Prechemotherapy Nursing Assessment Guidelines—*Continued*

Potential Problems/ Nursing Diagnosis	Physical Status Assessment Parameters/ Signs and Symptoms	Drug- and Dose-Limiting Factors
B. Alteration in comfort related to chemotherapy-induced hemorrhagic cystitis	• Hematuria; proteinuria • Development of oliguria or anuria • High-risk factors: Preexisting renal disease Concurrent treatment with nephrotoxic drugs (esp. aminoglycoside antibiotics)	• Notify oncologist and hold *cis*-platin, streptozocin Anuria x 24 hours • Notify oncologist and hold antineoplastic agents
Nervous system A. Impaired sensory/motor function related to chemotherapy-induced: 1. Peripheral neuropathy 2. Cranial nerve neuropathy	Paresthesias (numbness, tingling in feet, fingertips) • Trigeminal nerve toxicity (severe jaw pain) • Diminished or absent deep tendon reflexes (ankle and knee jerks) • Motor weakness, slapping gait, ataxia • Visual and auditory disturbances	Presence of any neurologic S/s: • Notify oncologist and hold vinca alkaloids, *cis*-platinum, hexamethylmelamine, procarbazine until differential diagnosis established
B. Impaired bowel and bladder elimination related to chemotherapy-induced autonomic nerve dysfunction	• Urinary retention • Constipation, abdominal cramping and distention • High-risk factors: Changes in diet or mobility Frequent use of narcotic analgesics Obstructive disease process	Presence of any neurologic S/s: • Notify oncoloist and hold vinca alkaloids until differential diagnosis established

TABLE 7–5 ■ Prechemotherapy Nursing Assessment Guidelines—*Continued*

Potential Problems/ Nursing Diagnosis	Physical Status Assessment Parameters/ Signs and Symptoms	Drug- and Dose-Limiting Factors
Reproductive system A. Altered sexuality patterns related to body image changes and decreased level of sexual excitement	Side effects of chemotherapy: • Alopecia • Weight loss related to nausea/vomiting • Diarrhea • Fatigue • Decreased libido	Most chemotherapy agents have the potential to cause this problem, although this is not a drug- or dose-limiting side effect.
B. Alterations in the ability to achieve sexual fulfillment	Side effects of chemotherapy: • Dryness of vaginal mucosa secondary to decreased estrogen levels • Inflammation and ulceration of vaginal mucosa (mucositis) secondary to stem cell injury Other possible factors: • Altered role function • Fear • Fatigue • Decreased libido • Anxiety • Lack of privacy • Anger • Medications/alcohol/analgesics Side effects of chemotherapy: • Temporary impotence possibly related to fatigue • Pain	Some chemotherapy agents or the psychosexual sequelae of the disease may cause this potential problem, although this is not a drug- or dose- limiting side effect.

TABLE 7–5 ■ Prechemotherapy Nursing Assessment Guidelines—*Continued*

Potential Problems/ Nursing Diagnosis	**Physical Status Assessment Parameters/ Signs and Symptoms**	**Drug- and Dose-Limiting Factors**
C. Sexual dysfunction	Side effects of chemotherapy: • Temporary or permanent sterility Ovarian fibrosis with decrease in estrogen levels, decrease in number of available ova, especially with higher-dose alkylating agents and age over 39 Atrophy of endometrial lining of uterus Irregular menses or amenorrhea (may be reversible under 30 years of age) • Potential for mutation of available ova (especially by alkylating agents) Spontaneous abortion, stillbirth, birth defects May have normal children who should be followed by a pediatric oncologist • Temporary or permanent sterility Damage and destruction of testicular germ cells and epithelium of seminiferous tubules Oligospermia or azoospermia 90–120 days after treatment begins; normal sperm levels may be achieved several years after therapy Testosterone levels may not be altered • Possible sperm mutation Spontaneous abortion, stillbirth, birth defects	Some chemotherapy agents cause sexual infertility: chlorambucil doxorubicin cytarabine procarbazine vinblastine

TABLE 7–5 ■ Prechemotherapy Nursing Assessment Guidelines—*Continued*

Potential Problems/ Nursing Diagnosis	Physical Status Assessment Parameters/ Signs and Symptoms	Drug- and Dose-Limiting Factors
	Normal children have been fathered; child should be closely followed by pediatric oncologist	
D. Alterations in fetal development	Possible side effects of chemotherapy • Drugs cross placental barrier • Antimetabolites (e.g., MTX) and alkylating agents most harmful • First trimester: drugs can cause cellular damage and destruction, leading to spontaneous abortion • Second, third trimester: cellular destruction leads to low birth weight or premature infant, stillbirth, birth defects, great potential for development of malignancy; there may be mutation of ova of female child Access options regarding alternative methods of family planning • Foster parenthood • Adopting • Provide information on sperm banking	

TABLE 7–5 ■ Prechemotherapy Nursing Assessment Guidelines—*Continued*

Potential Problems/ Nursing Diagnosis	Physical Status Assessment Parameters/ Signs and Symptoms	Drug- and Dose-Limiting Factors

Key: Hgb = hemoglobin; Hct = hematocrit; BP = blood pressure; WBC = white blood cell; SOB = shortness of life; S/s, signs and symptoms; LDH = lactate dehydrogenase; SGOT = aspartate transaminase; alk phos = alkaline phosphatase; PFT = pulmonary function test; CXR = chest x-ray study; EKG = electrocardiogram; ECHO = echocardiogram; MTX = methotrexate; MUGA = multigated angiogram; CHF = congestive heart failure; XRT = radiation therapy; I&O = intake and output; 5-FU = 5-fluorouracil; BM = bowel movement; 6-MP = 6-mercaptopurine; dx = diagnosis; hx = history.

Sources: Data from Gullatte, M. M. (Ed.) (2001). *Clinical guide to antineoplastic therapy: A chemotherapy handbook.* Pittsburgh: Oncology Nursing Society; Brown, K. A., Esper, P., Kelleher, L. O., et al. (2001). *Chemotherapy and biotherapy: Guidelines and recommendations for practice.* Pittsburgh: Oncology Nursing Society; Barton Burke, M., Wilkes, G., & Ingwersen, K. (1996). *Cancer chemotherapy: A nursing process approach* (2nd ed.). Sudbury, MA: Jones & Bartlett Publisher.

workplace. OSHA uses the term *hazardous drugs* rather that cytotoxic agents. For purposes of this chapter, we use the term hazardous drugs. The hazardous drugs are agents that elicit side effects that can cause (a) genetic mutation, (b) secondary cancers, (c) fetal malformation, and (d) fertility impairment. Concern is extended not only to hazardous drugs but also to the excreta of patients receiving the hazardous drugs. The accepted time frame for special handling of bodily fluids after receiving chemotherapy is 48 hours. This includes urine, feces, emesis, and sweat. Special precautions should be implemented when any of these body fluids are handled. Personal protective equipment should be worn when bathing patients or handling body fluids if these tasks are performed within the 48 hours of receiving hazardous drugs. Soiled linen should be placed in specially marked, nonpermeable laundry bags and washed separately from other linen. When possible, disposable equipment (urinal, bedpan) should be used, and this should be discarded with the other hazardous waste. There are several routes by which exposure to hazardous drugs may occur: (a) inhalation, (b) absorption, and (c) ingestion. Refer to Table 7–6 for safety measures related to each route of exposure.

Safety barriers effective in decreasing exposure to hazardous drugs include using a biologic safety cabinet, wearing personal protective equipment, washing hands before and after preparation and administration, and adhering to institutional policies and procedures for safe handling and disposal of hazardous drugs. The effectiveness of all safety measures is related not only to the development of, but also the adherence to, established policies and procedures. Remember that occupational exposure may occur at any point when safe handling guidelines are omitted or not followed fully during the preparation, administration, or disposal process. Policies should be reevaluated annually to ensure appropriateness, given current information. Health care workers should always stay informed and should educate patients and their families about exposure risks and ways to maintain a safe environment.

Whenever hazardous drugs are handled, care should be taken to avoid spills. Should a spill occur, a spill kit should always be available in the areas of storage, preparation, and administration of hazardous drugs. Staff must be knowledgeable regarding the location of the spill kit as well as the safe way to clean up spills. This applies to patients receiving hazardous drugs at home as well. The patient and family should know to report spills, have a spill kit available, and how to clean spills. When a spill is being cleaned up, personal protective equipment should be worn. This includes a gown with long sleeves to the wrist, double gloves, respiratory protection, and an eye shield. See Table 7–7 for the contents of spill kits.

TABLE 7-6 ■ Routes of Exposure: Safe Handling of Hazardous Drugs

Routes of Exposure	Examples	Safety Measures
Ingestion within the preparation/ administration area	Eating, drinking, smoking, accidental needle stick	No eating, drinking, or smoking. Store food/drink away from drugs. Follow organizational guidelines.
Absorption	Spillage, leakage, applying make-up, IV poles/pumps, arm of chair/patient seat used while receiving drug, receptacle/counter drug was placed on during administration/check-off	Wash hands before and after each contact with drug. Wear PPE during preparation, administration, and disposal of drug. Do not apply make-up or lotion in work area. Implement safe handling precautions when exposed to or handling body excreta. Place soiled linen in specially marked, nonpermeable laundry bags. Use needleless systems and closed-system devices. Clean work surface area with approved solution. Place plastic absorbent pad under patient's arm to absorb leakage.
Inhalation	Open drug containers Uncovered disposal containers Breaking open ampules Needle withdrawal from vial Drug transfer between containers Expelling of air from syringe with hazardous drug Contaminated articles stored in closed containers	Remove IV bag with tubing intact. Open ampule when under the BSC. Wear PPE attire. Prepare hazardous drugs in BSC. Adhere to institutional policies and procedures for handling hazardous drugs.

Key: IV = intravenous; PPE = personal protective equipment; BSC = biologic safety cabinet.

Sources: Data from Gullatte, M., (2001). Principles and standards of chemotherapy administration. In M. Gullatte (Ed.), *Clinical guide to antineoplastic therapy: A chemotherapy handbook* (pp. 40–43). Pittsburgh: Oncology Nursing Society. Polovich, M. (Ed.). (2003). *Safe handling of hazardous drugs.* Pittsburgh: Oncology Nursing Society.

TABLE 7–7 ■ Spill Kit Contents

1 gown (disposable, nonpermeable, cuffed)	1 respirator mask approved by National Institute of Occupational Safety and Health
1 pair of shoe covers	1 disposable dustpan
2 pair of appropriate-thickness chemotherapy-type gloves	1 plastic scraper
1 pair of utility gloves	1 sharps container
1 pair of splash goggles	

Table 7–8 demonstrates various points during the handling and disposal process where exposure may occur. Also listed are general safety measures that may be used to decrease risk of exposure or contamination. These are by no means all-inclusive but are intended to serve as a guide to prompt you in identifying other exposure potentials and in establishing effective safety barriers.

■ Conclusion

Nurses who treat patients with antineoplastic agents realize that their practice is both an art and a science. The actual administration of these agents requires skilled techniques and a thorough understanding of the tasks involved in specific administration procedures.

Given appropriately, these agents can potentially save lives, increase quality of life, and reduce overall mortality from most cancers. Given incorrectly and without the proper understanding of the potential risks and implications for administration, these same agents can be lethal to the provider as well as to the patient.

The Oncology Nursing Society (*www.ons.org*) and the Association of Pediatric Oncology Nurses recommend that only registered nurses, who have received both didactic and supervised clinical experience, administer cancer chemotherapy. This training should be authenticated in writing and a copy maintained on file for each nurse. Additionally, patients should be taught about the chemotherapy regimen that they are going to receive and should give their written informed consent to treatment. This teaching should be documented in the patient's record for communication and legal purposes.

The role of the nurse administering chemotherapy has expanded to include administration of the agents, educating patients and family, precepting other nurses, and managing side effects of that treatment.

TABLE 7-8 ■ Points of Exposure: Safe Handling of Hazardous Drugs

Points of Exposure	General Safety Measures
Preparation	Identify designated preparation area.
	Use biologic safety cabinet (BSC).
	Establish and adhere to institutional policy for spillages.
	Maintain spill kit on site.
	Gather all needed supplies before entering hood.
	Use closed-system device.
	Wear personal protective equipment.
	Change gloves hourly and on contamination.
	Terminal clean work area and BSC.
	Maintain disposal receptacle near BSC.
	Line BSC surface with plastic absorbent pad.
	Wash hands before and after replacing gloves.
Handling/Transport	Know and adhere to hazardous drug policies and procedures.
	Wear personal proactive equipment.
	Transport drugs in plastic sealed bags.
	Wash hands on completion of each task.
Administration	Use locking connections.
	Wear pesonal protective equipment.
	Gather needed supplies before beginning treatment.
	Wash hands before and after each treatment.
	Spike IV bags in BSC.
	Use plastic absorbent liner under IV and syringe connection sites for leakage.
	Wrap sterile gauze around injection ports during intravenous (IV) push to decrease spray potential.
	Never recap needles.
	Never expel air or prime IV tubing/syringe outside the BSC.
	Remove personal protective equipment and place in a sealed plastic bag.
Disposal	Drug, supplies, human fluids.

Sources: Data from Gullatte, M., (2001). Principles and standards of chemotherapy administration. In M. Gullatte. (Ed.), *Clinical guide to antineoplastic therapy: A chemotherapy handbook* (pp. 40–43). Pittsburgh: Oncology Nursing Society. Polovich, M. (Ed.). (2003). *Safe handling of hazardous drugs*. Pittsburgh: Oncology Nursing Society.

■ Resources

- American Cancer Society: 800-ACS-2345 or *www.cancer.org*
  - *Chemotherapy: A guide for patients and their families,* a free pamphlet available online at *www.cancer.org* or by calling 800-ACS-2345.
  - *Cancer Drug Database,* a resource with over 250 drugs related to cancer treatment available at *www.cancer.org.*
  - *American Cancer Society patient education guide to oncology drugs,* second edition, was written for the health care professional to use as an educational tool for their patients. The book is easy to read and provides instruction sheets in print and on CD-ROM, customizable for the patient on more than 200 forms of cancer medication. This complete reference answers frequently asked questions in a language that is easy to understand. A comprehensive range of drug side effects is discussed in detail.

Bibliography

Adams, V. R., & Bence, A. K. (2003). Guide for the administration and use of cancer chemotherapeutic agents 2003. *Oncology special edition: The annual clinical reference.* New Jersey: Novartis Oncology.

Barton Burke, M., Wilkes, G., & Ingwersen, K. (1996). *Cancer chemotherapy: A nursing process approach* (2nd ed.). Sudbury, MA: Jones & Bartlett Publishers.

Brown, K. A., Esper, P., Kelleher, L. O., et al. (2001). *Chemotherapy and biotherapy: Guidelines and recommendations for practice.* Pittsburgh: Oncology Nursing Society.

Gullatte, M. M. (Ed.) (2001). *Clinical guide to antineoplastic therapy: A chemotherapy handbook.* Pittsburgh: Oncology Nursing Society.

Jemal, A., Tiwari, R., Murry, T., et. al. (2004). Cancer statistics, 2004. *CA A Cancer Journal for Clinicians. 54* (1), 8.

Occupational Safety and Health Administration. (1995). *Work-practice guidelines for personnel dealing with cytotoxic (antineoplastic) drugs.* Washington, DC: Office of Occupational Medicine, Directorate of Technical Support, Occupational Safety and Health Administration.

Peters, B. G. (1998). *Pocket Guide to injectable chemotherapeutic agents: Drug information and dosages.* Pennsylvania: Rhone-Poulenc Rorer Oncology.

Polovich, M. (2003). *Safe handling of hazardous drugs.* Pittsburgh: Oncology Nursing Society.

Wilkes, G., Barton Burke, M., & Ingwersen, K. (1999). *1999 Oncology Nursing Drug Handbook.* Sudbury, MA: Jones & Bartlett Publishers.

CHAPTER

8

Radiation Therapy

Marilyn L. Haas

Historical Overview

The evolution of radiation oncology began more than 100 years ago. Crediting Wilhelm Roentgen with his discovery of x-rays in 1895, scientists began working with the new radiologic technology for therapeutic uses, including treating cancers. Emil Grubbe treated the first breast cancer patient by applying the tissue-damaging therapy to ulcerate the area of disease. Soon afterward, improvements in equipment allowed radiation to penetrate the skin to deeper cancerous tumors. However, radiation directed by the orthovoltage machines also damaged surrounding healthy tissues (especially lung and bowel) and could be life-threatening to the patient. The concept of giving radiation in smaller, divided doses was then introduced. Advances in equipment technology combined with the science of radiobiology have led to the delivery of radiation therapy (RT) with greater therapeutic benefits and minimized toxicity as a result of the sparing of healthy tissues. Today, approximately 60% of all adults with cancer will be treated with RT sometime during the oncology continuum.

Rationale of Treatment

Biologic Effects

RT uses high-energy ionizing radiation to kill cancer cells. It is considered a local therapy because cancer cells are destroyed only in the anatomic area being treated. The radiation causes breakage in one or both strands of the DNA molecule inside the cells, thereby preventing the cell's ability to grow and divide. Although cells in all phases of the cell cycle can be damaged by radiation, the lethal effect of radiation may not be apparent until after one or more cell divisions have occurred. Although normal cells can also be affected by ionizing radiation, they are usually better able to repair the DNA damage than are cancer cells.

Principles of Radiation Therapy

The dose of radiation administered is determined by numerous factors, including the radiosensitivity of the tumor, the normal tissue tolerance, and the volume of tissue to be irradiated. The Gray, the Systeme Internationale unit, has now replaced the Rad (radiation absorbed dose) as the accepted term for radiation dosage. One Gray (Gy) = 100 rads; therefore, 1 cGy = 1 rad.

A radiosensitive tumor is one that can be eradicated by a dose of radiation that is well tolerated by the surrounding normal tissues. The sensitivity of tumor cells to the effects of radiation is also dependent on the presence of oxygen. Killing hypoxic cells requires two to three times the dose of radiation required to achieve the same therapeutic effect in well-oxygenated cells. Cells become hypoxic when tumor growth exceeds the blood supply and the central core of the tumor becomes necrotic. New strategies are being developed to increase the radiosensitivity of these hypoxic, resistant cells either with chemicals that mimic the presence of oxygen or with hyperthermia (the use of heat).

The dose of radiation that can be delivered to a tumor is limited by the radiation tolerance of the adjacent normal tissues. This limit is the point at which normal tissues are irreparably damaged. The maximum dose of radiation that can be administered to parts of the body varies with the tissue involved. For example, the maximum tissue tolerance (T/D 5/5 volume) of the parotid gland would be a dose of 3200 cGy, versus the 6000 cGy dose volume that the whole rectum could tolerate.

Because administration of the tumor-lethal dose of radiation in a single treatment would result in unacceptable toxicity or even death, the total prescribed dose of radiation is usually divided into several smaller doses, or fractions. Treatments are usually given on a daily basis, 5 days per week. The length of treatment depends on the tumor location, size, and cell type. Gradual shrinkage of the tumor during treatment brings hypoxic cells closer to the vascular supply, where they become oxygenated and more susceptible to the effects of radiation.

For some tumors, a "boost" or "reduced field" of radiation is administered to complete the course of therapy. These treatments are delivered to limited areas within the treatment field that are at greatest risk for recurrence. In this way, the tumor can be treated with a higher dose than the normal surrounding tissues would tolerate or need. The boost may be administered externally or internally.

Purpose of Radiation Therapy

After cancer diagnosis and staging (determination of the extent of disease), the intent of RT should be clearly defined at the onset of the therapeutic interventions. RT can be selected for various purposes:

- Definitive treatment: RT is prescribed as the primary treatment modality, with or without chemotherapy, for the treatment of cancer. Examples include cancer of the head/neck, lung, prostate, bladder, or Hodgkin's disease.
- Neoadjuvant treatment: RT is prescribed before definitive treatment, usually surgery, to improve the chance of successful resection. Examples include esophageal or colon cancers.
- Adjuvant treatment: RT is given after definitive treatment (either surgery or chemotherapy) to improve local control. Examples include breast, lung, or high-risk rectal cancers.
- Prophylaxis: RT treats asymptomatic, but high-risk, areas to prevent growth of cancer. Examples include prophylactic cranial irradiation in lung cancer or central nervous system irradiation to prevent relapse of certain forms of leukemia.
- Control: RT is given to limit the growth of cancer cells to extend the symptom-free interval for the patient. Examples include pancreatic or lung cancers.
- Palliation: RT is given to manage symptoms of bleeding, pain, airway obstruction, or neurologic compromise to alleviate life-threatening problems in patients in whom cure is not the goal, or to improve the patient's quality of life. Examples include treating spinal cord compression or bone metastases, opening airways in pneumonia patients.

■ Planning and Simulation

The purpose of treatment planning is to determine the best way to deliver the radiation treatment and to limit the radiation dose to normal tissues. Pretreatment computed tomography (CT) is performed to identify both the tumor and the surrounding normal structures. A diagnostic x-ray machine, simulating an actual treatment machine, is used to visualize and define the exact treatment area. Today, many cancer centers have a combination CT and simulator. CT simulators increase speed, efficiency, and accuracy of treatment planning and delivery.

The radiation oncologist can use the outlining capabilities of the CT simulator to plan for a newer technique called conformal radiation therapy. Conformal irradiation—geometric shaping of the radiation beam that conforms with the beam's eye view of the tumor—follows the shape of the tumor. It may also involve aiming beams from several directions, thus sparing more of the surrounding critical structures than conventional RT (Figure 8–1). A more advanced method is intensity-modulated radiation therapy (IMRT). IMRT, which is an extension of conformal therapy, facilitates shaping of the intensity of the radiation beam itself. New multileaf collimators, located at the head of the linear accelerators, adjust to the shape of the tumor as they move in relation to the body to allow for a more precise dose distribution around the target site (Figure 8–2).

The medical physicist or dosimetrist uses information from the CT and simulates treatment plans. Once the treatment plan is selected by the radiation oncologist, the planning computer calculates the amount of time each beam should be on during treatment.

During the planning stage, temporary dye marks or small permanent tattoos about the size of a small freckle may be used to mark reference points on the skin. This facilitates correct alignment and positioning, so that the same area is treated exactly the same each day. In order to deliver treatments precisely, immobilization devices may also be used to support and assist the patient in maintaining an exact position during treatment.

■ Major Treatment Modalities

Radiation treatments can be administered externally or internally, depending on the location, size, and type of tumor. X-rays, radioactive elements, and radioactive isotopes are most often used. Some patients may receive both external and internal types of radiation treatments.

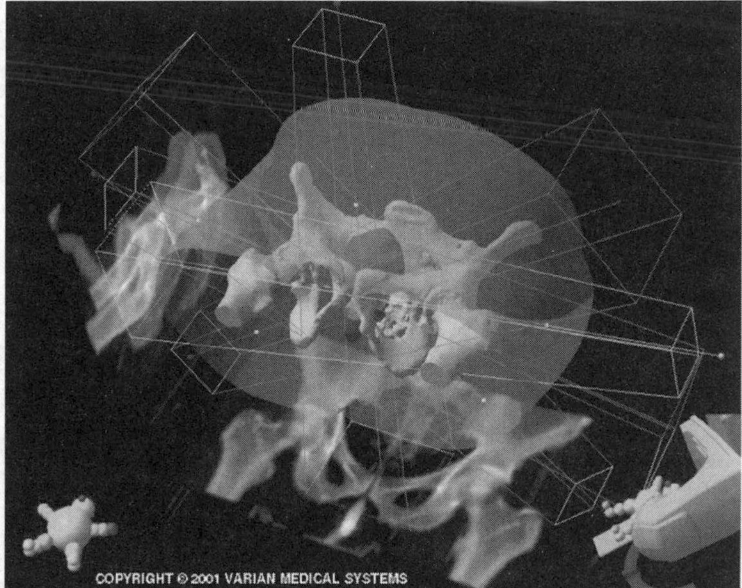

Helios™ Treatment Planning Systems Brochure: Geometric Planning with SomaVision™ - Targets and critical structures are contoured quickly with the advanced segmentation tools available in SomaVision. The physician may then enter a dose prescription and fractionation scheme and create the geometric treatment plan employing the powerful 3D visualization and virtual simulation tools in SomaVision.

Clinical description: Five field Helios IMRT beam arrangement for treating prostate viewed in three dimensions.

FIGURE 8–1 ■ Three-dimensional Conformal Treatment Planning of the Prostate.

Source: Photo courtesy of Varian Medical Systems, Palo Alto, CA. Copyright 2001. All rights reserved.

External-Beam (Teletherapy) Radiation Therapy

External radiation treatments, or teletherapy, are administered with machines that deliver high-energy radiation, usually directed at 80–100 cm from the target site. These machines vary according to the amount and the type of energy (electromagnetic or particulate) produced. The kind of machine used depends on the type and the extent of the tumor. The first megavoltage machine used cobalt 60. It has been replaced by newer machines called linear accelerators that deliver higher-energy beams of radiation and more precise treatments with less damage to superficial tissues (Figure 8–3). Placing lead or alloy blocks in the path of the beam spares normal structures, thus permitting higher doses to be given to the target site.

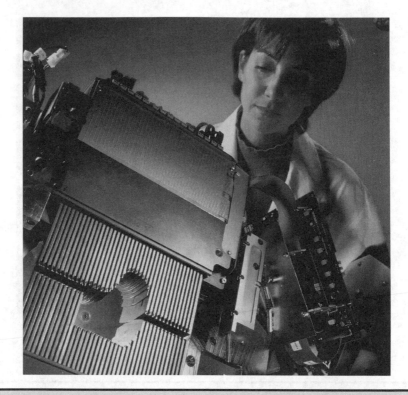

FIGURE 8-2 ■ Shaping the Beams with Intensity-modulated Radiation Therapy.

Source: Photo courtesy of Varian Medical Systems, Palo Alto, CA. Copyright 2001. All rights reserved.

Internal Therapy (Brachytherapy)

Internal radiation, or brachytherapy, is the use of radioactive isotopes for either temporary or permanent implants. Unlike external therapy, internal brachytherapy delivers the radiation in close proximity to the tumor. During brachytherapy, a radiation-producing source is implanted inside or placed next to the target tissue. Methods of delivering brachytherapy include intracavitary or interstitial placement of sealed radiation sources, instillation of colloidal solutions, and parenteral or oral administration of radioisotopes. Sealed radioactive sources are those encapsulated in a metal seed, wire, tube, or needle. Unsealed radioactive sources are prepared in suspension or solution.

Encapsulated radioactive isotopes are placed in body cavities or inserted directly into tissues with suitable applicators. The applicator is

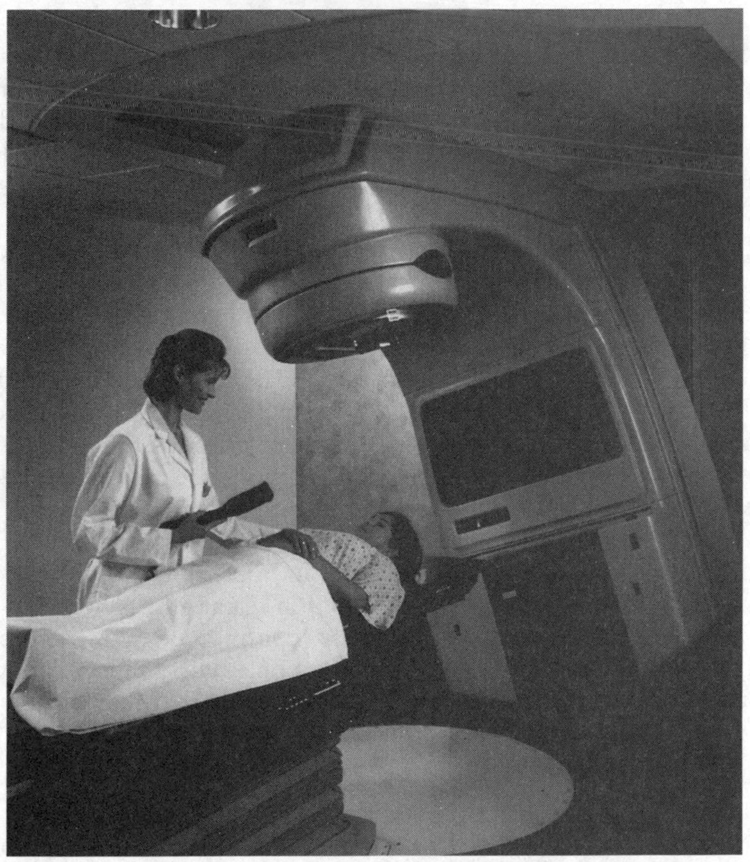

FIGURE 8–3 ■ A Linear Accelerator Is Used to Deliver External-beam Radiation Therapy.

Source: Photo courtesy of Varian Medical Systems, Palo Alto, CA. Copyright 2001. All rights reserved.

usually placed into the body cavity or tissue surgically or with the use of fluoroscopy. The applicators, usually plastic or metal tubes, may be sutured into or near the tumor. Later, the radioactive isotope is placed into the applicator. This "afterloading" technique is used to reduce the radiation exposure to hospital personnel. These implants provide radiation to a limited area while minimizing normal tissue exposure. Radioactive implants are used in the treatment of cancers of the tongue, lip, breast, vagina, cervix, endometrium, rectum, bladder, and brain.

Encapsulated sources may also be left within the patient as permanent implants. "Seeding" with small beads of radioactive material is an approach that can be used for the treatment of localized prostate cancers and localized but inoperable lung cancers. Together with the urologist (for prostate seed implants) or pulmonologist (for lung cancer), the radiation oncologist places the sources inside the tissue, providing a low-dose-rate brachytherapy. The patient's body attenuates, or blocks, most of the radiation, so the typical radiation precautions are usually not required afterward.

Radioactive isotopes can also be given orally or parenterally or instilled into intrapleural or peritoneal spaces. Thyroid cancer, for example, is frequently treated with oral administration of radioactive iodine 131. The period of greatest radioactivity for iodine 131 is 8 days. Other radiopharmaceuticals, such as samarium 153 (Quadramet) or strontium 89 (Metastron), can target areas where metastatic cells are attacking the bones and thereby relieve pain. These intravenous radioactive medications provide systemic radiation to the sites of bone metastases. Because the isotopes are present in blood and urine for up to a week after the injection, the patient is instructed on the precautions listed in Table 8–1. Occasionally, some patients note an increase in bone pain 2 or 3 days after the injection is given. This "flare" reaction usually lasts about 3 days. The nurse should instruct the patient to continue or even increase the use of pain medications if this flare reaction occurs. Blood counts are monitored for the mild bone marrow suppression that may occur.

Intraoperative Radiation

Intraoperative radiation therapy is the technique used to deliver radiation directly to the tumor or tumor bed during the course of surgery. Locally advanced nonmetastatic tumors of the gastrointestinal tract

TABLE 8–1 ■ Postprocedural Instructions for Patients Receiving Radioactive Isotopes

1. Drink extra fluids soon after receiving injection to flush isotopes out of the bladder.
2. When urinating, use toilet (no urinals) and flush the toilet twice after each use.
3. Wipe up any spilled urine with a tissue and flush it in the toilet.
4. Wash hands immediately after using the toilet.
5. Immediately wash clothing and linens that become stained with urine or blood. Wash these items separately from other clothes, and rinse thoroughly.
6. If you should cut yourself, wash away any spilled blood.
7. Inform dentist and/or pharmacist if you recently received this treatment because blood counts are affected.

and peritoneum can be treated with intraoperative radiation therapy. While the patient is under anesthesia, the surgeon locates the tumor, and either before or after excision of the tumor, the patient is transported to the radiation treatment room, where external-beam RT is delivered from a linear accelerator. Normal tissues surrounding the tumor are shielded from the radiation with the use of special cones and devices. Once treatment is delivered, the patient returns to the operating suite for surgical closure.

Stereotactic Radiosurgery

Stereotactic radiosurgery (SRS) is not really "surgery" because no incision is made and no removal of tissue takes place. The term *radiosurgery* describes a way to deliver a large dose of radiation to a very specific target within the brain while delivering only a small dose of radiation to surrounding normal brain structures. This is accomplished by directing many small beams at the target from different directions.

This treatment is delivered on an outpatient basis. SRS requires the highly coordinated efforts of a neurosurgeon, radiation oncologist, radiation physicist, nursing personnel, and diagnostic radiologists. Treatment is usually administered as a single treatment, compared with conventional external-beam irradiation, which is usually performed daily over a period of several weeks. Two different delivery systems are available (gamma knife or linear accelerator [linac]) and produce equivalent outcomes. Figure 8–4 shows a patient undergoing SRS with the use of the linear accelerator.

SRS allows the radiation oncologist and the neurosurgeon to effectively treat tumors that are situated deep in the brain and are either impossible to remove or that cannot be removed without damaging too much of the normal brain. Some patients have other medical problems (e.g., severe coronary disease or lung problems) that prevent them from undergoing conventional surgery. Still others prefer this less invasive approach rather than undergoing conventional brain surgery. SRS offers a nonsurgical alternative to these patients.

The technique is well suited to various malignant and benign brain tumors, such as arteriovenous malformations, acoustic schwannomas, meningiomas, brain metastases, glioblastoma, and some other rare types of tumors. Generally speaking, SRS is best given for tumors that are less than 3 cm in diameter, are well-circumscribed, and are well seen on CT or magnetic resonance imaging, and have the potential to respond to a single, large dose of radiation.

Although most patients tolerate this procedure very well, they may experience minor headaches, pin-site soreness, nausea, or possibly seizures. Generally, all patients feel fatigue after the procedure. Long-term

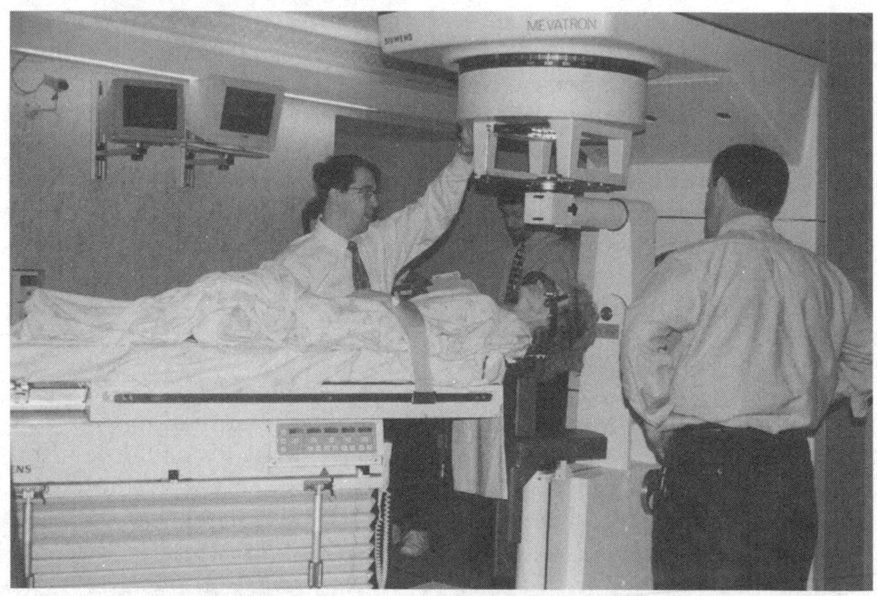

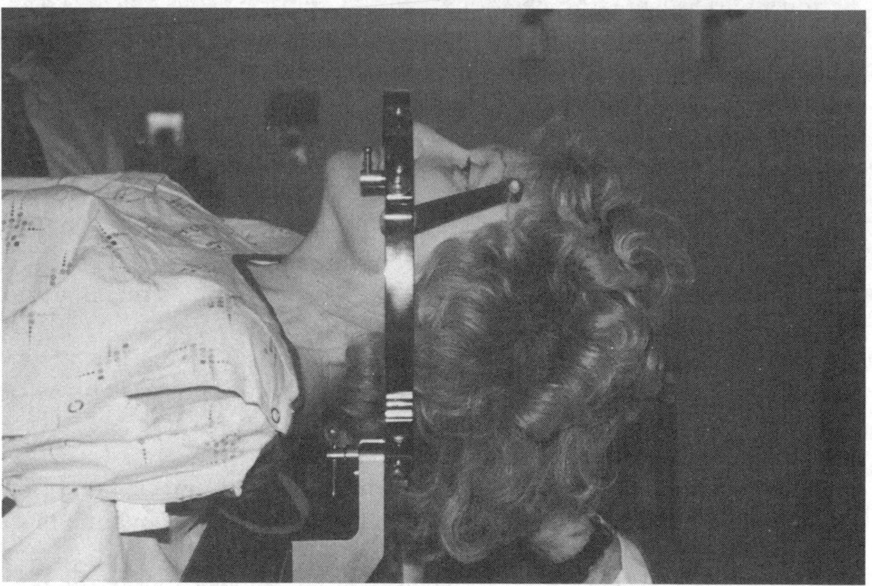

FIGURE 18–4 ■ A Linear Accelerator Is Used to Deliver Stereotactic Radiosurgery.

Source: Photo courtesy of Mountain Radiation Oncology.

risks depend on the size and the location of the tumor. These side effects may include asymptomatic or symptomatic cerebral edema, cranial nerve involvement (3–7), cognitive dysfunction, radionecrosis, or hormonal deficiencies.

■ The Role of the Nurse

Patients can be frightened by the concept of radiation, making assessment of the patient's and family's treatment knowledge and coping skills very important. Nurses can provide information about the use of RT in the treatment of cancer, the process of treatment planning, the treatment schedule, the self-care activities the patient can perform to control treatment side effects, and any radiation safety precautions. Inquiring about past experiences and coping abilities helps identify measures that have previously been effective for the patient. Giving time for the patient and family to talk about concerns related to illness and treatment is also beneficial.

Complications from RT are classified into three different phases: acute, subacute, and late effects. Acute phase side effects occur during or shortly after treatment. Two common acute symptoms that patients experience when receiving external RT are skin reactions and fatigue. Acute radiation reactions, such as skin reactions, occur during the course of therapy and generally resolve 2–4 weeks after the completion of therapy. Subacute effects usually occur 1–6 months after the completion of treatments and resolve over the next few months. Subacute effects may include radiation somnolence. Late effects occur months or years after treatment and are typically permanent. Examples of late effects include telangiectasia of the skin, pneumonitis of the lung, and fibrosis of the colon.

Side effects result when normal tissues within the treatment area are damaged by the radiation. Skin toxicity, fatigue, and anorexia can occur with treatment to any site, whereas other toxicities occur when specific areas of the body are treated (Table 8–2). The severity of side effects depends on volume of tissue treated, total dose, daily dose (fractionation) of therapy, method of treatment, and certain patient factors.

Nursing care involves assessment and intervention to prevent or minimize the occurrence of the side effects and to provide relief of symptoms that do occur. Table 8–3 lists nursing measures to manage side effects associated with RT.

TABLE 8–2 ■ Major Acute and Late Side Effects of Radiation Therapy

Site	Acute	Late
Skin	Mild to brisk erythema Dry desquamation Moist desquamation Alopecia (temporary)	Telangiectasias Fibrosis Necrosis Alopecia (permanent)
Brain	Cerebral edema manifesting headaches, nausea, vomiting limb weakness, mental changes visual changes, speech changes Seizures	Radiation necrosis Cerebral atrophy Cranial neuropathy Endocrinopathies Radiation myelopathy
Oral cavity	Mucositis/stomatitis Acute xerostomia Taste changes Pharyngitis	Osteoradionecrosis Chronic xerostomia Trismus
Lung	Increasing cough, dyspnea Pain (tumor) Esophagitis Radiodermatitis Hoarseness	Pneumonitis Fibrosis Esophageal stricture Hoarseness Spinal cord myelopathy
Breast	Radiodermatitis Breast pain, tenderness, swelling	Tanning Firmness, fibrosis Shrinkage Telangiectasias Lymphedema
Prostate	Diarrhea Tenesmus Proctalgia Rectal bleeding Erectile dysfunction	Persistent bowel changes of diarrhea, fistula formation, perforation, bleeding, incomplete bowel mucosa healing
Ovary	Hot flashes Vaginal dryness Dyspareunia	
Vagina	Vaginal dryness Dyspareunia Mucus drainage	Thinning, atrophy Adhesions Shortening, narrowing
Bladder	Frequency, urgency, dysuria hesitancy Hematuria Incontinence	Hematuria from mucosal inflammation/ telangiectasia
Colon	Abdominal cramping Diarrhea	Fibrosis Diarrhea

TABLE 8-2 ■ *Continued*

Site	Acute	Late
Rectum	Tenesmus Rectal pain Stool incontinence Mucus discharge Perianal pruritus	Fistulas Fibrosis Proctitis Adhesions Stenosis

Source: Data from Perez & Brady, 1998; Dow, K., Bucholtz, J., Iwamoto, R., Fieler, V., & Hilderley, L. (Eds.). (1997). *Nursing care in radiation oncology.* Philadelphia: W.B. Saunders; Watkins-Bruner, D., Bucholtz, J., Iwamoto, R., & Stohl, R. (Eds.). (1998). *Manual for radiation oncology nursing practice and education.* Pittsburgh: ONS Press; Held-Warmkessel, 2001; Haas, M. (2002). Contemporary Issues in Lung Cancer. Sudbury, MA: Jones & Bartlett.

■ Radiation Safety

External radiation does not require any special radiation safety behaviors by the patient. The patients are not radioactive and can participate in their normal activities of daily living. However, with internal irradiation, patients may require special radiation precautions based on the principles of time, distance, and shielding. Health care personnel should limit the amount of time spent in close proximity to the patient, minimize the time spent in the room, and use lead shielding as appropriate.

Patients receiving internal irradiation via either sealed or unsealed sources are generally physically isolated from other patients and staff members in a private room. Children younger than 18 years of age and pregnant women are not permitted in the room.

With sealed sources, body fluids, and materials used by the patient are not radioactive and do not require special handling precautions. Bed rest may be required to prevent dislodging of the radioactive source. Once the implant is removed and returned to the lead-lined container, the patient is no longer radioactive.

In patients treated with unsealed radioactive isotopes, secretions may be contaminated with radioactive material. Health care personnel should wear gloves when handling these secretions, and, when possible, disposable items (e.g., eating utensils, urinals) should be used. Nondisposable items (e.g., equipment, linens) should be placed in plastic bags and left in the patient's room to be checked for radioactivity and removed when permissible. These patients may be discharged from the hospital when it is determined that the total body retention of the isotope is at a safe level.

TABLE 8-3 ■ Nursing Measures to Manage Side Effects Associated with Radiation Therapy

Radiodermatitis (Skin Reaction)

1. Assess skin within the treatment area for erythema, dry (peeling) or moist desquamation, and pain.
2. Instruct patients about the care of their skin markings and not to remove temporary markings made for treatment purposes.
3. Suggest washing the treated area only with tepid water and a soft washcloth.
4. Suggest avoiding soaps, deodorants, powders, perfumes, cosmetics, heavily scented lotions, and skin preparations within the treatment area. Each radiation oncology facility recommends their preferred skin care product.
5. Instruct patients to wear loose-fitting clothing, preferably cotton, over treatment area.
6. Teach about avoiding things that produce extreme temperatures, such as hot water bottles, electric heating pads, and hot and cold packs; these must not be applied to the treatment area.
7. Recommend protecting the treatment area from the sun, wind, and cold, and utilizing protective clothing. After treatment, if sun exposure to the treatment area is unavoidable, suggest using a sun screen with a sun protection factor of 15–30. Inform patients that increased skin sensitivity within the treatment area may be a permanent outcome of irradiation.
8. If erythema or dry desquamation occurs, suggest using a moisturizing lotion. If moist desquamation occurs, suggest using hydrogels.

Fatigue

1. Assess level of fatigue and hemoglobin/hematocrit levels if indicated.
2. Determine activities that increase fatigue.
3. Identify activities that conserve energy. Suggest rest periods throughout the day.
4. Assist patient and family in obtaining resources for transportation, chores, and meal preparation.
5. Ensure optimal nutritional status.

Anorexia

1. Assess nutritional status, food intake, and weight.
2. Suggest small, frequent meals and high-protein and high-calorie foods and snacks.
3. Suggest using nutritional supplements as needed.
4. Make referrals to dietitian.

Oral Stomatitis

1. Assess oral cavity at least daily.
2. Review mouth care: brush teeth after each meal, floss teeth once a day (if tolerated).

TABLE 8–3 ■ Nursing Measures to Manage Side Effects Associated with Radiation Therapy—*Continued*

3. Suggest rinsing mouth with warm saline every 1–2 hours or as needed.
4. When mouth is tender, encourage the patients to select soft, nonirritating foods and fluids and to avoid alcohol.
5. Encourage topical anesthetics or analgesics as ordered before meals to improve comfort while eating.
6. Offer smoking cessation programs because smoking is an irritant and retards healing.

Dysgeusia (Taste Changes)

1. Assess for taste changes and food aversions.
2. Recommend experimenting with a variety of foods to find ones that provide some satisfying taste.
3. Suggest performing mouth care before meals.

Xerostomia (Dry Mouth)

1. Assess for amount and consistency of saliva.
2. Inspect oral cavity for signs of infection.
3. Recommend soft and moistened foods.
4. Suggest fluids with meals and snacks.
5. Suggest using saliva substitutes (many over-the-counter products, not requiring prescription) as needed.

Pharyngitis and Esophagitis

1. Assess for sore throat, esophagitis, and difficulty swallowing.
2. Recommend soft, nonirritating foods.
3. Encourage use of topical anesthetics or analgesics before meals as ordered.
4. Suggest avoiding drinking alcohol.
5. Offer smoking cessation programs.

Cough

1. Assess for cough, fever, chills, or sweats.
2. Ensure use of cough medications or antibiotics as ordered.
3. Encourage fluid intake as tolerated.
4. Encourage warm saline gargles as needed.

Nausea and Vomiting

1. Assess for nausea and vomiting, dehydration, and weight loss.
2. Prophylactically use antiemetic for treatments that are emetogenic.
3. Use antiemetic as needed.

(continued)

TABLE 8-3 ■ Nursing Measures to Manage Side Effects Associated with Radiation Therapy—*Continued*

4. Monitor hydration status and encourage fluids.
5. Encourage small, frequent meals.
6. Encourage resting after meals.
7. Teach imagery or relaxation techniques.

Diarrhea

1. Assess for diarrhea, dehydration, and weight loss.
2. Recommend a low-residue diet when diarrhea occurs.
3. Encourage use of antidiarrheal medications as needed.
4. Monitor hydration status.
5. Assess perianal tissues for excoriation.

Cystitis

1. Assess for dysuria, frequency, and urgency.
2. Assess for possible bladder infection if symptoms begin early.
3. Encourage fluid intake.
4. Encourage use of antispasmodics/analgesics as ordered.

Source: Haas, M. (2002). Contemporary Issues in Lung Cancer. Sudbury, MA: Jones & Bartlett.

Watkins-Bruner, D., Bucholtz, J., Iwamoto, R., & Stohl, R. (Eds.). (1998). *Manual for radiation oncology nursing practice and education.* Pittsburgh: ONS Press.

Watkins-Bruner, D., Moore-Higgs, G., & Haas, M. (Eds.). (2001). *Outcomes in radiation therapy.* Sudbury, MA: Jones & Bartlett.

■ Conclusion

Nursing care of the person receiving RT involves provision of symptom management and patient and family education. The radiation oncology nurse can identify resources for the patient and family in the community. Receiving RT affects the family's financial, time, energy, and emotional resources. By providing care that is attentive to psychosocial as well as physical needs, the radiation oncology nurse assists the patient and family in adapting to the illness and its treatment.

■ Resources

"Understanding Radiation Therapy: A Guide for Patients and Families" available online at American Cancer Society web site *www.cancer.org* or by calling 800-ACS-2345.

Bibliography

Dow, K., Bucholtz, J., Iwamoto, R., Fieler, V., & Hilderley, L. (Eds.). (1997). *Nursing care in radiation oncology*. Philadelphia: W.B. Saunders.

Haas, M. (2002). Contemporary Issues in Lung Cancer. Sudbury, MA: Jones & Bartlett.

Watkins-Bruner, D., Bucholtz, J., Iwamoto, R., & Stohl, R. (Eds.). (1998). *Manual for radiation oncology nursing practice and education*. Pittsburgh: ONS Press.

Watkins-Bruner, D., Moore-Higgs, G., & Haas, M. (Eds.). (2001). *Outcomes in radiation therapy*. Sudbury, MA: Jones & Bartlett.

CHAPTER

9

Hematopoietic Stem Cell Transplantation

Madeline O'Connor

Recent advances in hematopoietic stem cell transplantation (HSCT) have moved this treatment from a reluctantly offered therapy used when all other options had failed to an integral part of the therapeutic plan to manage certain malignant and nonmalignant diseases. The intent of HSCT is twofold: (a) a supportive measure and (b) a potentially curative intervention. As a supportive measure, HSCT is used to restore the patient's own bone marrow (BM) after intense myelotoxic therapies are used in an attempt to eradicate the cancerous process. As a potentially curative intervention, HSCT is used to eliminate and replace malignant cells with healthy donor stem cells capable of regenerating the recipient's hematopoietic system.

Recent statistics provided by the International Bone Marrow Transplant Registry demonstrate a wide range of both hematologic and nonhematologic malignancies treated with HSCT (Figure 9–1). As shown in this figure, many malignancies are treated with autologous or allogeneic transplantation. Autologous HSCT is primarily used with nonhematologic malignancies, such as solid tumors, whereas allogeneic HCST is the preferred mode of treatment for hematologic malignancies. Other applications of allogeneic HSCT include the treatment of nonmalignant diseases, such as sickle cell disease, severe combined immunodeficiency syndrome, osteogenesis imperfecta, Wiskott-Aldridge syndrome, severe aplastic anemia, and other congenital diseases primarily treated in the pediatric setting.

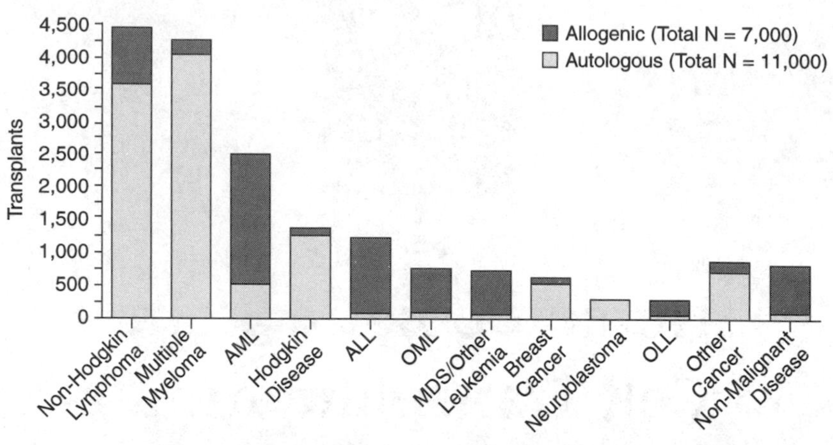

FIGURE 9–1 ■ Indications for Blood and Marrow Transplantation in North America, 2001.

Source: IBMTR/BMTR summary slides from IBMTR/ABMTR February 2002 newsletter (volume 9, issue, February 2002) and 2001 Statistical Center Report of Survival Statistics for Blood and Marrow Transplants.

The purpose of this chapter is to provide a review of current terminology and principles of HSCT and practice issues encountered by nurses caring for patients with malignant diseases who receive HSCT. Most nurses who deal with HSCT used in this patient population are oncology nurses or transplantation-specific nurses. The increased use of HSCT and the late effects associated with this procedure, such as second cancers, skin disorders related to chronic graft-versus-host disease (GvHD), cataracts, infertility, and psychosocial problems, require that nurses in various clinical settings have a better understanding of the complexities of HSCT treatment and the multisystem effects on patients.

■ Anatomic Sources of Hematopoietic Stem Cells

Bone marrow is the soft, spongy matter stored in the bones and is a rich source of hematopoietic stem cells (HSCs). The process for harvesting (collection of cells) BM involves a sterile surgical procedure whereby large-bore needles are repeatedly inserted into the posterior iliac crests after the patient has received general anesthesia. Depending on the size of the donor and the recipient, the amount of BM usually obtained during a harvest is between 0.5 and 1 L.

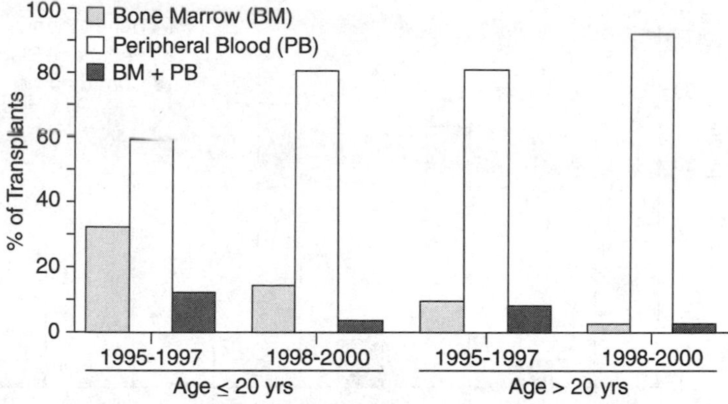

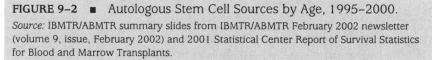

FIGURE 9–2 ■ Autologous Stem Cell Sources by Age, 1995–2000.
Source: IBMTR/ABMTR summary slides from IBMTR/ABMTR February 2002 newsletter (volume 9, issue, February 2002) and 2001 Statistical Center Report of Survival Statistics for Blood and Marrow Transplants.

Peripheral Blood is the blood circulating through the vasculature. HSCs are not found in peripheral blood in a steady-state condition. In order to mobilize (expand and increase) circulating HSCs to provide a number sufficient for transplantation, the donor receives hematopoietic growth-stimulating factors (typically granulocyte colony-stimulating factor) over a period of 4–5 days. Laboratory tests are then performed to determine whether the donor's peripheral blood CD34+ cell numbers are adequate for harvest. If both are adequate, the donor undergoes an apheresis procedure using a device similar to the one used for platelet collection. Most donors need to undergo only one or two apheresis procedures to provide the cell doses needed for transplantation. For this procedure, the donor's blood is circulated through a large-gauge intravenous catheter attached to a continuous-flow cell separator device for a period of 3–4 hours. This device carefully extracts the necessary stem cells and returns the remaining blood cells and plasma back to the donor.

Historically, BM was the primary source of HSCs for transplantation, but the use of peripheral blood stem cells (PBSCs) is now becoming the conventional standard (Figures 9–2 and 9–3). One reason is that PBSC harvests do not carry the risks, side effects, and high costs inherent in the surgery and anesthesia required for BM harvests. Clinical advantages of peripheral blood over BM as a source of stem cells are demonstrated in both autografts and human leukocyte antigen

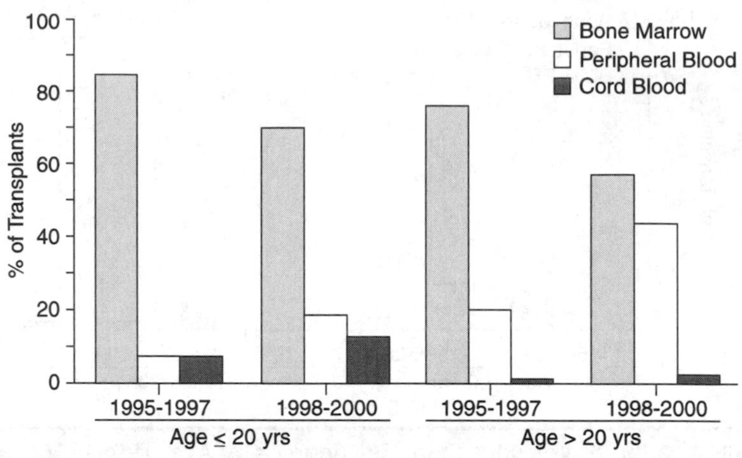

FIGURE 9–3 ■ Allogenic Stem Cell Sources by Age, 1995–2000.
Source: IBMTR/ABMTR summary slides from IBMTR/ABMTR February 2002 newsletter (volume 9, issue, February 2002) and 2001 Statistical Center Report of Survival Statistics for Blood and Marrow Transplants.

(HLA)-matched siblings. Recipients of PBSC grafts have an earlier absolute neutrophil count recovery with no clinically significant difference in the rates of acute GvHD (aGvHD) or overall survival. This is clinically significant because a faster absolute neutrophil count recovery indicates that the patient's immune system is regenerating and functioning, reflecting the patient's own ability to fight infection, which is a common and potentially fatal complication of HSCT. Clinical disadvantages of PBSC include an increased risk of chronic GvHD and the need for central venous access in younger patients.

Cord blood is the blood (rich in stem cells) removed from the umbilical vein of a neonate soon after delivery. Harvesting of these cells carries little to no risk to the neonate donor. Cord blood used for HSCT is obtained anonymously from cord blood banks.

A benefit of cord blood HSCs is the immaturity of the neonatal cells. Neonates have not developed a significant immune system and have few mature, functional T cells. Therefore, the incidence of GvHD is less likely with cord blood transplantation. However, contamination of maternal T cells in neonatal blood can induce alloreactivity, resulting in some GvHD responses. Another benefit is that neonatal donor products are less likely to transmit cytomegalovirus (CMV) and Epstein-Barr virus. Because neonatal donors have not been exposed to environmental sources of these viruses, infections that can be detrimental to HSCT-immunocompromised recipients are less likely to occur.

Although little to no alloreactivity of these donor cells has advantages in terms of GvHD, a lack of alloreactivity diminishes any chance of inducing a positive graft-versus-malignancy effect. Other drawbacks with the use of cord blood include a slower time to engraftment which puts the recipient at a higher risk for infections. An additional risk is the impossibility of knowing whether a neonatal donor has any type of genetic disease that could compromise the HSCT recipient over time. Finally, cord blood products are donated anonymously to cord blood banks, so if the recipient experiences graft insufficiency or graft failure, the transplantation team would be unable to return to the donor for any additional cells.

■ Human Leukocyte Antigen Matching

HLAs are the fundamental components of the major histocompatibility complex in humans. They are proteins imbedded into and onto the surface of essentially all human cells, including white blood cells. These proteins are genetically programmed with antigenic properties so that they can help the immune system discriminate self from foreign cells.

Although the HLA typing system is complicated and intricate, the primary screening for histocompatibility takes place through the evaluation of the HLA genes contained within chromosome 6. The three most important HLA loci are HLA-A, HLA-B and HLA-DR. Each person has two sets of these genes. One set is inherited from each parent and is referred to as a haplotype. When a patient has been HLA tested in preparation for allogeneic transplantation, medical personnel will look for a donor who has an HLA type that most clearly corresponds to the patient's. The greater the HLA donor/patient similarity or "match" for the six loci, the less risk that the donor cells will trigger an immunologic response from the host cells. The greater the HLA disparity (typically less than a five out of six match), the greater the chance for immune reactions, which significantly increase the risk of transplant-related morbidity and mortality.

■ Types of HSCTs

Autologous transplantation involves patients donating and later receiving back their own stem cells. This is a transplantation option that is primarily used for solid tumors, such as breast cancer and brain tumors, in which the multiple high doses of radiation therapy and/or chemotherapy required to reduce or eradicate the tumor often result in severe toxic effects on marrow or complete myeloablation. Autologous transplantation may be used for hematologic malignancies if the patient has no alternative donor source or if the regimen-related toxicities associated with allogeneic transplantation challenge the overall risk/benefit ratio. This added risk may be caused by advanced age or clinically significant comorbid conditions, such as congestive heart failure, renal failure, cardiomyopathy, or hepatic insufficiency.

Autologous stem cell harvest, whether BM or PBSC, occurs after the initiation of the initial conditioning regimen. The patient receives granulocyte colony-stimulating factor to help stimulate production and mobilization of his or her own HSCs. Once these cells are obtained, they are processed and cryopreserved for later reinfusion back to the patient. After the myelotoxic therapy has been completed, the healthy autologous stem cells are used in a *rescue* infusion to help replace the patient's own damaged or destroyed marrow. The goal is that the patient would be able to regenerate and ultimately restore normal BM function with the help of the infusion of his own HSCs.

Allogeneic transplantations use stem cells from a non-self donor. Four types of allogeneic donor sources are syngeneic, HLA-matched sibling, unrelated donor (matched or mismatched), and mismatched family donor.

Syngeneic

The source of HSCs is a genetically identical monozygotic twin. This type of transplantation carries the lowest risk for GvHD because the host would not recognize the donor cells as foreign and would not mount any type of immune response against the transplanted graft.

HLA-Matched Sibling

The donor is an HLA fully matched (HLA identical) brother or sister. Patients who have a sibling from the same parents have a one in four chance of matching on all six HLA antigens. HLA-matched siblings are generally the first choices for allogeneic donor selection because of the favorable HLA match and the availability and willingness of the donor.

Unrelated Donor

Stem cell products are obtained from volunteer donors unknown to the recipient. Two types of unrelated donors are used for HSCT: matched unrelated donors (unrelated donors matched with the recipient on all six HLA loci) and mismatched unrelated donors, which differ at one of the six loci (5/6 match). Volunteer donor BM or PBSCs mismatched at 4/6 would not be used for HSCT because of the increased potential for graft rejection or GvHD.

Unrelated BM, PBSC, and cord blood products are obtained through the National Marrow Donor Program (NMDP). The NMDP is a federally funded, nonprofit organization that arranges the collection, storage, and if available, the matching of unrelated volunteer donors from an international database for patients in need of a transplant who do not have a compatible family donor available. In order to initiate the search process, transplantation team members initially contact the NMDP with the required transplantation candidate's information, including HLA typing data, disease, disease status, and other pertinent information. The average time to transplant is 3 months, although some HSCT candidates may never find a compatible donor through these international databases.

HLA-Mismatched Family

Mismatched family donors (MFD) are closely related family members (parents, siblings, first cousins) of the recipient. These donors have an HLA mismatch in 3 (sometimes 2) of the 6 loci.

The acceptability, and success, of mismatched family donor transplants are currently being explored in clinical trials. Most patients have a mismatched family donor who is available and willing to donate. If successful, this greatly expands the availability of donors. Although the higher degree of HLA incompatibly increases the risk for GvHD in the recipients of these transplants, the reality is that most patients with malignancies requiring transplantation do not have a matched sibling donor available and do not have time to wait for matches with unrelated donors through the registries. Mismatched family transplantations currently have a greater morbidity and mortality rate than HLA-matched transplantations, but this is still a practical and promising treatment option for patients with life-threatening diseases. It is often the only option for surviving devastating malignancies for patients who have no alternate donor source.

■ Donor Requirements

Before consideration as a source of HSCs, all donors must complete a questionnaire that assesses their high-risk health-related behaviors. This is similar to the questionnaire used for all blood product donors. A series of blood tests are performed to evaluate the presence of the following infectious diseases: human immunodeficiency virus types 1 and 2, hepatitis B virus, hepatitis C virus, *Treponema pallidum* (syphilis), and human T-cell lymphotropic virus types I and II (FDA 21 CFR 1271). CMV and Epstein-Barr virus testing is not required but are performed by many institutions because of the exacerbated risk posed by these viruses in the immunocompromised recipient. All testing must be conducted using screening devices licensed, approved, or cleared by the US Food and Drug Administration.

Once the infectious disease testing has been completed and donor candidacy established, individuals considered for BM harvest need to meet the eligibility requirements for surgery and general anesthesia. Although PBSC collection does not require the use of general anesthesia, contraindications to this type of procedure would include known sensitivity to growth-stimulating factors, presence of autoimmune diseases with inflammatory components, or known high risk of thrombotic complications. The lower and upper age limit for HSC donation may vary by institution, depending on the clinical condition of the donor.

■ HSCT: Pretreatment and Infusion of Cells

Informed Consent

HSCT is not a medical situation requiring immediate decisions from patients, families, and medical practitioners; rather, it is a treatment option that adult cancer patients have the right to decide to pursue or not. Medical personnel are required to obtain informed consent from patients or their authorized representative, as with all medical interventions.

Informed consent is an ongoing process that begins when the transplantation team introduces the concept of HSCT to the patient. The consent document contains information detailing what is involved in the transplantation, the potential benefits and risks of the treatment, and alternatives to this procedure. No assurance about the procedure's ability to correct the immunodeficient state or cure the underlying malignancy can be included in the consent form, because this may be misleading and may provide false hope. Patients are typically given time to review the consent form and discuss their options with family and friends before making any final decisions regarding transplantation.

The HSCT Procedure

On the day of the transplantation, cryopreserved autologous cells are transported to the patient's room and thawed at the bedside in a room-temperature water bath until they are ready for infusion. If allogeneic cells are used, they are normally infused "fresh," meaning that the product has been harvested, processed, and infused within 24 hours of collection. Anaphylactic reaction may occur with either autologous or allogeneic HSC infusions. The causative factor for most intra- and posttransplantation reactions in autologous HCST recipients is the cryopreservative agent dimethyl sulfoxide (DMSO). For allogeneic HSCT, a small amount of residual donor red blood cells in the product may cause a hemolytic reaction once it is infused into the patient. In order to lower the risks of any infusion-related hypersensivity, HSC recipients are premedicated with a combination of steroids, diphenhydramine, and acetaminophen.

The volume of cells infused and the required infusion time for autologous and allogeneic donor products vary by patient/donor weight and by institutional standard operating procedures. For most institutions, HSCs are infused through a central line over a period of approximately 15–60 minutes, depending on the type of product and product volume in relation to patient body weight. Unmanipulated donor cells are administered by intravenous piggyback into a 0.9% normal saline line over a longer period of time because of their larger total fluid volume. Since HSC processing selects particular cells for infusion, the end product is often significantly reduced. Therefore, manipulated products are typically delivered in a syringe and administered by slow intravenous push. Patients are typically awake and alert during all allogeneic and autologous infusions. Some patients may need to receive anxiolytics, depending on their level of concern about the infusion procedure.

The type of transplantation is an important predictor of transplantation-related morbidity and mortality (Table 9–1). Autologous transplants carry a low risk of transplantation-related complications, whereas the allogeneic procedures, especially with HLA-mismatched donor/recipients, have a higher potential for significant, even fatal, HSCT-related toxicities. The primary allogeneic HSCT-related complications (Table 9–2) are GvHD and graft failure. Other serious complications of transplant (Table 9–3), including infection, veno-occlusive disease (VOD), and disease relapse, can occur in autologous and allogeneic transplant recipients and are described in the following sections.

TABLE 9–1 ■ Transplantation-Related Morbidity Risk Factors

- Type of transplantation: autologous or allogeneic (if allogeneic—degree of donor/patient HLA conformity)
- Pretransplantation immunoablative therapy
- Patient's primary diagnosis
- Prior treatment

Key: HLA = human leukocyte antigen.

TABLE 9–2 ■ Transplantation-Induced Complications
• Graft-versus-host disease
• Graft failure
• Toxicity of the induction process

TABLE 9–3 ■ Anticipated Toxicities from Transplantation
• Infection
• Hemorrhagic cystitis
• Pneumonitis
• Cardiomyopathy
• Increased liver function enzymes
• Altered renal function

Early Complications

Acute Graft-versus-Host Disease

The basic pathology of GvHD, a potentially fatal complication of HSCT, is that the transplanted donor T cells detect host antigen cells as foreign and therefore mount an immunologic attack on these cells. This reaction induces a disease process manifested by mild to major tissue damage in specific areas of the body, including skin, liver, and gastrointestinal tract. aGvHD, by definition, occurs during the first 100 days after transplantation, although most cases are typically noted 5–40 days after transplantation.

In its early stages, acute GvHD can be difficult to diagnose because its early signs and symptoms (mild rash, diarrhea, and increased liver function test results) can be attributed to numerous other disorders. Symptoms may progress to severe skin excoriation resembling second-degree burns, major gastrointestinal hemorrhage, hepatic insufficiency, and ultimately, hepatic failure. Although aGvHD may be definitively diagnosed by the clinical assessment of the presenting signs and symptoms, the diagnosis frequently requires confirmation through the use of biopsies.

Patients who receive allogeneic HSC products undergo prophylactic immunosuppressive treatment on or about the time of the initiation of the transplantation infusion to prevent aGvHD. If GvHD is diagnosed, additional immunosuppressants, usually steroids, are added to the patient's medication regimen, as are other supportive measures specific to the site or organ affected by the disease. Although aGvHD can be self-limiting and can be controlled to some extent with the use of current preventive and supportive measures, it remains a serious complication with devastating effects on patients.

Primary and Secondary Graft Failure

Engraftment is considered the time period when the recipient accepts the donor cells into their bone marrow space and these cells begin to replicate and proliferate throughout their body. The average time to engraftment is about 14 days for autologous transplantations and from 14–21 days for allogeneic transplantation recipients.

Frequent blood tests (e.g., complete blood counts) for graft function must be conducted in the first 100 days after transplantation to evaluate engraftment and graft stability.

One major, often life-threatening, complication for transplant recipients is graft failure, sometimes referred to as graft rejection. There are two types of graft failure: primary graft failure, which occurs when a patient never engrafts the transplanted cells, and secondary graft failure, which occurs when the patient initially engrafts and then subsequently loses the graft. Patients with graft failure are at risk of infection because of their sustained lack of a competent immune system and of hemorrhage due to persistent thrombocytopenia. The primary causes for graft failure are concurrent infections and insufficient number of cells in the donor product required for engraftment in the recipient. The treatment for graft rejection is administration of additional HSC infusions, or "boosts." Graft failure requires an additional transplantation procedure, but the conditioning regimen may be reduced.

Infection

One of the most common and often most serious complications of autologous and allogeneic HSCT is infection. Transplantation patients are profoundly immunocompromised because of the intense chemotherapeutic regimens and radiation treatments they must undergo, with allograft recipients being much more affected than autologous recipients. During the initial 30-day time period after transplantation, bacterial infections are the primary pathogens noted. Prophylactic broad-spectrum antibiotic treatments are initiated early and need to be reassessed with each episode of fevers and culture results.

Viral infections that occur in HSCT recipients can result from exposure to a new virus or reactivation of latent viruses, such as herpes simplex virus, varicella zoster virus, and CMV. Reactivation of CMV can occur at approximately 3 months after transplantation and can cause severe, even fatal, pulmonary and hepatic complications. Treatment includes antiviral agents, such as acyclovir and ganciclovir, as well as supportive measures specific to the site or organ affected by the virus.

Fungal infections pose a significant risk for morbidity and mortality in HSCT recipients. *Candida,* part of the normal flora of the oropharynx, vagina, and gastrointestinal tract, can proliferate in the immunocompromised patient, infecting numerous body systems. *Aspergillus* infections primarily target the lung, causing pneumonia. Treatment for fungal infections would include the administration of intravenous antifungals, such as fluconazole and amphotericin B.

Veno-Occlusive Disease

Veno-occlusive disease (VOD) is a significant cause of morbidity and mortality for patients undergoing allogeneic HSCT and is seen less commonly after autologous HSCT. VOD is a regimen-related toxicity that primarily affects the liver but may also affect the lungs. It is believed to be caused by chemotherapy- or radiation-induced damage to the epithelial cells of the hepatic blood vessels. VOD may respond to supportive measures, such as fluid restriction and diuresis, or it may result in hepatic failure and death. Although there is no proven method for preventing or treating VOD, ongoing clinical trials are using heparin and novel biologic agents to try to reduce the incidence and severity of this potentially fatal disease.

Disease Relapse

Despite intense chemotherapeutic and radiation treatments, many aggressive malignant diseases recur or *relapse* with the same or greater intensity as occurred before transplantation. Treatment options for patients who experience relapse can include palliative care (no further curative treatment), further chemotherapy, second transplantation (if the patient qualifies), or donor lymphocyte infusions.

■ Late Effects of HSCT

As the number of transplant survivors increases, the late effects of HSCT and its related therapies are being more clearly brought to light. Most of the late effects are known sequelae of the chemotherapy and radiation treatment (see Chapter 7, Chemotherapy and Chapter 8, Radiation Therapy). A late-onset form of GvHD is a transplantation-

TABLE 9–4 ■ Late Effects of HSCT-Related Therapy

- *Neurologic complications*—numbness and tingling in extremities, or seizure disorders due to cranial radiation, chemotherapy, or disease metastasis to the brain.
- *Cataract formation*—secondary to radiation treatment and steroid administration used to prevent GvHD; progressive and typically requires surgery to correct vision.
- *Thyroid dysfunction (principally hypothyroidism)*—secondary to radiation treatment of the thyroid gland; treatment includes thyroid hormone replacement therapy.
- *Osteoporosis*—due to a combination of steroid use, underlying disease, and/or calcium depletion; causes significant bone pain. Prevention and treatment have traditionally included hormone replacement therapy (HRT) and calcium supplements. However, because of the recent concerns about HRT, other options for treatment of osteoporosis after HSCT are being examined.
- *Growth hormone deficiency (GHD)*—noted in children who have received radiation treatment; may also be a side effect of busulfan; when diagnosed early, GHD can be treated effectively with growth hormone replacement and ongoing monitoring of blood levels and growth status.
- *Infertility*—a complication of both radiation therapy and/or chemotherapy, specifically, the conditioning agent busulfan.
- *Second malignancy*—seen in patients who received radiation therapy; most often occurs 10–15 years after transplantation.

Key: HSCT = hematopoietic stem cell transplantation; GvHD = graft-versus-host disease.

specific complication that may be debilitative and may continue to afflict the patient for years after transplantation. Other late complications include disease relapse and onset of a second malignancy (Table 9–4).

Chronic GvHD

When symptoms of GvHD occur and are diagnosed 100 days or more after transplantation, the condition is referred to as chronic GvHD (cGvHD). cGvHD usually occurs in the first 2 years after transplantation but may be diagnosed even later.

The symptoms of cGvHD (Table 9–5) can progress and cause severe debilitation. When cGvHD is suspected, physical therapy and occupational therapy should be initiated early to improve joint movement. Particular attention to skin care and oral hygiene can help prevent infections. Patients with cGvHD are considered to be functionally asplenic and typically require penicillin prophylaxis. Pharmacologic intervention includes administration of steroids or other immunosuppression to control the alloreactivity.

TABLE 9–5 ■ Symptoms of Chronic Graft-Versus-Host Disease

- Dry eyes
- Dry mouth
- Oral mucosa changes
- Rash
- Hardening of the skin
- Stiff joints
- Elevated liver function enzymes
- Thrombocytopenia
- Pulmonary abnormalities

The Role of the Nurse

Nursing care of the patient treated with HSCT is both challenging and rewarding. The gravity of the underlying illness, compounded by the severe toxicities related to an aggressive transplantation procedure, requires that nurses be well prepared. Initially, HSCT patients can be seriously ill, and their tenuous status warrants one-on-one nursing care during the immediate posttransplantation period. Nursing efforts to assess and manage pain are particularly critical. A common source of pain during the immediate posttransplantation period is mucositis (see Chapter 24, Gastrointestinal Symptoms). Patients who experience mucositis can have such severe oropharyngeal and gastrointestinal mucosal bleeding or swelling that prophylactic intubation may be considered.

The transplantation procedure is a frightening experience for patients and their families. It is a long, often painful process during which the recipients' and their families' lives are completely disrupted—emotionally, logistically, and financially. Nurses can help facilitate the coping process for both the patient and the family and set up additional supportive services with other transplantation team members, such as chaplains, social workers, and psychiatry staff.

Ethical Issues with HSCT

Examples of ethical dilemmas specific to HSCT are listed in Table 9–6.

TABLE 9–6 ■ Ethical Issues to Consider in the Transplantation Setting

- Disagreement about treatment between minors and their guardians
- Cost of the procedure
- Aggressiveness of the therapy in a high-risk patient

Conclusion

Although HSCT has improved survival rates in patients with malignancies and other catastrophic illnesses over the past 3 decades, outcomes remain suboptimal. Novel clinical applications are continually being discovered and tested in clinical trials. Current debates within the transplantation research community serve to fuel new ideas and refine current methodologies in the clinical trial setting. Future research efforts will focus on reducing the toxicities of existing therapies, diminishing the GvHD potential while maximizing the graft-versus-malignancy effect, and extending the treatment option to patients with other life-threatening illness who may also benefit from HSCT.

Resources

- National Marrow Donor Program (NMDP) 3001 Broadway Street Northeast Suite 500 Minneapolis, MN 55413-1753
  In the United States and Canada, call toll free: 800-MARROW2 (1-800-627-7692)
  Outside the United States, call: 612-627-5800
  URL: *www.marrow.org*
- International Bone Marrow/Autologous Bone Marrow Transplant Registries
  IBMTR/ABMTR Statistical Center Health Policy Institute at the Medical College of Wisconsin 8701 Watertown Plank Road P.O. Box 26509 Milwaukee, WI 53226 Telephone: 414-456-8325 Fax: 414-456-6530E-mail: *ibmtr@mcw.edu* URL: *www.ibmtr.org*
- Ronald McDonald House Charities
  (provides lodging for families of seriously ill children being treated away from home)
  URL: *www.rmhc.org*

- American Cancer Society Hope Lodges
  (provides temporary housing for cancer patients undergoing outpatient treatment)
  Telephone: 800-ACS-2345 to inquire about this or similar housing services in your area

Bibliography

Buchsel, P. C., Kapustay, P. M. (2000). (Eds.). *Stem cell transplantation: A clinical textbook*. Pittsburgh: Oncology Nursing Press, Inc.

Ho, A. D., Haas, R., Champlin, R. E. (Eds.). (2000). *Hematopoietic stem cell transplantation.* New York: Marcel Dekker.

Steen, R. G., Mirro, J. (Eds.). (2000). *Childhood cancer: A handbook from St. Jude Children's Research Hospital with contributions from St. Jude clinicians and scientists*. Cambridge, MA: Perseus, Inc.

Biologic Therapy

Terri Ades

Biologic therapy, immunotherapy, or biotherapy uses certain components of the body's immune system as a cancer treatment. This can include stimulating the person's own immune system or using an outside source, such as a synthetic protein. Immunotherapy is sometimes used by itself, but it is most often used as an adjuvant to the primary therapy.

Although the thought of using the immune system to fight cancer is appealing, immunotherapy currently has a small role in treating the most common types of cancer. However, important progress has been made in this field in the past few years. Many researchers are optimistic that more effective immunotherapies can be developed that will have better patient outcomes.

■ Types of Immunotherapy

Active immunotherapies stimulate the body's immune system to fight the disease, whereas passive immunotherapies use immune system components (e.g., antibodies) created outside of the body. Types of immunotherapies include vaccines, monoclonal antibody therapy, and nonspecific immunotherapies and adjuvants.

Cancer Vaccines

Cancer vaccines are active specific immunotherapies that contain cancer cells, parts of cells, or pure antigens that cause the body to produce antibodies and/or killer T cells. Although cancer vaccines have shown some promise in early clinical trials, none have been approved for cancer treatment in the United States.

Monoclonal Antibody Therapy

Monoclonal antibody therapy is a passive immunotherapy that involves the production of antibodies outside the body. The antibodies are referred to as *monoclonal* (sometimes abbreviated as MoAbs, or MAbs) because they are all produced from a single cloned cell. Monoclonal antibodies can be made that react with specific antigens on certain types of cancer cells.

Clinical trials of monoclonal antibody therapy are in progress with almost every type of cancer, and the US Food and Drug Administration (FDA) has approved several for the treatment of certain cancers (Table 10–1).

Some monoclonal antibodies, called naked MAbs, do not have any drug or radioactive material attached to them. Alemtuzumab (Campath), an antibody against the CD52 antigen present on both B cells and T cells, is used to treat B-cell chronic lymphocytic leukemia in patients who have not responded to chemotherapy.

TABLE 10–1 ▪ Monoclonal Antibodies Approved by the US Food and Drug Administration for Cancer Treatment

MAb Name/ Type	Trade Name	Used to Treat	Year Approved
Rituximab (naked)	Rituxan	Non-Hodgkin's lymphoma	1997
Trastuzumab (naked)	Herceptin	Breast cancer	1998
Gemtuzumab ozogamicin (conjugated)	Mylotarg	Acute myelogenous leukemia	2000
Alemtuzumab (naked)	Campath	Chronic lymphocytic leukemia	2001
Ibritumomab tiuxetan (conjugated)	Zevalin	Non-Hodgkin's lymphoma	2002
Tositumomab (conjugated)	Bexxar	Non-Hodgkin's lymphoma	2003

Conjugated monoclonal antibodies are joined to drugs, toxins, or radioactive atoms and used as delivery vehicles to take those substances directly to the cancer cells. The MAb attaches itself to a cancer cell with a matching antigen and delivers the toxic substance to where it is needed most, minimizing damage to normal cells in other parts of the body. Conjugated antibodies generally cause more side effects than do naked antibodies.

Conjugated MAbs are also sometimes referred to as "tagged," "labeled," or "loaded." They can be "tagged" with chemotherapy agents or with radioactive particles. Radiolabeled and chemolabeled MAbs are now being tested in clinical trials for use in treating many types of cancer. Radiolabeled antibodies are also being used to detect areas of cancer spread in the body. The two radiolabeled antibodies that have been approved by the FDA to detect cancer are OncoScint (for colorectal and ovarian cancer) and ProstaScint (for prostate cancer).

In 2002, the FDA approved the first radiolabeled MAb to treat cancer outside of clinical trials. Ibritumomab tiuxetan (Zevalin) delivers radioactivity directly to cancerous B lymphocytes. It is now used to treat recurrent B cell non-Hodgkin's lymphoma. A second radiolabeled MAb, tositumomab (Bexxar), is used to treat certain types of non-Hodgkin's lymphoma that have not responded to rituximab (Rituxan) or chemotherapy.

Immunotoxins have been made by attaching monoclonal antibodies to bacterial toxins, such as diphtherial toxin and pseudomonal exotoxin, or to plant toxins such as ricin A and saporin. Immunotoxins studied in clinical trials have shown some early promise in shrinking a few cancers, particularly lymphomas.

The only immunotoxin thus far to receive FDA approval for treating cancer is gemtuzumab ozogamicin (Mylotarg). It contains a toxin called calicheamicin that is attached to an antibody directed against the CD33 antigen, which is present on most leukemia cells. Gemtuzumab is used to treat acute myelogenous leukemia in people who have not responded to chemotherapy.

Other targeted therapies that contain toxins are also being delivered to cancer cells by growth factors that attach to cancer cell receptors. The only growth factor/toxin currently approved by the FDA is denileukin diftitox (Ontak). It consists of the cytokine interleukin-2 (IL-2) attached to a toxin from the germ that causes diphtheria. Denileukin diftitox is used to treat cutaneous T-cell lymphoma.

Nonspecific Immunotherapies and Adjuvants

Nonspecific immunotherapies stimulate the immune system in a very general way. Some nonspecific immunotherapies can be given as main therapies by themselves or as an adjuvant to enhance immune system function.

Cytokines play a crucial role in regulating the growth and activity of other immune system cells and blood cells. Some cytokines, known as hematopoietic growth factors, help the bone marrow in the production of new blood cells after chemotherapy has destroyed them (see Table 7–2):

- Granulocyte colony-stimulating factor (also called G-CSF, filgrastim, or Neupogen) stimulates the bone marrow to make granulocytes. Pegfilgrastim (Neulasta) is a longer-acting form.
- Granulocyte-macrophage colony-stimulating factor (also called GM-CSF, sargramostim, or Leukine) promotes production of both granulocytes and macrophages.
- Erythropoietin (epoetin alfa, Procrit, Epogen) causes the bone marrow to produce erythrocytes. Darbepoietin (Aranesp) is a longer-acting form.
- Interleukin-11 (IL-11, oprelvekin, Neumega) promotes the production of platelets.

Interleukins

When interleukin-2 (IL-2) was approved by the FDA in 1992 for the treatment of metastatic renal cell (kidney) cancer, it became the first true immunotherapy approved for use alone in treating advanced cancer. Since that time, it has also been approved to treat metastatic melanoma. Other interleukins, such as IL-4 and IL-12, are now being studied in cancer, both as adjuvants and as stand-alone agents.

Interferons

This family of cytokines affects cancer cells by one of several mechanisms—directly slowing the growth of cells in many cancers; slowing angiogenesis producing more antigens, making them easier for the immune system to recognize and destroy; or enhancing natural killer cell and other immune system cell function. The FDA has approved interferon alfa for use in hairy cell leukemia, chronic myelogenous leukemia, follicular non-Hodgkin's lymphoma, cutaneous (affecting the skin) T-cell lymphoma, renal cell cancer, melanoma, and Kaposi's sarcoma.

Adjuvants Other than Cytokines

Levamisole, a drug first used against parasitic infections, can activate T lymphocytes. It has recently been found to improve survival rates in people with colorectal cancer when it is used together with chemotherapy.

Bacille Calmette-Guérin is a bacterium related to the tubercle bacillus. It infects human tissues, attracts immune system cells to areas of infection, and activates the immune system. FDA has approved it as a treatment for superficial bladder cancer. Its usefulness in other cancers as a nonspecific adjuvant is also being tested.

■ Side Effects

Compared with side effects of standard chemotherapy, the side effects of biologics are generally related to flulike symptoms and allergic reactions. Potential side effects include fever, chills, weakness, headache, nausea, vomiting, diarrhea, fatigue, hypotension, and rash. Some biologics can cause leukopenia and thrombocytopenia similar to that occurring in chemotherapy. Most side effects do not last long after the treatment stops, but fatigue can last longer. Side effects of IL-2, although similar, can be severe and also include weight gain, confusion, irregular heartbeat, chest pain, and serious heart problems. Neuropathies can occur, although rare, as a long-term effect of interferons. Nursing care during treatment is highly supportive and anticipatory, with ongoing assessment of side effects, initiation of measures to prevent effects, and symptom management once they do occur (see Unit V chapters on specific symptoms, as well as Chapter 7, Chemotherapy).

■ The Role of the Nurse

Because most of the biologics are still being studied, many patients being treated with biologic therapy are enrolled in clinical trials. (For more information on clinical trials, see Chapter 7.) Although these therapies are usually administered at the sponsoring cancer treatment center, patients usually receive some medical care in their community. The nurse's role in the community includes assessment of the current cancer treatment status and of the presence of side effects, implementation of care instructions from the cancer treatment center, and dialogue with the treatment center regarding patient status and care measures.

Patients receiving biologic therapy in a clinical trial have likely already received standard therapy and now are facing a disease recurrence or advanced disease. A psychosocial needs assessment can identify patient and family needs regarding social support and psychological adjustment (see Chapter 35, Psychosocial-Spiritual Responses to Cancer and Treatment: Living with Cancer).

Resources

- Call the American Cancer Society at 1-800-ACS-2345 and ask for patient information on immunotherapy or access the same information on the web site at *www.cancer.org.*
- The National Cancer Institute has an excellent patient booklet explaining the immune system and immunotherapy called *Understanding your immune system.* It can be ordered at *www.cancer.gov.*

Bibliography

Bast, R. C., Kufe, D. W., Pollock, E., Weichselbaum, R. R., Holland, J. F., Frei, E. (Eds.), *Cancer medicine* (5th ed.). Baltimore: Williams & Wilkins, 2000.

DeVita, V. T., Hellman, S., & Rosenberg, S. A. (Eds.), *Cancer: Principles and practice of oncology* (6th ed.). Philadelphia: Lippincott-Raven, 2001.

Greten, T. F., & Jaffee, E. M. (1999). Cancer vaccines. *Journal of Clinical Oncology, 17,* 1047–1060.

Rosenberg, S. A. (Ed.), *Principles and practice of the biologic therapy of cancer* (3rd ed.). Philadelphia: Lippincott, Williams & Wilkins, 2000.

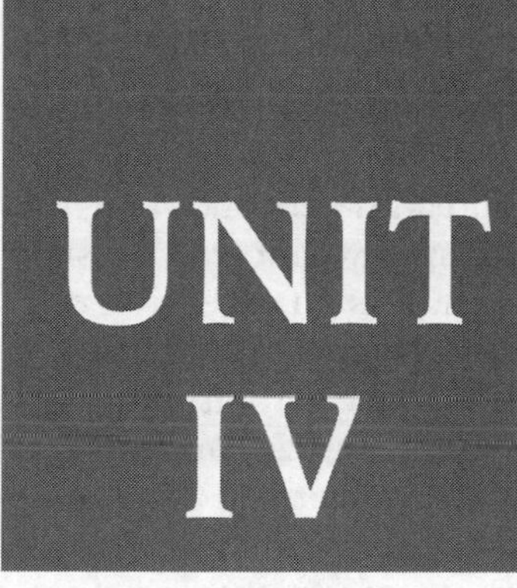

UNIT IV

Cancer Sites

Ann Reiner

Cancer is not just one disease, but many. As this unit will explore, different cancers pose specific challenges to treatment plans and prognosis, depending on where a cancer originates, where it has spread, and whether it has returned after treatment. Knowing specific information about a cancer's original location, current location, and extent of growth assists in the understanding of treatment possibilities and expected survival. Specific terms are used to describe these characteristics of cancers.

■ Primary

The primary site of a cancer refers to the particular organ in which the cancer begins. For example, if a cancer is identified as prostate cancer, pathologists have determined that the specific characteristics of the particular cancer cells most fit with a cancer starting in the prostate gland. Curative treatment is directed to the original site of a cancer. If a cancer starts in the colon and has not spread to any other part in the body, then surgical removal of the affected colon could very well provide long-term remission from the cancer.

■ Metastasis

Cancer can spread from its original location to other parts of the body by either direct extension or metastasis. Microscopic evaluation of the cancer cells that have spread determines that these cancer cells are like those in the original or primary cancer. Metastatic cancer is not considered to be a second cancer. It is an extension or a persistence of the primary cancer. Certain cancers, such as lung and ovarian, are often diagnosed after they have spread from their primary location.

Cancer spreads by direct extension, through the lymph nodes, or via the bloodstream. When cancer cells spread into the surrounding tissues, it is called *local invasion* or *extension by direct spread*. Regional metastasis refers to the spread of the original cancer to other body parts in the same general area, but not necessarily adjacent to the original cancer. An example is breast cancer that has spread from the breast to lymph nodes in the underarm area. Distant metastasis pertains to cancer cells most like the original cancer appearing in another area of the body that is not contiguous. An example of distant metastasis is colon cancer that has spread to the lungs. Every cancer has a distinct pattern of metastasis.

The exact mechanism of metastasis is still not understood; however, it is known that cancer cells spread via the body's blood and/or lymph systems. Treatment of metastatic cancer is designed to stop further spread and growth of the cancer. Long-term remission is dependent on the level of metastasis, with treatment being less likely to eliminate distant metastasis.

■ Recurrence

If after initial treatment a cancer returns at its original or a metastatic site, it is said to have recurred. Recurrence suggests that initial treatment did not control the cancer's growth. It has a profound psychosocial impact on the patient and family, because long-term remission is highly unlikely. Treatment is directed at controlling the cancer's further growth and spread, as well as managing the disease and treatment -related symptoms.

■ Second Primary

Some individuals experience more than one cancer. Long-term side effects of certain cancer treatments can cause the development of a second primary cancer, although this is rare. Radiation therapy used to treat upper body lymphoma has been implicated in the development of breast cancer. Treatment is designed around the nature of the new primary cancer, not the original cancer.

CHAPTER

11

Breast Cancer

Lorraine M. Hutson

■ Incidence

Breast cancer remains the most commonly occurring noncutaneous malignancy in women and is still second to lung cancer an as overall cause of cancer-related deaths. Over the past 2 decades, the incidence of breast cancer has increased by an average of 1%–2% annually. The American Cancer Society estimates that 211,300 cases of breast cancer will have been diagnosed and 40,200 will have died of the disease in the year 2003. The good news is that even though the incidence of the disease has increased, the mortality rates have decreased significantly. Detecting the disease in its earliest stage increases the chance that it will be cured. Most women who are diagnosed with, and treated for, localized breast cancer have a 98% chance of living disease free at 10 years. The goal of treatment remains cure of the disease through improved screening, enhanced diagnostic tools, and application of more precise therapy.

This good news for breast cancer survivors and those at risk for developing the disease does not apply to all American women (see Chapter 2, Epidemiology of Cancer, and Chapter 4, Culturally Competent Care)—there are differences in outcomes within minority groups in the United States. Western Black and Hispanic white women with breast cancer tend to present with more advanced stages of disease and have poorer survival rates than non-Hispanic whites. This discrepancy has prompted increased research efforts focused on identifying factors that attribute to differences in stage at presentation among ethnic populations.

Risk Factors

It is difficult to estimate an exact risk that an individual will develop breast cancer. One in eight women will develop breast cancer during their lifetime, but no one specific cause of the disease has been identified. Many factors may increase the risk of disease development. The primary risk factors are female gender, increasing age, family history, gene mutations, and biopsy history. Additional risk factors include early menarche, late menopause, nulliparity, delayed or postponed pregnancy, long-term exposure to exogenous estrogens, postmenopausal obesity, high-fat diets, alcohol consumption, and exposure to ionizing chest wall radiation. Age still remains the most significant risk factor for the development of breast cancer; as one ages, the risk of developing breast cancer increases.

The hormone environment is acknowledged as the most significant factor in the development of the disease. Women are 100 times likelier to develop the disease than men; men do get breast cancer, but they represent approximately 1% of the reported cases. It is thought that estrogen and increased exposure to estrogen may provoke the development of the disease; this hypothesis is strengthened when a known breast cancer that is hormone receptor positive can be manipulated into suppression by estrogen blockade.

The significance of early menarche, late menopause, and delayed or no pregnancies on an increased risk of the disease is an important factor in risk counseling. The rationale is that the longer cells are exposed to estrogen, the higher the risk for disease development. Uncertainty remains about the effects of exogenous estrogen effects on the development of breast cancer. Recent clinical trials have reported that combined (estrogen plus progestin) hormone replacement therapy increases the risk of developing the disease.

Breast cancer—like colon, lung, and prostate cancer—is a cancer of aging. The longer one lives, the more one is at risk for the development of the disease. Most breast cancers are diagnosed in women aged 60 years or more. Most of these breast cancers are less aggressive, respond to therapy better, and have an overall lower chance of recurring that breast cancers that are diagnosed in younger women. The risk of breast cancer is greatest in developed countries, such as North America and Northern Europe. Asian countries, especially Japan, have a lower incidence of breast cancer than the United States. However, with immigration of Japanese women to America, the incidence of breast cancer increases in each generation of Japanese American descendents. Daughters born to second-generation Japanese American women have an equal incidence of the disease as their American counterparts. Adoption of a more typical Western diet is thought to be significant, but other variables, such as tobacco and alcohol use, decreased exercise, and increased use of hormonal agents, may also increase risk in these women.

Family history may contribute to the potential risk of developing breast cancer. The risk of breast cancer, based on family history alone, can be either overestimated or underestimated without careful assessment of the individual family pedigree. The importance of age of onset, number of primary relatives, bilaterality of disease, and presence of other malignancies (ovarian, colon, and prostate) are to be considered when a person's risk of disease is estimated.

The modified Gail model estimates a woman's risk for developing breast cancer on the basis of age, menarche, primary relatives with breast cancer, number of breast biopsies, and ethnicity. Those women with a 1.7% 5-year actuarial risk of breast cancer according to the Gail model are strongly counseled to go further for genetic testing, consideration of chemotherapy for risk reduction, and strategies of estrogen blockade, oblation, prophylactic surgery, and/or close surveillance.

When there is an identified increased risk based on family pedigree, a genetic evaluation to determine the presence of gene mutations is considered. Two breast/ovarian cancer susceptibility genes have been identified, mapped, and cloned. The first gene mutation identified is known as *BRCA1* (BReastCAncer number 1) and is found on chromosome 17, and *BRCA2* (BReastCAncer number 2) is found on chromosome 13. Mutations of genes generally require physical, environmental, and genetic influences that result in the development of cancer. When there are known inherited gene mutations, there is a very strong likelihood that cancer will develop. Women who have inherited the *BRCA1* or *BRCA2* gene mutation have a 50%–80% risk of disease development in their lifetime. Male breast cancer is associated with the *BRCA2* gene mutation and is also associated with a family history of premenopausal or early-onset breast cancer.

In women who have a personal history of breast cancer, whether invasive or noninvasive, the risk for developing a second primary breast cancer increases by as much as 15%. There is also an approximate 1%–2% increased risk in women who have prior-diagnosed ovarian and endometrial malignancies. Women who have undergone previous breast biopsies that show cell proliferation but no clear malignancy may be at an increased risk for breast cancer, especially where there is cellular atypia along with hyperplasia. Atypical hyperplasia has some of the cellular characteristics of in situ carcinoma and is often seen as a marker for tumor development. Along the histologic continuum in the natural history of the disease, atypical ductal hyperplasia may precede ductal carcinoma in situ. Therefore, the individual diagnosed with in situ disease is at risk for developing invasive breast cancer. This is also true for lobular carcinoma in situ, a neoplastic process that is associated with an increased risk of carcinoma.

As stated earlier, a carcinogenic effect is associated with ionizing radiation. Mantle irradiation for Hodgkin's disease increases the risk of development of breast cancer by more than 4%. The results from the Late Effects Study Group indicate that women who received mantle irradiation in their second or third decade of life have an increased risk of developing breast cancer by the age of 40. The overall risk associated with prior mantle irradiation at a young age is 75 times greater than the risk of breast cancer in the general population. The radiation received from screening and diagnostic x-rays is minimal and is not associated with an increased risk of breast cancer.

Estimating the risk of developing breast cancer is difficult because most breast cancers are not related to any risk factors other than gender and advancing age. The identification of risk factors can encourage screening and earlier detection and can subsequently reduce the mortality from the disease. Risk-reduction counseling should include a determination of the individual's qualitative and quantitative risk for developing breast cancer. Public education can heighten awareness of the need for screening and early detection. Identification of actual or potential risk factors for breast cancer can encourage early access to evaluation.

■ Detection

The clinical breast examination (CBE) and annual mammography together are used to screen for breast cancer (see Chapter 3, Cancer Screening, Early Detection, Risk Reduction, and Genetic Counseling). There is controversy regarding the cost-effectiveness of screening in women younger than 40. However, most breast health experts support the current American Cancer Society recommendations listed in Table 11–1 and, in addition, also consider known risk factors when making screening recommendations.

Mammography is still the gold standard in breast imaging screening. It allows high-quality imaging with a minimum of radiation exposure. It is also the most cost-effective screening tool. The goal of screening is to detect a breast cancer before it becomes clinically evi-

TABLE 11–1 ■ American Cancer Society Recommendations for Early Breast Cancer Detection

- Women aged 40 years and older should have a screening mammogram every year and should continue to do so for as long as they are in good health.
- Women in their 20s and 30s should have a clinical breast examination (CBE) as part of a periodic (regular) health exam by a health professional, preferably every 3 years. After age 40, women should have a breast exam by a health professional every year.
- BSE is an option for women starting in their 20s. Women should be told about the benefits and limitations of BSE. Women should report any breast changes to their health professional right away.
- Women at increased risk should talk with their doctor about the benefits and limitations of starting mammograms when they are younger, having additional tests, or having more frequent exams.

dent; a palpable lesion discovered by expert CBE can be as small as 1 cm. Mammography can identify lesions that are less than 1 cm, and it also identifies calcifications. Although they are sometimes found in benign breast lesions, calcifications are often the first sign of breast cancer, especially ductal carcinoma in situ.

■ Diagnosis

Defining a breast lesion involves a multistep process, using CBE, mammography, ultrasounds, and invasive procedures for tissue analysis. The diagnosis of breast cancer requires attention to detail. Patients present with various clinical manifestations that are not easily segregated into either benign or malignant categories. It is the job of a prudent practitioner to piece everything together to determine the next step (Table 11–2).

Staging

The TNM system developed by the American Joint Committee of Cancer is the system used to stage breast cancer. This system uses an algorithm of combining tumor size (T) with nodal involvement (N) with the presence of disease spread (metastasis, M) to determine the stage of the disease. Accurately staging breast cancer is perhaps the most significant component in treatment decision making.

Breast cancer is divided into several different histologic types (Table 11–3). Understanding the pathobiology of these tumors and

TABLE 11–2 ■ Diagnostic Procedure Used to Detect Breast Cancer

- Diagnostic imaging
  - Mammography
  - Ultrasound
  - Magnetic resonance imaging
- Fine-needle aspiration
- Core needle biopsy
- Incisional and excisional biopsy

TABLE 11–3 ■ Stage of Breast Cancer

Stage 0	Tis	N0	M0
Stage I	T1	N0	M0
Stage IIA	T0-1	N1	M0
	T2	N0	M0
Stage IIB	T2	N1	M0
	T3	N0	M0
Stage IIIA	T0-2	N2	M0
	T3	N1-2	M0
Stage IIIB	T4	N0-2	M0
Stage IIIC	Any T	N3	M0
Stage IV	Any T	Any N	M1

their clinical manifestations will assist a prudent clinician in diagnosing breast cancer. Most breast cancers are adenocarcinomas. There are two main types of mammary adenocarcinomas: ductal and lobular. Each of these types may be invasive or in situ (noninvasive). About 85% of in situ breast cancers are ductal carcinoma in situ, and the remainder are lobular carcinoma in situ. Invasive ductal carcinoma represents approximately 75% of all cases of invasive breast cancer; invasive lobular carcinoma accounts for another 10%. The remaining histologic types of invasive breast cancer include tubular, medullary, mucinous, and papillary carcinomas, which are notable for their relatively favorable prognosis, and a few types that are much less common (Table 11–4). Inflammatory carcinoma is not really a histologic type but denotes the spread of cancer within lymphatic channels of the skin of the breast. Paget's disease indicates breast cancer cells within the epidermis of the nipple. Paget's disease of the nipple may be entirely in situ or may be associated with an underlying invasive breast cancer.

TABLE 11–4 ■ Types of Breast Cancer

In situ carcinomas	DCIS, LCIS
Invasive carcinomas	Ductal, lobular, tubular, medullary, papillary, mucinous, inflammatory
	Other (adenoid cystic, secretory, squamous cell, phyllodes tumors, primary breast lymphomas)

Key: DCIS = ductal carcinoma in situ; LCIS = lobular carcinoma in situ.

TABLE 11-5 ■ Tumor Grade and Differentiation

Tumor Grade	Tumor Differentiation
Grade 1	Well differentiated
Grade 2	Intermediate differentiation
Grade 3	Poorly differentiated

The tumor types are further divided into grades of differentiation. Cellular differentiation describes the degree to which the tumor histologically resembles normal breast tissue (with regard to tubule formation and the size and shape of individual cells) and the rate at which the tumor is dividing and replicating. In addition to stage, tumor grade is sometimes an important variable during therapeutic decision making (Table 11–5).

Other characteristics of the tumor are associated with either favorable or unfavorable behavior. Hormone receptor status of the tumor is important in predicting which patients will respond to hormone manipulation. Tumors that are better differentiated and lower grade usually are estrogen and/or progesterone receptor positive, are associated with better outcome, and have potentially lower relapse rates. These tumors respond to estrogen blockade. In contrast, an overabundance of the oncogene HER2/*neu* tends to be associated with higher-grade, hormone-refractory tumors, with higher rates of relapse. Overabundance of HER2/*neu* is also important in predicting therapeutic response to trastuzumab (Herceptin).

■ Treatment

A multidisciplinary approach to breast cancer treatment includes a combination of surgery, radiation therapy, chemotherapy, and hormonal therapy. Treatment decisions for breast cancer are influenced by many factors: the clinical presentation of the patient, a complete review of breast imaging, a histologic review of the pathology, and a careful evaluation of the patients desires.

Local Control

The goal of local therapy is to control the disease in the breast. Either breast-conserving surgery followed by radiation therapy or mastectomy alone can accomplish this. When lumpectomy is the surgical option chosen and adequate margins are surgically achieved, radiation therapy follows. For patients for whom mastectomy is chosen as the surgical option, unless there is significant bulky disease in the breast (T3) or lymph nodes (greater than three lymph nodes involved), no radiation therapy is necessary. Mastectomy is also recommended for patients who have undergone prior mantle radiation therapy, are pregnant, or have other contraindications to radiation therapy.

Surgical evaluation of the regional axillary nodes is important for staging and for guiding decisions about systemic therapy, and it is also part of local control of the disease. It includes axillary clearance by complete lymph node dissection, lymphatic mapping, sentinel lymph node mapping, and biopsy. Historically, axillary clearance is achieved through surgical resection of at least 10 lymph nodes from level 1 and two lymph nodes of the ipsilateral axillary basin. In certain circumstances, sentinel lymph node mapping and biopsy comprise acceptable surgical therapy. Sentinel node identification is an intraoperative procedure that identifies the first nodes in the axillary basin. It is hypothesized that if the first node is free of metastatic disease, then the remaining nodes are also. This procedure can save the patient from a more extensive complete node dissection that carries a high risk of postoperative complications and lymphedema.

After adequate surgery with clear surgical margins, the long-term local recurrence rate is approximately 30%. Radiation therapy following lumpectomy reduces the risk of local recurrence to about 10% and in general is very well tolerated. The radiation treatments are usually scheduled daily for 30 treatments (5 days per week) and last approximately 6 weeks. Side effects of radiation therapy include skin changes, fatigue, and radiation-induced pneumonitis (see Chapter 8, Radiation Therapy). Although the risk of local recurrence after mastectomy is lower than that after breast-conserving therapy (even with radiation therapy), numerous studies have documented that survival rates are equivalent. For this reason, most breast specialists and patients prefer breast-conserving therapy unless there is some contraindication to this choice.

Chemotherapy

For early breast cancer, the aim of therapy is to achieve a long, disease-free survival. Depending on the stage of disease, systemic chemotherapy is added in order to potentially increase the rate of cure. This is called *adjuvant therapy* and is given to treat microscopic disease when there is substantial risk of recurrence or metastasis. Deciding which chemotherapeutic treatment regimens should be used is an arduous task for the clinician and the patient. Chemotherapy given for breast cancer, like other malignancies, may have many side effects. Weighing the side effect profile of certain combination agents against the benefit and the risk of relapse drives the treatment decision and recommendations. Several regimens are used to treat breast cancer, and for the most part, all have equal benefit and side effects. Combination therapy is mostly used to treat invasive breast cancer. Agents that are most active in breast cancer include antitumor antibiotic anthracyclines (doxorubicin, epirubicin), alkylating agents (cyclophosphamide), antimetabolites (methotrexate, 5-fluorouracil), and microtubular inhibitor taxanes (paclitaxel, docetaxel). Side effects of chemotherapy are discussed in Chapter 7 (Chemotherapy).

When breast cancer relapses, the goal of therapy is disease control. Treatment of metastatic or stage IV disease is individualized to the patient and to the extent of disease and prior treatment history. Agents used in the treatment of metastatic disease include the antimetabolites gemcitabine, capecitabine, and vinorelbine. Trastuzumab is a monoclonal antibody used in patients whose tumor overexpresses the HER2/*neu* oncogene.

Hormonal Therapy

Adjuvant hormonal manipulation is another treatment option for certain patients with early-stage breast cancer. Certain tumors contain receptor sites that respond to estrogen. Tumors that are estrogen receptor positive depend on estrogen for growth. Therefore, tumor growth is inhibited when the effect of estrogen on the cell is blocked. This is achieved by either stopping estrogen from attaching to cells or stopping the production of estrogen completely. Tamoxifen is a selective estrogen receptor modulator that blocks the cellular receptor site from estrogen, thereby limiting estrogen's effect on tumor cells. It is used in pre- and postmenopausal women as well as men to treat breast cancer. For postmenopausal women with nonfunctioning ovaries, estrogen is produced by converting adrenal androgens to estrogens in the presence of the enzyme aromatase. Anastrozole is a nonsteroidal aromatase inhibitor that inhibits this synthesis by blocking aromatase, thereby stopping estrogen's production in the adrenal glands. Anastrozole is beneficial only in the postmenopausal female, whose ovaries are either nonexistent or nonfunctioning, whereas tamoxifen is beneficial in premenopausal women, postmenopausal women, and men with breast cancer.

As with all medications, there are side effects from hormonal manipulation. Suppressing estrogen's effects on tumor cells also suppresses the potential benefits of estrogen. Hot flashes are the most frequent complaint with all hormonal therapy. Other side effects are nausea, vomiting, fluid retention, weight gain, vision changes, cognitive changes, and mood disorders (see Unit V, Symptom Management, for specific symptom management). Tamoxifen also carries a risk of more worrisome adverse effects. A higher risk of endometrial cancer is associated with tamoxifen therapy and is usually seen in long-term usage. Blood clots can also be associated with tamoxifen use. Anastrozole is thought to be associated with a high risk of osteoporosis and a higher risk of fracture.

Rehabilitation

Survival rates for those with breast cancer are at an all-time recorded high. Survival rates for early-stage disease after appropriate therapy can reach 98% at 10 years. Therefore, women and men are living long enough to experience the long-term effects of the disease and its subsequent treatment. These effects are multidimensional and, in concert, can often negatively affect the life of the survivor (see Chapter 36, Cancer Survivorship).

There are certain body image issues specific to breast cancer survivors. Loss of a breast or both breasts certainly is a constant reminder of the disease, no matter how long one has survived. Reconstruction efforts are much more refined these days, but there are limitations, and the cosmetic outcome never completely replaces the natural breast. Lymphedema is a common side effect after lymph node dissection and is especially risky for those whose therapy includes radiation therapy to the axilla. The risk of lymphedema is lifelong, and the effects of the syndrome are everlasting and for the most part not reversible if caught late. Women who have been treated for breast cancer are at higher risk for osteoporosis because the protective effects of estrogen are limited by chemotherapy-induced early menopause or estrogen blockade. Residual fatigue can linger for several months and even years after treatment is complete.

Coping with the diagnosis and treatment of breast cancer is only half the battle. Assimilating breast cancer into a life is a task some find difficult, if not impossible. The psychological effects of the disease affect all aspects of the person as well as the social and family circle. Body issues may affect the person's sense of self and sexuality and therefore limit intimacy (see Chapter 33, Sexuality). Finding clothing to fit after mastectomy is difficult for many. The fear of recurrence or relapse is an arduous task to overcome for most. Annual examination often brings on so much anxiety for some patients that they have several sleepless nights before the mammogram and CBE. Anxiety and depression are common emotional reactions within the breast cancer survivor populations.

The cost of breast cancer diagnosis and treatment presents a financial burden for many patients. Treatment for breast cancer can take as long as a year from the actual diagnosis. Therefore, there may be extended periods of employment interruptions. Sympathetic employers are certainly a benefit for those lucky enough to have them. For those who do not have an understanding work environment or have to change jobs because of physical limitations, the financial implications can be devastating. This can result in significant psychosocial problems and can affect the patient's quality of life. In addition, preexisting conditions affect the person's insurability. All these impose undue stress on the individual and can create psychological pathology.

■ Conclusion and The Role of the Nurse

It is important to understand the natural history of breast cancer. By doing so, one can fully appreciate the impact of the diagnosis, treatment, and symptom sequelae of survivorship. Nurses are in the best position to address most needs of the breast cancer patient and survivor. Assessment of physical, psychological, social, and economic concerns during screening for the disease, diagnosis of breast cancer, and monitoring for recurrence is a therapeutic goal of the nursing profession. Education and patient advocacy are nursing tasks that can increase patient empowerment. Helping patients make the best, most informed treatment decision can affect treatment outcomes and quality of life.

■ Resources

American Cancer Society Programs, *www.cancer.org* or 800-ACS-2345

- Reach to Recovery: Designed to help people cope with their breast cancer experience, this program has provided more than 30 years of service in the fight against breast cancer. Reach to Recovery volunteers are breast cancer survivors who are trained to offer support at various points along the breast cancer continuum: diagnosis; decision making about treatment; dealing with treatment and its side effects; returning to a full, active life; or confronting any long-term effects including a possible recurrence of the disease.

- Look Good . . . Feel Better: In partnership with the Cosmetic, Toiletry and Fragrance Association Foundation and the National Cosmetology Association, this free program is designed to teach women with cancer beauty techniques to help restore their appearance and self-image during chemotherapy and radiation treatments.

American Cancer Society Publications, *www.cancer.org* or 800-ACS-2345

- American Cancer Society. (2004). *A breast cancer journey: Your personal guidebook* (2nd ed.). Atlanta, GA: Author.
- Breast Reconstruction After Mastectomy, *www.cancer.org/docroot/CRI/content/CR_I2_6X_Breast_Reconstruction_After_Mastectomy_5.asp*
- NCCN Breast Cancer Treatment Guidelines for Patients, *www.cancer.org/docroot/CRI/content/CRI_2_4_7x_NCCN_Breast_Cancer_Treatment_Guidelines_for_Patients_2003.asp* or *www.nccn.org/patient_gls/_english/_breast/index.htm*

  "tlc": "tlc" is a "magalog" designed to provide needed medical information and special products for women newly diagnosed with breast cancer and breast cancer survivors. The magalog features articles that focus on medical questions specific to breast cancer and also has a Question & Answer section. "tlc" features a variety of hats, caps, turbans, hairpieces, swimwear, bras, prostheses, and breast forms. Many products are also appropriate for any woman experiencing treatment-related hair loss. Free copies are available by calling 800-850-9445.

BreastCancer.org, a nonprofit organization for breast cancer education, *www.breastcancer.org*

The Susan G. Komen Breast Cancer Foundation, *www.komen.org*

Bibliography

AJCC Cancer Staging Manual (6th ed., 2002, pp. 257–281). Philadelphia: Lippincott-Raven.

Breast Cancer Facts & Figures 2002–2003. American Cancer Society. *www.cancer.org.*

Groenwald, S., Frogge, M., Goodman, M., & Yargro, C. (Eds.). (1997). *Cancer nursing: Principles and practice.* Boston: Jones & Bartlett.

Li, C., Malone, K., & Daling, J. (2003). Differences in breast cancer stage, treatment, and survival by race and ethnicity. *Archives of Internal Medicine, 13,* 49–56.

Practice guidelines in oncology. Breast cancer. Version 2.2003. (2002). National Comprehensive Cancer Network (NCCN). *www.nccn.org.*

CHAPTER

12

Colorectal Cancer

Deborah Berg

■ Incidence

Colon cancer is a malignancy primarily located in the colon, while rectal cancer refers to a tumor in the rectum. The term *colorectal* is often used to generally describe these malignancies. Colorectal cancer (CRC) is one of the most prevalent cancers and is a major health problem. It is the third most common cancer in both men and women, after lung and prostate cancer in men and lung and breast cancer in women. CRC is second only to lung cancer in its mortality. This year, it is estimated that about 147,500 individuals will be afflicted with this disease, with an annual death rate of about 57,000. The incidence has been declining in recent years, perhaps because of increased screening and polyp removal. Mortality is also declining, reflecting the decrease in incidence, perhaps the fact that more tumors are found at an earlier stage, and improvements in treatment (see Chapter 2, Epidemiology of Cancer).

CRC is primarily a disease of the older adult, with the average age at diagnosis of 67 years; > 90% of individuals are older than 50 years at the time of diagnosis, whereas < 6% are younger than 50. Overall, African Americans have the highest incidence and mortality rates, 8% higher than whites, 15% higher than Asian/Pacific Islanders, and about 25% higher than Hispanics and American Natives (Indian and Alaskan) (see Chapter 4, Culturally Competent Care).

Risk Factors

The two major risk factors for CRC are increasing age and personal or family history of predisposing diseases of the large intestine. The risk of developing CRC begins to increase after the age of 40, rises sharply after the age of 50, peaks between 65 and 74 years, and then stabilizes around the age of 80. Personal history of adenomatous polyps in the colon or rectum, previous history of CRC, and inflammatory bowel disease, such as ulcerative colitis and Crohn's disease, are all associated with a higher risk of CRC. Familial factors include a family history of CRC and polyposis syndromes, most commonly familial adenomatous polyposis (FAP), hereditary nonpolyposis colorectal cancer (HNPCC), and the *APC I1307K* mutation noted in Ashkenazi Jews of European descent. The risk of CRC is doubled if an individual has a first-degree relative (parent or sibling) with CRC. Although the genetic polyposis syndromes are generally rare, for individuals who have the genetic predisposition, the probability of developing CRC is high (70% risk in those with familial adenomatous polyposis and 100% risk in those with hereditary nonpolyposis colorectal cancer).

Other risk factors are behavioral, nutritional, and environmental. A high-fat diet inadequate in fruits and vegetables; alcohol consumption; cigarette smoking; obesity; and sedentary lifestyle are all implicated in the development of CRC. Approximately 70% of cases of CRC are believed to be sporadic, 15%–25% report a positive family history of CRC, and the remaining 5% are considered related to an inherited genetic mutation.

Prevention, Screening, and Early Detection

Prevention

CRC is a preventable malignancy. Preemptive surgical excision of adenomatous polyps prevents the development of CRC by eliminating the primary precursor lesion. CRC develops slowly over many years—starting first as a small benign polyp that progresses to an invasive tumor under the influence of genetic alterations. If the polyp is removed, the sequence is broken and the CRC does not develop.

Modifying behavioral factors can also decrease the likelihood of developing CRC (see Chapter 3, Cancer Screening, Early Detection, Risk Reduction, and Genetic Counseling). The American Cancer Society recommends that individuals lower their risk by managing factors within their control, such as eating a diet low in animal fat, drinking alcohol in moderation, quitting smoking, maintaining a healthy weight, and participating in regular exercise. Although considered controversial, current research does not support the protective effect of increased fiber in the diet.

Observational studies suggest that regular use of aspirin, nonsteroidal anti-inflammatory drugs, and the cyclooxygenase-inhibitor celecoxib may reduce CRC risk through a reduction in polyp formation. However, the dose and the duration of use of the agents have not been defined. Some evidence also suggests that taking a daily multivitamin containing folic acid and increasing calcium intake, either in supplements or in the diet, are beneficial. The antioxidants carotene, vitamin C, and vitamin E do not demonstrate a protective effect against CRC. Estrogen hormone replacement therapy in postmenopausal women may reduce the risk of CRC, but its benefits must be weighed against its risks for breast and uterine cancers. In addition to the reduction in risk of CRC, many of the behavioral recommendations may confer other health benefits, such as a decrease in the risk of heart disease. Continued research to provide more definitive information on how to prevent CRC is underway.

■ Screening and Early Detection

Many risk factors cannot be controlled through behavioral changes, making screening and early detection crucial to the improvement in survival. The National Cancer Institute estimates that 20,000 to 30,000 lives could be saved each year if screening and early detection methods were utilized. Unfortunately, according to the Centers for Disease Control and Prevention, in 2001, only 40% of individuals aged 50 years or older reported undergoing any recent screening test for CRC.

Screening tests are performed to find cancer before the onset of symptoms; however, the same tests are used to detect cancers early if symptoms are reported to the health care provider (see Chapter 3, Cancer Screening, Early Detection, Risk Reduction, and Genetic Counseling). The tests are fecal occult blood test, flexible sigmoidoscopy, colonoscopy, and double-contrast barium enema. All of these screening tests are considered cost effective by national standards (Table 12–1).

Fecal occult blood test is a noninvasive chemical test used to detect hidden blood in a sample of stool. Studies have shown it to be an inexpensive effective screening method that, when performed annually by the patient at home, reduces CRC incidence by 20% and mortality by about 30%. However, false-positive or false-negative results are often due to concomitant medications (aspirin, nonsteroidal anti-inflammatory drugs, vitamin C, antacids), foods with peroxidase activity (red meat, tomatoes, turnips, horseradish), preexisting conditions (bleeding hemorrhoids,

TABLE 12–1 ■ American Cancer Society Recommendations for Early Detection of Colorectal Cancer

Beginning at age 50, both men and women should follow one of these five testing schedules:

- Yearly fecal occult blood test (FOBT)
- Flexible sigmoidoscopy every 5 years
- Yearly fecal occult blood test plus flexible sigmoidoscopy every 5 years[a]
- Double-contrast barium enema every 5 years
- Colonoscopy every 10 years

People should begin colorectal cancer screening earlier and/or should undergo screening more often if they have any of the following colorectal cancer risk factors:

- Personal history of colorectal cancer or adenomatous polyps
- Strong family history of colorectal cancer or polyps (cancer or polyps in a first-degree relative younger than 60 or in two first-degree relatives of any age)
- Personal history of chronic inflammatory bowel disease
- Family history of hereditary colorectal cancer syndromes (familial adenomatous polyposis and hereditary nonpolyposis colon cancer)

[a]The combination of FOBT and flexible sigmoidoscopy is preferred over either test alone. All positive results should be followed up with colonoscopy.

diverticulosis), and/or nonbleeding cancerous lesions. A positive fecal occult blood test is followed up with a colonoscopy.

Flexible sigmoidoscopy is an invasive endoscopic procedure allowing direct visualization of the rectum and lower colon up to the splenic flexure. Because the sigmoidoscopy is only 60 cm long, it is effective in seeing less than half of the colon; fortunately, almost 50% of all CRC tumors are found in this limited area, so the method is effective. If any abnormality is found, the full colon is assessed for additional lesions.

Colonoscopy, an invasive endoscopic procedure necessitating conscious sedation, allows direct visualization of the entire large intestine. This procedure, which is extremely sensitive at detecting abnormalities, is used for both screening and diagnosis. Adenomatous polyps and suspected malignancies can undergo biopsy and, if appropriate, can be excised during the same procedure. Limitations of colonoscopy include an inability to identify small polyps or lesions hidden within colonic folds and, at times, the technical inability to reach the cecum.

Double-contrast barium enema, a radiographic procedure, involves x-ray studies of the colon after the patient drinks a barium-containing liquid and air has been instilled into the colon to press the barium against the colonic mucosa. Poor bowel preparation, difficulty in detecting small lesions, poor visual quality within the rectum, and other issues lower the sensitivity of this procedure.

Emerging screening technologies include virtual colonoscopy, molecular screening of the stool, and a disposable miniature video camera imbedded in an ingestible capsule. Although there are insufficient data to recommend these tests, the goal is to find tests that are more sensitive and more palatable to the individual and demonstrate a higher utilization and compliance rate. Individuals with genetic syndromes should also consider genetic counseling and testing.

■ Diagnostic Evaluation

CRC is often asymptomatic until the tumor is well advanced, thereby causing disruption in the flow of stool or organ dysfunction that is induced by metastatic disease. Signs and symptoms vary depending on the location of the tumor within the colon because of the anatomic structure of the colon and the biologic formation of stool. General signs and symptoms commonly associated with CRC are bleeding from the rectum; blood in the stool; change in bowel habits; change in size, shape, or color of stool; tenesmus; abdominal cramping or pain; or loss of energy.

With symptoms or suspicion of CRC, the health care provider conducts a complete medical history and physical examination with a focus on the abdominopelvic area. These may provide physical evidence of the disease and help determine any familial/genetic or other identifiable risk factors. A colonic examination is necessary to determine the primary site of disease, with the specific examination selected being based on the suspected location of the lesion. Biopsy of suspicious lesions and pathological analysis are mandatory for a final diagnosis. Most CRCs are moderately to well-differentiated adenocarcinomas.

After the cancer diagnosis is confirmed, additional testing is required to determine all sites of disease. Chest x-ray study, computed tomography of the abdomen and pelvis, and transrectal ultrasound (for rectal tumors) are performed; magnetic resonance imaging and positron emission tomography are optional. General blood tests identify anemia and liver dysfunction, if present. Carcinoembryonic antigen and CA 19-9, useful tumor markers, are often elevated in CRC and may have prognostic value at diagnosis or disease recurrence. They are not useful screening tools, because they are not elevated solely as a result of CRC.

Staging

Accurately determining the extent of the cancer staging is critical to establish both therapeutic strategies and prognosis. The staging of CRC is based on three key elements: depth of tumor penetration through the bowel wall, presence or absence of lymph node involvement (including number of positive lymph nodes), and whether or not the cancer has metastasized to distant areas. The two most common staging schemas are the Duke's staging system and the American Joint Commission on Cancer tumor node metastasis system. The tumor node metastasis system is recommended because it is internationally accepted and provides the most prognostic detail. Table 12–2 compares the two common schemas. The stage of disease at the time of diagnosis is the most important prognostic factor and thus has implications for long-term outcome. Individuals diagnosed at a localized stage (tumor confined within the colon or rectum) have a 90% chance of living 5 years, which decreases to 65% if there is regional disease (tumor that has spread to regional lymph nodes) and to 9% when the cancer has metastasized to distant sites. Thirty-seven percent of individuals present with localized disease, 37% present with regional disease, and 25% present with metastatic disease. Other factors favoring good outcome include well or moderately differentiated tumor and microsatellite instability. Factors denoting a poor outcome include poorly differentiated tumors, lymphatic or vascular invasion, regional lymph node metastasis, obstruction or perforation at diagnosis, and specific genetic abnormalities (e.g., *p53* mutations, deleted in colon cancer gene loss, K-*ras* mutations, and allele loss on chromosome 18q). Age, gender, status of symptoms, site of disease, perineural invasion, and preoperative carcinoembryonic antigen level, and other factors have not produced consistent data regarding outcome.

▪ Pathophysiology

Oncologists have a clear understanding of the natural history, biologic features, and many of the genetic abnormalities associated with CRC. Under normal conditions, the biologic cycle of cellular division, proliferation, differentiation, and death of colonic epithelial cells is strictly balanced. Any disruption in this balance can result in overproliferation of cells or lack of cellular death, leading to the development of an adenomatous polyp on the mucosal wall. Without intervention, either surgery or chemoprevention, the initially benign polyp continues to enlarge, growing slowly in a predictable way. However, with genetic mutations accumulated over time, the cells transform into cancerous cells and, on reaching a critical mass, begin to invade the colonic wall

TABLE 12–2 ■ Duke's Staging System and the American Joint Commission on Cancer (AJCC) Tumor Node Metastasis (TNM) System

Tumor (T)

Descriptor	Definition
Tis	Carcinoma in situ
T1	Tumor invades through mucosa into submucosa
T2	Tumor invades through submucosa into muscle layer (muscularis propria)
T3	Tumor invades through muscularis propria into the subserosa or into non-peritonealized tissue or perirectal tissue
T4	Tumor perforates completely through the colonic/rectal wall into visceral peritoneum or directly invades or adheres to other organs or structures

Lymph Node (N)

Descriptor	Definition
NX	Regional lymph node cannot be assessed because of incomplete information
N0	No regional lymph node involvement
N1	Cancer cells found in 1-3 regional lymph nodes
N2	Cancer cells in more than 4 regional lymph nodes

Metastasis (M)

Descriptor	Definition
MX	Distant metastasis can not be assessed because of incomplete information
M0	No positive distant spread found
M1	Distant spread is present

Stage	TNM Descriptors			Duke Stage Correlation
0	Tis	N0	M0	___
I	T1-2	N0	M0	A
II	T3-4	N0	M0	B
III	Any T	N1	M0	
	AnyT	N2	M0	C
IV	AnyT	AnyN	M1	___ (later called D)

Source: Adapted from American Joint Committee on Cancer (AJCC). (2002). *AJCC cancer staging manual* (6th ed., pp. 113–123). New York: Springer.

and metastasize. On average, it takes about 10 years from the formation of a polyp to the development of cancer.

The patterns of metastasis and disease failure are different between colon and rectal cancers as a result of their anatomic location within the abdomen and pelvis and their respective venous circulation. Colon tumors are higher in the abdomen, and the circulation drains into the portal system. Therefore, the most common site of metastasis is the liver. Rectal tumors are low in the pelvis, and the circulation drains by way of the inferior vena cava. Therefore, pulmonary metastasis is common. Moreover because of these same anatomic reasons, rectal tumors are three times likelier to recur in locoregional lymph nodes, whereas colon tumors often recur at a distant site. These differences in patterns of metastasis and disease failure dictate treatment strategies.

■ Treatment Strategies

Surgery

The primary management of CRC is excision of the involved segment of the large intestine with disease-free margins, the corresponding mesentery, and the adjacent lymph nodes (see Chapter 6, Surgical Oncology). Tumors may be excised endoscopically or by open laparotomy, depending on the location and the clinical stage of disease. The decision of which surgical procedure should be used also depends on whether the tumor is within the colon or the rectum and its exact location within the colon or rectum. The standard procedure for colon cancers is a partial colectomy with an end-to-end anastomosis. A low anterior resection with total mesorectal excision and coloanal anastomosis is considered the standard procedure for rectal tumors. The amount of colon removed depends on the mesenteric nodal resection. However, for rectal cancer, there must be at least a 2-cm surgical margin and a complete excision of the mesorectum.

Maintaining functional capacity is a primary goal, especially with rectal cancers. Newer technologies and improved surgical techniques spare sphincter functioning. As a result, only one in eight individuals undergoing surgery require a permanent colostomy. A temporary colostomy may be used to allow for healing of a segment of intestine; this is then reversed once healing has occurred, and normal bowel flow resumes. Surgery may also be performed for palliation: reduction of tumor size/burden, pain and pressure relief, and bleeding control. If the disease is localized at the time of diagnosis, the chance of cure with surgery alone is high. If there is regional disease, adjuvant chemotherapy is recommended (See Table 12–3 for CRC surgical complications.).

TABLE 12–3 ■ Surgical Complications[a]

• Infection: wound, intra-abdominal abscess, urinary, pulmonary	• Abdominal distention
• Pain	• Paralytic ileus
• Fluid and electrolyte imbalance	• Clotting disorders
• Anastomotic leak	• Urinary retention
• Poor wound healing	• Impotence

[a]See unit V.

TABLE 12–4 ■ Radiation Therapy Side Effects[a]

Acute	Chronic
• Local skin reactions	• Fibrosis
• Diarrhea	• Long-term pigmentation changes
• Myelosuppression	• Atrophy
• Proctitis	• Organ or sexual dysfunction
• Cystitis	• Ulceration
• Fatigue	• Necrosis
	• Late cystitis

[a]See unit V.

Radiation Therapy

Radiation therapy is an important therapeutic modality in the treatment of rectal cancers (see Chapter 8, Radiation Therapy). In colon cancer, radiation therapy has a limited value because of possible damage to adjacent organs and the small intestine. In rectal cancers, radiation therapy given either before or after surgery reduces the locoregional recurrence rate. Radiation therapy may be given alone or in combination with surgery or chemotherapy. Preoperative radiation therapy is often used to shrink unresectable lesions. Postoperative radiation therapy given concurrently with chemotherapy improves disease recurrence and survival better than radiation therapy or surgery alone. The specific combination of chemotherapy agents and the sequence of radiation therapy plus chemotherapy are being investigated in ongoing clinical trials. Currently, radiation therapy at doses of 45–55 Gy plus 5-fluorouracil (5-FU)-based chemotherapy given as a continuous infusion is recommended. Radiation therapy also has palliative benefits as a means to control pain, treat bowel obstruction, and bleeding in patients with advanced disease (See Table 12–4 for potential acute and long-term effects of radiation therapy.).

Chemotherapy

Chemotherapy for the treatment of CRC is being actively studied (see Chapter 7, Chemotherapy). For years, the only active agent was 5-FU, but now there are new effective chemotherapy agents and novel molecularly targeted agents that may provide further clinical advances. Guidelines available from the National Comprehensive Cancer Network assist practitioners in selecting treatment regimens for patients with colon and rectal carcinomas.

Since the 1990s, adjuvant chemotherapy given after surgery has been recommended for colon cancer with regional involvement (stage III). 5-FU plus leucovorin has been the standard regimen; however, a new combination of 5-FU, leucovorin, and oxaliplatin (FOLFOX4) may prove more beneficial. To date, the FOLFOX4 regimen appears to delay disease recurrence better than a standard 5-FU plus leucovorin regimen, but its effect on overall survival is unknown. Additional clinical research with other chemotherapy combinations has completed accrual and is awaiting analysis. In early-stage rectal cancer, adjuvant chemoradiation therapy regimens are standard, as discussed under radiation therapy.

Similar chemotherapy regimens are administered to patients with metastatic disease, regardless of whether the tumor originated in the colon or rectum. These regimens can prolong survival and provide palliative benefits. Currently, there are three new agents approved by the US Food and Drug Administration (FDA) for the treatment of advanced CRC: irinotecan, capecitabine, and oxaliplatin. The FDA has recognized 5-FV plus leucovorin in combination with either oxaliplatin or irinotecan as the regimens that prolong survival in individuals with metastatic CRC. Data suggest that survival is increased when patients are treated with oxaliplatin, irinotecan, and 5-FV (three agents with differing mechanisms of action); both sequences are similar and achieve survival in the range of 20 months. Capecitabine, an oral agent, is recommended for patients for whom the health care provider would typically recommend single-agent 5-FU, but it has not demonstrated a survival benefit. Recent results of a randomized clinical trial comparing the antivascular endothelial growth factor inhibitor bevacizumab plus IFL versus IFL plus placebo have demonstrated a benefit with bevacizumab plus IFL. The benefit was multifold—an improvement in tumor shrinkage, a longer duration before disease recurrence, and an increase in overall survival. This is the first research to demonstrate a survival benefit in CRC with the use of an antiangiogenesis agent. The FDA will be reviewing these data to determine whether bevacizumab should be commercially available.

TABLE 12–5 ■ Chemotherapy Side Effects[a]

• Nausea and vomiting	• Peripheral neuropathy
• Diarrhea	• Hand-foot syndrome
• Myelosuppression	• Thromboembolic events
• Hair loss	

[a]See unit V.

There are several treatment options for patients who have metastatic disease isolated to the liver: surgery, regional chemotherapy, or intralesion therapy. Excision of the lesions is recommended if there are discrete lesions and no extrahepatic disease. Approximately 10% of patients with liver metastasis are eligible for curative resection. Another option is the infusion of chemotherapy directly into the liver; hepatic artery infusion (HAI) which delivers a higher concentration of chemotherapy to the liver lesions than could be delivered systemically. The role of this option remains controversial. Hepatic artery infusion is effective at shrinking tumors, but in most studies, it has not had an impact on overall survival. Targeted intralesion therapy, such as selective internal radiation therapy, ethanol injections, radiofrequency ablation, chemoembolization, and cryotherapy, are additional treatment options. All methods use a local approach to destroy the cancer cells and are beneficial in patients with small, discreet tumors isolated to the liver. Radiofrequency ablation uses heat, ethanol injections use absolute ethanol, chemoembolization uses a foreign substance "soaked" with chemotherapy, and cryosurgery directly freezes the lesion to kill the cancerous cells. The only intralesion option that is FDA approved is selective internal radiation therapy. This new technique selectively delivers high doses of radiation therapy in small, biocompatible microspheres to liver tumors, but it has not demonstrated an improvement in overall survival when compared with systemic chemotherapy. (See Table 12–5 for possible side effects of chemotherapy for CRC.)

■ Rehabilitation and Long-Term Follow-Up

In early-stage CRC, the period after the completion of primary treatment is a time of adjustment. Patients begin to feel physically well, and their patterns of activity begin to return to more normal levels. They may have a sense of loss or anxiety related to less contact with their health care provider (see Chapter 27, Anxiety and Depression in the Oncology Setting). Posttreatment surveillance is important to identify additional tumors early. The American Society of Clinical Oncology recommends a physical examination every 3–6 months for 3 years, then yearly; colonoscopy within 1 year after diagnosis, then every 3–5 years; and carcinoembryonic antigen determinations every 2–3 months for 2 years, then at the physician's discretion.

The greatest risk for recurrence is within the first 5 years. Recurrence may be more traumatic than the initial diagnosis, as the patient realizes the initial treatment failed to completely control the disease. Coping strategies in patients with recurrent or newly metastatic disease are tested because there is much uncertainty about the future (see Chapter 36, Cancer Survivorship).

Regardless of the stage of disease, there may be perceived or real difficulties and concerns regarding employment, insurability, and management of short- and long-term complications of therapy. A collaborative approach to care is important. Identification of rehabilitation needs and referrals to appropriate services and agencies may be necessary. Social work may assist with insurance, employment discrimination, local community resources, and psychological support.

■ The Role of the Nurse

CRC presents nurses with many challenges along the continuum of prevention, early detection, and treatment. Proactive counseling of patients and their family members about healthy life style choices could help reduce their risk of CRC. A risk assessment tool, such as the "Your Cancer Risk" tool available at *www.yourcancerrisk.harvard.edu* can help stratify individuals into average-, moderate-, or high-risk categories. This delineation then helps the health care professional tailor information to the person's needs. Professional and community education programs, especially for socioeconomically disadvantaged and minority populations, that promote healthy choices and describe the early signs and symptoms of CRC and the benefits, the schedule, and the value of regular CRC screening, provide further opportunities to make an impact in this disease.

During the diagnostic period, most nurses serve as advocates and informational resources. Advance-practice nurses are active in the diagnostic process by completing medical histories and performing physical examinations, and some are certified to perform sigmoidoscopies. All involved nurses provide instruction as to the rationale for specific diagnostic procedures and any required pre- and postprocedure preparations. Listening to concerns regarding the diagnostic evaluation is also essential. Care of the patient during treatment is collaborative among the health care team. The nursing focus is to design a plan of care in which therapy is administered as prescribed, complications are minimized, and independent self care is promoted. Age-appropriate and culturally sensitive materials are used to educate the patient on the treatment plan, rationale, potential schedule, and side effects. Reinforcing coping strategies as the patient grieves over loss of health, change in body image, possible alterations in sexual function, and fear of death are also pivotal responsibilities.

The side effects of chemotherapy are drug, dose, schedule, and patient dependent. Two important patient-dependent factors are comorbid diseases and the individual's overall functional (performance) status. Age alone is not an adverse factor because there is growing evidence that elderly patients can receive the same therapeutic benefit as younger patients when they are grouped by functional status. The focus is on the patient's physical and metabolic needs, preventing complications, reinforcing self-care symptom management strategies, and providing emotional support. The nurse must frequently evaluate the impact of the disease and treatment on the patient and their significant others and then make adjustments in the plan of care as appropriate.

■ Conclusion

The care of patients with CRC is an exciting and challenging field. Promotion of American Cancer Society screening guidelines can decrease the incidence of this disease while improving survival rates through early detection. Clinical trials offer the hope for new treatment regimens. Therefore, educating patients about this therapeutic option is a critical element in improving CRC care and long-term outcomes. The nurse must be knowledgeable about CRC and its evolving management, skilled in symptom management, and supportive and attentive to the needs of the patient and family. The nurse has a pivotal role in prevention, diagnosis, treatment, and rehabilitation of the patient with CRC.

■ Resources

American Cancer Society, *www.cancer.org* or 800-ACS-2345

- "Colorectal Cancer Treatment Decision Tool," *www.cancer.org/docroot/ETO/eto_1_1a.asp*

- "What Should You Ask Your Doctor About Colon and Rectal Cancer," *www.cancer.org/docroot/CRI/content/CRI_2_4_5X_What_should_you_ask_your_doctor_about_colon_and_rectum_cancer.asp?sitearea=*
- NCCN Colon and Rectal Cancer Treatment Guidelines for Patients, *www.cancer.org/downloads/CRI/nccn_colorectal_guide.pdf*

American Gastroenterological Association, *www.gastro.org*
Colon Cancer Alliance, *www.ccalliance.org/*
Colorectal Cancer Network, *www.colorectal-cancer.net*
National Colorectal Research Alliance, *www.eifoundation.org/national/nccra/splash/index.html*
United Ostomy Association, *www.uoa.org* or 800-826-0826
"Your Cancer Risk" Assessment Tool, *www.yourcancer.harvard.edu*

Bibliography

American Cancer Society. (2003). *American Cancer Society Cancer facts and figures 2003*. Atlanta: author.

Berg, D. T. (2003). *Pocket guide to colorectal cancer*. Boston: Jones & Bartlett Publishers.

Ellenhorn, J. D., Coia, R., Alberts, S. R., Hoff, P. M. (2002). Colon, rectal, and anal cancers. In R. Pazdur, L. R. Coia, W. J. Hoskins, L. D. Wagman. (Eds.), *Cancer management: A multidisciplinary approach* (6th ed., pp. 295–330). Melville, NY: PRR.

National Comprehensive Cancer Network (NCCN). 2003. *The complete library of NCCN clinical practice guidelines in oncology*. Rockledge, PA: author.

CHAPTER

13

Prostate Cancer

Maureen E. O'Rourke

Prostate cancer remains the most frequently diagnosed male cancer in the United States, with 230,110 new cases estimated to be diagnosed in 2004. Prostate cancer accounts for one third of all male cancer deaths; 29,900 deaths are expected to occur in the United States in 2004. Five-year survival rates have steadily improved since 1974 for both whites and African Americans; however, African-Americans continue to have lower 5-year survival rates for all stages of prostate cancer. The relative 5-year survival for all races within the United States is 97%: 98% for whites and 93% for African Americans.

■ Incidence

Prostate cancer is the sixth most common cancer worldwide. Within the Unites States, prostate cancer incidence increased steadily from 1988 to 1992, coinciding with the advent of widespread prostate cancer screening using the prostate-specific antigen (PSA) test. From 1992 to 1995, however, sharp declines in incidence were noted, followed by a gradual leveling off from 1995 to 1999. Current estimates suggest that about 17% of all men living within the United States will experience prostate cancer in their lifetime (see Chapter 2, Epidemiology of Cancer).

Risk Factors

More than 80% of all prostate cancers are diagnosed in men 65 years of age or older, making age an especially significant risk factor. Autopsy studies have demonstrated that at least 30% of men over the age of 50 have some evidence of adenocarcinoma of the prostate, and by the age of 90 years, that percentage rises to 57%. Risk is also linked with race and ethnicity. The highest incidence rates worldwide are among African Americans. Hormonal factors have been suggested as an explanation for the differences in incidence and mortality rates. Higher rates of bioavailable testosterone have been noted among African Americans, and they also have a higher incidence of mutations in prostate cancer susceptibility genes. Different ethnic groups experience different rates of incidence. Americans of Northern European origin have higher rates of incidence than Native-Americans, Mexican-Americans, or Chinese-Americans. Prostate cancer is rare in developing countries. Japanese have one of the lowest incidence rates; yet, on moving to the Unites States, incidence rates after two generations approach those of whites.

Although much has been written linking prostate cancer with diet and lifestyle, no conclusive evidence exists at this point. Associations have been noted between high-fat diets and high rates of prostate cancer. Some experts believe that men who have high fat intake coupled with a low fiber intake have double the lifetime risk. Diets high in vitamins E and D, selenium, and lycopene have been suggested to be protective. Occupational exposure to chemicals/pesticides through farming and exposure to cadmium though welding or battery manufacturing have also been linked with an increased risk of prostate cancer. Job-related physical activity has been investigated as a factor associated with incidence levels; however, although aerobic activity is associated with lower levels of circulating testosterone, no conclusive evidence has been found.

A variety of genetic links have been suggested (see Chapter 1, The Biology of Cancer). A possible susceptibility locus has been noted on chromosome 1, and this is thought to be responsible for up to 33% of all hereditary prostate cancers. However, at present, heredity is estimated to account for only 3% of prostate cancers overall. Some genetic mutations associated with the development of breast cancer have also been implicated in prostate cancer, including the genes *BRCA1* and *BRCA2*. Strong familial associations have been noted, although it remains unclear whether these are purely genetic links or some combination of environmental and genetic factors. Men with a first-degree relative, such as their brother or father, affected by prostate cancer are two to three times likelier to develop the disease themselves. Men with a first-degree relative and a second-degree relative affected are six times likelier to develop prostate cancer themselves.

The literature contains a variety of other suspected linkages, although associations are weak and inconclusive or show no association.

■ Detection

Screening Tests

At both the national and the international levels, there continues to be a high level of controversy surrounding the issue of prostate cancer screening. The controversy focuses on one central issue, an understanding that screening can and does reveal clinically insignificant tumors that are subsequently treated, resulting in significant treatment-related side effects and diminished quality of life (see Chapter 3, Cancer Screening, Early Detection, Risk Reduction, and Genetic Counseling). Although there is disagreement among major health care groups, the current American Cancer Society guidelines regarding testing for early-stage prostate cancer were updated in 2001 and are summarized in Table 13–1.

The pros and cons of prostate cancer screening have been detailed in numerous scholarly publications and in the lay literature. Each man must essentially decide whether or not to screen for himself after consultation with his physician or nurse practitioner. Some of the factors cited in favor of prostate cancer screening include the fact that advanced prostate cancer is not curable. Men who are screened have a greater likelihood of being diagnosed at an earlier stage that is more

TABLE 13–1 ■ American Cancer Society Prostate Cancer Screening Guidelines

- The PSA test and the DRE should be offered annually, beginning at age 50, to men who have a life expectancy of at least 10 years.
- Men at high risk (African American men and men with a strong family history of one or more first-degree relatives diagnosed with prostate cancer at an early age) should begin testing at age 45.
- Men at average risk and high risk should be provided with information about what is known and what is uncertain about the benefits and limitations of early detection and treatment of prostate cancer so that they can make an informed decision about testing.

Key: DRE = digital rectal examination; PSA = prostate-specific antigen.

conducive to cure. Factors that have been cited in the arguments against routine screening include (a) the fact that many men die *with* the disease and not *of* the disease, and (b) the lack of clear scientific evidence to conclude that screening does in fact decrease a man's risk of dying from prostate cancer.

The general accepted definition for a normal PSA is less than or equal to 4.0 ng/ml. Although the PSA test is prostate specific, it is not cancer specific—elevations may not be related to prostate cancer. Some elevations are secondary to benign prostatic hypertrophy or prostatitis. PSA increases with both age and prostatic volume. Use of the percent-free PSA test and the PSA velocity has improved the sensitivity and specificity of testing. Age- and race-specific PSA values have also been suggested for improving sensitivity and specificity.

Digital rectal examination (DRE) testing by trained professionals can detect prostate abnormalities, including nodules, asymmetry, swelling, and changes in texture. Although this procedure is simple and inexpensive, only the posterior and lateral regions of the prostate gland can be palpated. One in four prostate cancers is detected in men with normal PSAs and abnormal DREs.

■ Diagnosis

Most prostate cancers arise from the outer peripheral zone of the gland, distant from the urethra. For this reason, men with early-stage prostate cancer are often symptom free. As the disease progresses, however, symptoms caused by obstruction, such as decreased urinary stream force, urinary hesitancy, incomplete emptying of the bladder, and increased urinary frequency, may result. Progression may also cause blood in the semen with decreased ejaculatory volume and, less commonly, impotence. Bone pain, hematuria, and anemia are signs of advanced disease.

As in the case of any malignancy, diagnosis is definitively established only by biopsy. Men go for an evaluation either because of bothersome symptoms or because of an elevated PSA or digital rectal examination indicative of a problem. In the presence of symptoms or questionable screening test results, a biopsy is generally performed. Biopsies are performed transrectally under transrectal ultrasound to facilitate visualization of the gland. A spring-loaded biopsy gun is used to obtain multiple samples (generally six to 13) from all regions of the prostate gland. The procedure is performed on an outpatient basis. Patient education at this time includes instruction that hematuria and hematospermia may occur for several days to several weeks after the procedure. Men should be instructed to contact their urologist if elevated temperature, excessive or prolonged bleeding, or increased urinary difficulties occur.

Other diagnostic tests may be used. Magnetic resonance imagining may be used to evaluate extracapsular penetration beyond the prostate gland itself, and possible lymph node metastasis. Computed tomographic scans may also be used to evaluate prostate size and lymph node status. Radionucleotide bones scans are generally performed only if the PSA levels are > 10 ng/ml. These scans are performed to assess possible bone metastasis, but they are interpreted with caution because they may yield false-positive results, signaling activity at sites of old trauma or arthritis.

Staging

As for all types of cancer, prostate cancer is staged as a means of describing the extent of the disease and determining the appropriate type of therapy. The American Joint Committee on Cancer has recently updated the tumor, node, metastasis staging system for prostate cancer (T refers to the primary tumor itself, N is the level of lymph node involvement, and M refers to the metastatic status).

Prostate cancer is graded according to the level of cellular differentiation noted among the malignant specimens taken from biopsies. Currently, the most common system employed for the grading of prostate cancer is the Gleason score. Two grades are assigned. The two most common malignant cellular patterns noted under microscopic examination are graded on a scale of 1–5. Grades for the two patterns are then summed to yield the Gleason score. Total scores range from 2–10, with higher scores indicating more aggressive disease and subsequently poorer prognosis.

■ Treatment and The Role of the Nurse

At the present time, men are generally presented with three main treatment options for early-stage prostate cancer: radical prostatectomy, radiation therapy (external-beam and/or brachytherapy), or the "watchful waiting" or expectant management approach. Cryotherapy is becoming more available in some regions, although it remains investigational as a first-line therapy and without solid long-term outcome data. Neoadjuvant hormonal therapy may be offered before surgical or radiation therapy treatments (Table 13–2).

TABLE 13-2 ■ Treatment Options

Stage I disease (T1, N0, M0, grade 1)
- Close Observation, including PSA testing biannually or annually
- For young patients: aggressive treatment, generally radical prostatectomy

Stage II disease (T1a, b, c, ; N0; M0; grade 2, 3, 4)
- Radical prostatectomy
- External-beam radiation therapy or interstitial radioisotope implants
- Watchful waiting or expectant management
- Cryosurgery (under investigation)

Stage III disease (T3, N0, M0, any grade)
- External-beam radiation therapy (with or without hormonal therapy)
- Asymptomatic patients with comorbid conditions: Watchful waiting
- Hormonal therapy

Stage IV disease (T4, N0, M0, any grade; any T, N1, M0; any T, any N, M1)
- Hormonal therapy/orchiectomy
- Chemotherapy for hormone-resistant disease
- External-beam radiation therapy for selected patients with M0 disease
- Watchful waiting for selected asymptomatic patients
- Palliative radiation therapy for bone metastasis
- Systemic radioisotopes for generalized bone pain

Key PSA = prostate-specific antigen.

Source: Reprinted from Table 1, *Seminars in Oncology Nursing,* V17: 109, O'Rourke, ME: "Decision making and prostate cancer treatment: A review. 2002 Elsevier Inc, with permission from Elsevier."

Treatment Decision Making

A multitude of factors are involved in decision making about treatment selection for early-stage cancer. It is critical that the process of deciding on the most appropriate prostate cancer treatment is a truly collaborative process between the patient, his partner, and the health care team. At present, there is no true consensus within the scientific community as to which, if any, treatment is optimal for early-stage prostate cancer. The ultimate decision is affected by medical considerations and patients' unique preferences. Numerous medical decision-making guides have been developed both for physicians and men and their partners. Key factors in these decision-enhancement models include patient age, projected survival, coexisting medical conditions, stage of disease, and Gleason score. Patient factors include their personal preferences and biases toward or against particular treatment modalities, personal and vicarious experiences with cancer and cancer treatments, concerns about potential side effects of therapy and their effects on quality of life, costs of treatment and lost work time, and tolerance of uncertainty.

Data from the National Cancer Institute Surveillance, Epidemiology, and End Results program demonstrated that in the mid-1990s, approximately 48% of men were treated with radical prostatectomy, 23% with radiation therapy, 19% with watchful waiting, and 11% with hormonal therapy. Treatment variations have been noted by age, with increasing numbers of men older than 70 years receiving external-beam radiation therapy (XRT), brachytherapy, or conservative management with the watchful waiting approach.

Treatment also varies by race. Older African American men are significantly less likely to receive any treatment at all (surgery, radiation therapy, or hormonal therapy). Although African American men as a group have a tendency toward more coexisting diseases, these treatment deficits were noted even after investigators controlled (note tense is past) for these conditions. Such racial disparities are of particular concern and signal an area where nurses can effectively intervene in the public education arena.

For all men, comprehensive, accurate information from credible sources is the critical factor in decision making. A trusting relationship with health care providers and assistance in sorting through the wide array of patient education products now available on the market and on the internet represent areas where nurses play a pivotal professional role.

Radical Prostatectomy

Within the United States, the mainstay of treatment is the radical retropubic prostatectomy, which includes complete removal of the prostate gland, with lymph node sampling. The anatomic nerve-sparing approach involves isolation of the neurovascular bundles responsible for innervation of the corpus cavernosa of the penis, which is necessary for erection, thereby improving the likelihood of maintaining potency after surgery.

Immediate nursing priorities focus on managing pain (see Chapter 23, Cancer Pain) and maintaining patency of the urinary catheter. Pain management may include the use of patient-controlled analgesia devices dispensing morphine. Ketorolac tromethamine is often used for pain management. Vigilant pain assessment is essential. The use of antispasmodics to relieve painful bladder spasms may also be indicated.

Nursing emphasis is also focused on the prevention of postoperative complications (see Unit V for specific symptoms), such as thrombophlebitis and pulmonary emboli. Early ambulation on the first postoperative day and performance of dorsiflexion exercises are advised. The use of an incentive spirometer, compression hose, or sequential compression devices may also be indicated. Pillow splinting may be helpful during coughing and deep-breathing exercises. Fluid intake should be encouraged in order to maintain a minimum urine output of at least 30 ml/hr. Rectal manipulation, including rectal temperatures and suppositories, should be avoided because of the close proximity of the prostate gland to the rectal wall and the risk of rectal injury.

Additional nursing priorities focus on patient and partner education. Management of the indwelling catheter in the home setting, including procedures for switching from the daytime leg bag to bedside drainage overnight, monitoring and reporting temperature elevations of 101°F, and avoiding lifting anything 10 pounds or greater should be emphasized before discharge and in follow-up phone contacts. Patients should also be instructed regarding maintenance of adequate fluid intake. Before discharge, patients should be instructed on the performance of Kegel exercises to strengthen pelvic floor muscles. A wide variety of incontinence products are available for men to accommodate full urinary incontinence or minor urinary dribbling. Scheduled urination may help men avoid overflow incontinence.

Radiation Therapy

Radiation therapy remains a viable potentially curative treatment option for men with early-stage prostate cancer and also has utility in the management of advanced disease for palliation of painful bone metastasis and other symptoms, such as urethral or rectal obstruction, lymphatic blockage, and spinal cord compression. Radiation may be delivered as a single modality or in combination with other treatment modalities (see Chapter 8, Radiation Therapy). XRT may be used after radical prostatectomy for patients at high risk for recurrence, such as those with high Gleason scores (7–10) and invasive disease beyond the prostate capsule. Radiation therapy may also be recommended for men experiencing locally recurrent disease, documented by a rising PSA level with or without symptoms.

Nursing considerations for men undergoing XRT focus on symptom management (see Unit V for specific symptoms). Acute side effects include diarrhea, proctitis, cystitis, fatigue, and local skin reactions. Adequate nutritional intake and hydration status are important nursing foci. Low-residue diets and antidiarrheal medications are indicated for these patients. Topical rectal steroid products may be prescribed to provide relief from proctitis, as well as sitz baths and water-based topical skin preparations for intragluteal skin fold irritation. Interventions to minimize fatigue include patient and family teaching regarding energy-conservation methods. Mild aerobic activity and planned rest periods can provide some symptom relief.

Radiation may also be delivered through the implantation of radioactive seeds directly into the prostate gland. This technique is referred to as brachytherapy (see Chapter 8, Radiation Therapy). Brachytherapy may be used as a solo treatment or in combination with XRT and/or hormonal therapy. For men with prostate cancer, brachytherapy is generally performed as a same-day surgery procedure under general or spinal anesthesia. Radioactive seeds are implanted into the gland itself through a perineal approach guided by transrectal ultrasound. The most common isotopes used include iodine 125 or palladium 103. The procedure itself takes 1–2 hours, and the patient is discharged to home at the end of the day. Patients may be discharged with an indwelling Foley catheter, generally for a period of 24–48 hours.

Nursing care includes teaching and management of symptoms similar to those associated with XRT: cystitis, proctitis, and fatigue. Additional considerations include assessment and teaching regarding potential infection and instruction regarding prophylactic antibiotic use. Perineal pain, ecchymosis, and scrotal edema may be treated with ice packs and analgesic administration. Instructions regarding radiation safety are another nursing priority.

Watchful Waiting or Expectant Management

Watchful waiting, also known as expectant management, observation, or surveillance, has been defined as initial surveillance followed by active treatment in the presence of bothersome symptoms. The rationale for this option for early-stage prostate cancer is based on the observation that prostate cancer incidence rates far exceed prostate cancer death rates, and the further observation that more men die with the disease than of the disease. Aggressive treatment is associated with significant negative effects on patient quality of life. To date, studies have failed to demonstrate conclusively that screening and early detection of prostate cancer lead to improved survival.

The goal of watchful waiting is to spare men with clinically localized disease the morbidity and mortality associated with aggressive treatment without compromising their survival. At this point, there is little scientific literature comparing quality of life between men with localized disease treated aggressively and men who opt for the watchful waiting approach.

There is no general consensus as to which men are appropriate candidates for watchful waiting. It is considered a plausible option for men with a life expectancy of 10 years or less; men with favorable pathological findings, such as low Gleason scores (< 7); and cancer involving less than three biopsy specimens. Other considerations include PSA levels of < 10 ng/ml and absence of palpable disease on DRE. Men with significant coexisting medical conditions are also candidates for this option. Men selecting this option would benefit from a high tolerance for uncertainty and a strong support system.

There is no accepted standard for the watchful waiting protocol itself. Men in the watchful waiting group of the Prostate Cancer Intervention Versus Observation Trial are followed every 3 months for the first year and every 6 months subsequently. At each visit, the men undergo a thorough assessment of their urologic symptoms; a physical examination, including a DRE; and PSA testing. An annual bone scan is also performed. If men experience symptoms, have new findings on DRE, or significant PSA changes, restaging is recommended with or using—not from a repeat transrectal ultrasound and biopsy.

Nursing considerations for men who select watchful waiting basically consist of continuous assessment of quality of life, including both the physiologic and the psychosocial dimensions. When possible, nurses should include the patient's partner in discussions and teaching regarding signs and symptoms that require reporting. Nurses should provide reassurance that although no active treatment is being used, the patient is not being neglected and vigilant surveillance is an acceptable option based on the current scientific knowledge. Encourage the use of supportive strategies, such as participation in a support group and use of spiritual resources. The nurse should reassure the patient and his partner that no decision is irrevocable, and treatment may be initiated if their desire or condition changes.

Hormonal Therapy

Hormone therapy is the treatment of choice for the management of metastatic prostate cancer and, in many cases, for the management of recurrent disease. The goal of hormonal treatment in these cases is palliation and prolonged survival. Neoadjuvant hormonal therapy is indicated in some cases to shrink the tumor before surgery or radiation therapy. Adjuvant hormonal therapy is an option for some men who have undergone prostatectomy or radiation therapy and have unfavorable prognostic factors suggesting that the cancer is likely to recur.

Hormonal therapy is based on the rationale that androgens regulate prostate tissue growth. Four major types of hormonal manipulation are used in the treatment of prostate cancer, each aimed at disruption of androgen stimulation: the bilateral removal of the testicles (orchiectomy) or the use of luteinizing hormone-releasing hormones (LHRH), antiandrogens, and estrogen therapy. Another approach is total androgen blockade via orchiectomy plus an antiandrogen, or the combination of an LHRH agonist with the use of an antiandrogen. Recently, intermittent or pulse hormonal therapy has been used in an effort to minimize patient side effects and forestall the development of hormone resistance.

Nursing care of men receiving hormonal therapy is aimed at patient education, psychosocial support, recognition of side effects, and effective symptom management. Body image changes and altered perceptions of masculinity are a potential issue for men undergoing hormonal therapy. Hot flashes, decreased libido (sexual drive), impotence, fatigue, and muscle wasting are associated with the use of LHRH agonists and orchiectomy. Antiandrogens may cause breast enlargement or tenderness, hot flashes, alterations in lipid profiles, loss of bone density, and anemia. Additionally, elevated liver enzymes, diarrhea, and ocular disturbances have been noted. Many medical approaches have been employed to alleviate hot flashes, with varying success: clonidine, low-dose megestrol acetate, cyproterone, and the antidepressant venlafaxine. Less traditional approaches include the use of acupuncture or soy and vitamin E preparations.

Rehabilitation

Rehabilitation issues relative to prostate cancer treatment center around two main long-term issues: the management of urinary incontinence and the management of impotence.

Urinary Incontinence Dysfunction in either the storage of urine or in the process of emptying urine can result in incontinence. Research has suggested that the most common cause of urinary incontinence after prostatectomy is sphincter insufficiency.

The actual incidence of urinary incontinence after prostatectomy or radiation treatments is difficult to determine in the literature, and reports vary from 2%–87%. This wide range is related to measurement methods and differences in definitions of incontinence. Urinary incontinence is particularly significant because it is associated with embarrassment and the potential for social isolation, diminished quality of life, and depression. Urinary incontinence may also be associated with skin breakdown. In one recent nursing study, men identified numerous problems associated with prostate cancer treatment-related incontinence, ranging from difficulties with odor and skin irritation to finding the right type of pad and disposing of pads when away from home.

Medical interventions for incontinence include the use of anticholinergic or alpha-sympathomimetic medications combined with pelvic floor strengthening exercises (Kegels). Persistent incontinence may require surgical intervention for the placement of an artificial sphincter. Other management strategies include the use of pads, scheduled bladder emptying, sitting to void to facilitate complete emptying, and use of penile clamps. Patients may benefit from restricting caffeine in their diets and maintaining a regular bowel schedule to decrease bowel pressure on the bladder.

Erectile Dysfunction and Impotence For both men and their partners, erectile dysfunction and impotence represent distressing treatment-related side effects (see Chapter 33, Sexuality). Numerous researchers have noted higher rates of impotence after radical prostatectomy than after XRT or brachytherapy. The use of the anatomical nerve–sparing radial prostatectomy technique is associated with lower rates of impotence. Brachytherapy is associated with the lowest rates of impotence when compared with other treatment modalities. Determinants of erectile function after treatment include pretreatment status, age, clinical and pathological stage of disease, and type of surgical approach used.

Patient assessment and education are primary nursing responsibilities. Both patients and their partners need assurance that this condition can be effectively dealt with and does not signal the end of their sexual relationship. Interventions are both medical and psychological. Strategies include the use of sildenafil (Viagra); the use of vasoconstrictive devices, such as penile vacuum pumps; and counseling. Other interventions include the use of intraurethral prostaglandin suppositories or the use of intercavernosal penile injections to attain erections. Lastly, erectile dysfunction may be treated surgically with penile implants that are either semirigid or inflatable.

■ Conclusion

Prostate cancer is a model of uncertainty in terms of prevention, screening, and treatment. Nurses are in a pivotal position to be leaders in the area of public education regarding these issues. The clear disparity in incidence and mortality rates among African Americans suggests an area for immediate nursing action. Care of patients undergoing treatment for prostate cancer must be family focused and requires expertise in symptom management and psychosocial support. Nurses have a strong history of dedication to these issues.

■ Resources

Organizations and Websites

- American Foundation for Urologic Disease: provides information on urologic conditions and a list of prostate cancer support groups. 800-828-7866 or *http://www.afud.org*
- National Association for Continence: provides information on continence. 800-252-3337 (1-800-BLADDER) or *http://www.nafc.org*
- US Too International, Inc.: prostate cancer information, support group information, hotline for questions. 800-80US-TOO, 1-800-808-7866 or *http://www.ustoo.com*
- American Cancer Society. 800-ACS-2345 or *http://www.cancer.org*
  - Man to Man: American Cancer Society program that provides information about prostate cancer and related issues for men and their partners in a supportive atmosphere. Some areas offer Side by Side, a group program for the partners of men with prostate cancer, and/or a visitation program in which a trained prostate cancer survivor provides support to a man newly diagnosed with prostate cancer.
  - "Ask the Expert" message board at *www.cancer.org:* men and their families can receive answers to their questions from the experts at the American Cancer Society.

Specific Publications

- Available from ACS by calling 1-800-ACS-2345:
  - *Sexuality & cancer: For the man who has cancer & his partner* (Booklet)
  - NCCN Prostate Cancer Treatment Guidelines for Patients (Booklet) and also available at *http://www.nccn.org/patient_gls/_english/_prostate/index.htm*
- Available from US Too International and the National Cancer Institute:
  Understanding treatment choices for prostate cancer. (NIH Publication # 00-4659)

Bibliography

Griffin, A. S., & O'Rourke, M. E. (2001). Expectant management of prostate cancer. *Seminars in Oncology Nursing, 17,* 101–107.

Iwamoto, R. R., & Maher, K.E. (2001). Radiation therapy for prostate cancer. *Seminars in Oncology Forum, 17,* 90–100.

O'Rourke, M. E. (2001). Decision making and prostate cancer treatment selection: A review. *Seminars in Oncology Nursing, 17,* 108–117.

Wallace, M., & Powel, L. L. (Eds.). (2002). *Prostate cancer: Nursing assessment, management, and care.* New York: Springer.

CHAPTER

14

Lung Cancer

Janet H. Van Cleave

Mary E. Cooley

Lung cancer is the second most common cancer and the number one cause of cancer death in both men and women in the United States. It is estimated that 173,770 new cases of lung cancer will be diagnosed in 2004, accounting for about 13% of cancers. An estimated 160,440 people are expected to die of the disease in 2004, making up 28% of all cancer deaths.

Lung cancer incidence and mortality rates pose a significant public health risk among all ethnic and racial groups. However, incidence and mortality rates are highest among whites and African Americans. Overall, the incidence rates in men have been decreasing over time but have remained stable among white and African American women during the 1990s. The average death rate was 40% higher for African American men than white men between 1995 and 1999, whereas there were no differences in death rates among African American and white women. Lung cancer occurs most often in older adults, peaking at age 75. It is the leading cause of cancer death in males aged 40 years and older, and it is the leading cause of cancer death in women aged 60 years and older. Mortality rates from lung cancer are high because the vast majority of cases are diagnosed at an advanced stage, when curative treatment is not available (see Chapter 2, Epidemiology of Cancer).

■ Risk Factors

Smoking tobacco is by far the most important risk factor associated with the development of lung cancer. In fact, smoking is responsible for causing approximately 90% of lung cancers. The risk of lung cancer increases with the number of lifetime cigarettes and the number of years one has smoked. Although some epidemiologic studies suggest that filtered cigarettes and lower-tar cigarettes slightly reduced the risk of lung cancer compared with unfiltered cigarettes, other studies have shown that when smokers choose lower-tar cigarettes they often compensate by inhaling more deeply and smoking more cigarettes. Smoking cessation at any age is associated with significant benefit. As the length of time from cessation of smoking increases, the risk of lung cancer decreases but remains elevated in former smokers.

Other common factors associated with the development of lung cancer include passive smoking and exposure to occupational and environmental carcinogens. Exposure to smoke from other people's cigarettes has been associated with increased risk for lung cancer. Workers exposed to tar and soot, arsenic, chromium, and nickel are also at increased risk for lung cancer. Asbestos is a well-established occupational carcinogen. Asbestos and cigarettes are independent causes of lung cancer but together work synergistically to greatly increase the risk for lung cancer. Exposure to radiation is also associated with an increased lung cancer risk (see Chapter 1, Biology of Cancer).

■ Prevention and Detection

Although many interventions have been investigated as strategies for decreasing the incidence of lung cancer, including dietary or nutritional changes, screening, and chemoprevention, the only proven prevention strategy is to avoid the initiation of smoking and promote the cessation of smoking among smokers. Smoking prevention interventions should be targeted toward children and adolescents because most smokers begin smoking before the age of 20. Antismoking strategies that have been successful include school programs emphasizing lifestyle skills training; brief, recurrent antismoking messages in the media; banning smoking in public places; and high excise taxes on tobacco products. Evidence suggests that a multilevel approach that combines a mix of educational, clinical, regulatory, economic, and social strategies is the best approach for reducing the use of tobacco. Other strategies to prevent lung cancer include adherence to industrial safety standards and control of environmental radon, asbestos, and other carcinogens.

Because a substantial portion of adults diagnosed with early-stage lung cancer can be cured, a high level of interest exists in identifying effective and practical screening methods that will increase the early detection of lung cancer. Currently, however, no effective screening test exists to detect lung cancer early enough to cure it. In the past, studies evaluating chest x-rays and sputum cytology have failed to demonstrate that screening with either of these methods improved lung cancer mortality. Low-dose computed tomography is a new method proposed for screening for lung cancer. Recent studies using this technology have been promising in detecting early-stage lung cancers, but concerns have been raised about overdiagnosis and inefficacy of treatment for disease detected through this method.

■ Clinical Presentation

More than 90% of adults with lung cancer are symptomatic at presentation of their disease. A minority of patients present with local symptoms related to the primary tumor, but most present with either nonspecific systemic or metastatic symptoms, as listed in Table 14–1. The most common sites of metastases are bones, liver, adrenal glands, pericardium, brain, and spinal cord. Paraneoplastic syndromes are common in lung cancer and include hypercalcemia, Cushing's syndrome, syndrome of inappropriate antidiuretic hormone, digital clubbing, pulmonary hypertrophic osteoarthropathy, and neurologic syndromes.

TABLE 14–1 ■ Initial Symptoms of Lung Cancer

Local Symptoms	Nonspecific Systemic or Metastatic Symptoms
• Cough	• Anorexia
• Dyspnea	• Weight loss
• Wheezing	• Fatigue
• Hemoptysis	• Clubbing
• Dysphagia	• Fever
• Hoarseness	• Bone pain
• Chest pain	• Headache
• Swelling face and arm	• Seizures
• Nausea/Vomiting	

Source: Adapted from Beckles, Spiro, Colice, & Rudd. (2003). Initial evaluation of the patient with lung cancer: Symptoms, signs, laboratory tests, and paraneoplastic syndromes. *Chest, 123,* 97S-104S. By permission of the publisher.

■ Diagnosis and Staging

Two types of lung cancer exist: non-small cell lung cancer (NSCLC) and small-cell lung cancer (SCLC). Because treatment differs greatly depending on the type and the stage of lung cancer present, the diagnostic work-up is designed to identify the specific type of lung cancer, the stage of disease, and the ability of the patient to tolerate treatment.

NSCLC represents 80% of lung cancers and consists of three main histologic groupings: squamous cell carcinoma, adenocarcinoma, and large-cell carcinoma. Squamous cell carcinoma occurs most frequently in the central zone of the lung. Currently, adenocarcinoma accounts for 40% of all cases of lung cancer. Most of these tumors are peripheral in origin, where they arise from alveolar surface epithelium or bronchial mucosal glands. Large-cell carcinoma is the least common of all NSCLC, making up approximately 15% of all lung cancers, and is decreasing in incidence because of improved diagnostic techniques.

The second major type of lung cancer is SCLC. Similar to the groupings of NSCLC, there are three histologic groupings in SCLC: pure small cell, mixed small-cell and large-cell carcinoma, and combined small cell. SCLC typically presents as a central lesion with hilar and mediastinal invasion and regional adenopathy.

Guidelines for the diagnostic work-up of patients with known or suspected lung cancer include a thorough history, physical examination, and standard laboratory tests to screen for metastatic disease. Differences in the diagnostic work-up include a more involved surgical work-up using mediastinoscopy in NSCLC to help determine whether or not surgery will be used to treat local disease, whereas a bone marrow biopsy may be necessary to adequately stage SCLC. Confirmation of the type of lung cancer by cytology is critical before treatment can be determined.

Staging for NSCLC is determined by use of the internationally accepted tumor, node, and metastasis staging system (Tables 14–2 and 14–3). A two-stage staging system developed by the Veterans Administration Lung Cancer Study Group is used to determine treatment and prognosis in SCLC. The stages for SCLC are limited-stage and extensive-stage disease. Patients with limited-stage disease have involvement restricted to the ipsilateral hemithorax that can be encompassed by a single radiation port, whereas those with extensive-stage disease have obvious metastatic disease or disease that cannot be encompassed within a radiation port.

The overall 5-year survival rate for all patients with lung cancer is 15%. However, 5-year survival rates for lung cancer depend on the histology and the stage of disease and ranges from approximately 1% to 60%.

TABLE 14-2 ■ AJCC TNM Definitions for Lung Cancers

Primary	**Tumor**
Tx	Primary tumor cannot be assessed, or tumor proved by the presence of malignant cells in sputum or bronchial washings but not visualized by imaging or bronchoscopy
T0	No evidence of primary tumor
Tis	Carcinoma in situ
T1	Tumor 3 cm or less in greatest dimension, surrounded by lung or visceral pleura, without bronchoscopic evidence of invasion more proximal than the lobar bronchus[a] (i.e., not in the main bronchus)
T2	Tumor with any of the following features of size or extent: More than 3 cm in greatest dimension Involving main bronchus, 2 cm or more distal to the carina Invading the visceral pleura Associated with atelectasis or obstructive pneumonitis that extends to the hilar region but does not involve the entire lung
T3	Tumor any size that directly invades any of the following: Chest wall (including superior sulcus tumors), diaphragm, mediastinal pleura, or parietal pericardium; or tumor in the main bronchus less than 2 cm distal to the carina but without involvement of the carina or associated atelectasis or obstructive pneumonitis of the entire lung
T4	Tumor of any size that invades any of the following: mediastinum, heart, great vessels, trachea, esophagus, vertebral body, carina or separate tumor nodules in the same lobe; tumor with a malignant pleural effusion[b]

Regional Lymph Nodes(N)	
NX	Regional lymph nodes cannot be assessed
N0	No regional lymph node metastasis
N1	Metastasis in ipsilateral peribronchial and/or ipsilateral hilar lymph nodes, and intrapulmonary nodes including involvement by direct extension of the primary tumor
N2	Metastasis in ipsilateral mediastinal and/or subcarinal lymph node(s)
N3	Metastasis to contralateral mediastinal, contralateral hilar, ipsilateral or contralateral scalene or supraclavicular lymph node(s)

(continued)

TABLE 14-2 ■ AJCC TNM Definitions for Lung Cancers—*Continued*

Primary	**Tumor**
Distant Metastasis (M)	
MX	Presence of distant metastasis cannot be assessed
M0	No distant metastasis
M1	Distant metastasis present

[a]Note: The uncommon superficial tumor of any size with its invasive component limited to the bronchial wall, which may extend proximal to the main bronchus, is also classified as T1.

[b]Note: Most pleural effusions associated with lung cancer are due to tumor. However, there are a few patients in whom multiple cytopathological examinations of pleural fluid are negative for tumor. In these cases, fluid is nonbloody and is not an exudate. When these elements and clinical judgment dictate that the effusion is not related to the tumor, the effusion should be excluded as a staging element and the patient should be staged as T1, T2, or T3.

Source: Used with the permission of the American Joint Committee on Cancer (AJCC), Chicago, Illinois. The original source for this material is the American Joint Committee on Cancer. (2002). *AJCC cancer staging manual,* (6th ed.). New York: Springer-Verlag. *www.springer-ny.com*

TABLE 14-3 ■ Stage Grouping

Stage	**TNM Subset**
0	Tis N0 M0
1A	T1 N0 M0
1B	T2 N0 M0
IIA	T1 N1 M0
IIB	T2 N1 M0
	T3 N0 M0
IIIA	T3 N1 M0
	T1 N2 M0
	T2 N2 M0
	T3 N2 M0
IIIB	Any T N3 M0
	T4 Any N M0
IV	Any T any N M1

Source: Used with the permission of the American Joint Committee on Cancer (AJCC), Chicago, Illinois. The original source for this material is the American Joint Committee on Cancer. (2002). *AJCC cancer staging manual,* (6th ed.). New York: Springer-Verlag. *www.springer-ny.com*

■ Treatment

Non-Small Cell Lung Cancer

Surgery is the treatment of choice for patients with early-stage NSCLC (stage I and II and some IIIA) who are able to tolerate surgery. A lobar or greater resection (lobectomy, pneumonectomy) rather than sublobar (wedge or bronchopulmonary segment) resections are recommended; however, a sublobar resection may be considered in patients who are unable to tolerate this type of surgery because of comorbidities. Patients with positive resection margins may be evaluated for additional treatment, which may include more surgery, radiation therapy, and possibly chemotherapy. For patients who are unable to undergo a complete resection of the chest wall tumor and mediastinal tumors, however, postoperative radiation therapy may provide a survival benefit. It is recommended that patients with centrally located clinical T3 NSCLC undergo surgical evaluation of their mediastinal lymph nodes before resection because identification of N2 lymph node disease precludes surgical resection as initial therapy in this setting. Radiation therapy is considered as primary treatment for individuals who have comorbidities (e.g., severe chronic pulmonary disease, cardiac disease) and who are poor surgical candidates (see Chapter 8, Radiation Therapy).

Patients with preoperatively identified stage IIIA lung cancer have a relatively poor prognosis with surgical resection alone. Several small clinical trials of induction chemotherapy (preoperative) have yielded conflicting results. Multidisciplinary evaluation is particularly important in this setting. At the present time, induction chemotherapy followed by surgery for stage IIIA disease is recommended only in the setting of a clinical trial. Incompletely resected patients and those with residual nodal disease found at surgery may be considered for postoperative radiation therapy.

It is recommended that otherwise healthy stage IIIB patients with clinical T4N0 NSCLC from either satellite tumor nodule(s) in the same lobe or carinal involvement be referred to a thoracic surgeon for a possible resection. Combined chemoradiotherapy for patients with stage IIIB disease without malignant effusions with good performance status, defined as normal activity or fatigue without any significant decrease in activity, is considered standard of care. Concurrent therapy is recommended in patients with good performance status and minimal weight loss; however, there is increased esophagitis with this method of therapy.

Patients with stage IV NSCLC have a poor prognosis, with a median survival time of 8–10 months, a 1-year survival rate of 30%–35%, and essentially no 5-year survival. Studies show small but consistent improvement in the survival of patients who have been treated with chemotherapy compared with those receiving best supportive care alone. The most important factor associated with a response to chemotherapy seems to be a good performance status. Thus, patients with good performance status are often offered chemotherapy containing a platinum-based regimen that includes one of the new agents (Table 14–4). Because advanced lung cancer is incurable with the use of present-day therapies, quality of life and patient preference—based measures are important outcomes when new treatments in clinical trials are assessed. Studies have revealed that most patients would not choose chemotherapy for a likely survival of 3 months or a < 10% improvement in the 1-year survival rate unless there is an improvement in quality of life.

Clinical research is investigating novel therapies that are specific to biologic mechanisms involved in the development of lung cancer. The biologic mechanisms include cellular communication process (signal transduction), growth factors, cell death (apoptosis), tumor suppressor genes, and new blood vessel growth that support tumors (angiogenesis). Although multiple drugs are in clinical trials, gefitinib (Iressa, ZD1839) is the first biologically targeted drug for lung cancer to be approved by the US Food and Drug Administration. It is an epidermal growth receptor—tyrosine kinase inhibitor and is indicated for use in patients with locally advanced and metastatic NSCLC who have not responded to either platinum-based and docetaxel chemotherapy.

Small-Cell Lung Cancer

SCLC tends to be more aggressive than NSCL. Distant metastasis at presentation is common in patients with SCLC. Thus, the primary treatment is usually combination chemotherapy alone or in combination with radiation therapy (see Table 14–4). However, limited-stage SCLC is potentially curable with combined chemotherapy and radiation therapy. Surgical resection may be considered in the rare patient with very limited SCLC, thus avoiding radiation therapy. Fifty percent to 60% of patients who achieve a complete response after induction chemotherapy will develop brain metastases within 2 years. The brain is the sole site of metastatic disease in 20%–30% of these patients. Therefore, patients who achieve complete remission are offered prophylactic cranial irradiation to reduce the risk of central nervous system failure, and improve survival. If patients experience relapse after an initial response to treatment or do not respond to the initial treatment, further chemotherapy is usually offered, depending on the patient's response and its duration following first-line treatment. It is recommended that elderly patients older than 70 years with good performance status and intact organ function receive platinum-based

TABLE 14-4 ■ Commonly Used Chemotherapy Regimens

Non-small cell lung cancer	*Small-cell lung cancer*	
Cisplatin Paclitaxel	Cyclophosphamide Doxorubicin VP-16	VP-16 Ifosfamide Cisplatin
Carboplatin Paclitaxel	Cyclophosphamide Doxorubicin Vincristine	Ifosfamide Carboplatin VP-16
Cisplatin Vinorelbine	Cisplatin VP-16	
Cisplatin Gemcitabine	Cisplatin Irinotecan	
Cisplatin Docetaxel		

Data from Murren, J., Glatstein, E., & Pass, H.I. (2000). Small cell lung cancer. In: V. T. Devita, S. Hellman, & S. A. Rosenberg (Eds.), *Cancer: Principles & practice of oncology* (6th ed.) Philadelphia: Lippincott and Socinski, M. A., Morris, D. E., Masters, G. A., & Lilenbaum, R. (2003). Chemotherapeutic management of stage IV non-small cell lung cancer. *Chest, 123,* 226S–243S. Noda et al., (2002). Irinotecan plus cisplatin compared with etoposide plus cisplatin for extensive small-cell lung cancer. New England Journal of Medicine, 346, 85-91.

The authors would like to thank Fran Cartwright-Alcarese PhD(c), A. Philippe Chahinian, M.D., Mitchell Machtay, M.D., and Scott Swanson M.D. for their thoughtful review and comments.,

chemotherapy. Those with poor prognostic factors, such as poor performance status and severe comorbidities, may still be considered for chemotherapy. If a complete response is achieved, elderly patients should also be offered prophylactic cranial irradiation.

■ Rehabilitation

Long-term survival for patients with stage I NSCLC can be as high as approximately 70% and can be 55% for those with stage II NSCLC. Surveillance and follow-up for patients who have undergone curative treatment consists of a medical history, physical examination, and imaging study (chest x-ray study or computed tomographic scan) every 6 months for 2 years and then annually. The patients are monitored carefully for symptoms that may signal recurrence and are advised to contact their health care provider if they notice any change in their symptoms (see Chapter 36, Cancer Survivorship).

Sarna and colleagues (2002) described quality of life in long-term survivors of NSCLC and found that most participants were hopeful after their treatment and viewed lung cancer as making a positive change in their lives. However, 22% of survivors had distressed mood, 13% continued to smoke, and 50% had moderate-to-severe pulmonary impairment. Being in the group with distressed mood was the most important predictor of quality of life. This finding suggests that assessment of emotional distress and treatment for depression is an important focus for interventions to improve the quality of life among long-term survivors (see Chapter 27, Anxiety and Depression in the Oncology Setting). In another study, Evangelista and colleagues evaluated the health perceptions and risk behaviors in lung cancer survivors. Seventy percent of participants reported their health to be good to excellent. Approximately half of the participants drank alcohol and were overweight, and 13% continued to smoke. Alcohol, the state of being overweight, smoking, and exposure to passive smoke were predictors of poor health status. Thus, although a substantial number of long-term survivors have adopted healthy lifestyles, a significant number have not, underscoring the need for interventions to decrease risk behaviors.

■ The Role of the Nurse

Clinical care for adults with lung cancer and their families spans the disease continuum from prevention through active treatment and recovery to progression of disease, supportive care, and hospice (see Chapter 37, End of Life). The focus for nursing care depends on the stage of the disease and the overall goals of care and may include interventions directed toward risk reduction through encouraging smoking cessation, providing education regarding the disease and its treatment, and promoting symptom management and psychosocial adjustment throughout the illness trajectory.

Smoking Cessation

Smoking cessation is the most effective strategy for decreasing the incidence of lung cancer. Even in those who develop lung cancer, smoking cessation after diagnosis is associated with decreased incidence of second malignancy and enhanced survival. Therefore, assessment and documentation of the smoking status for all patients are important parts of the nursing history. A four-step intervention strategy is recommended to aid smokers in their quit attempt (Table 14–5). For those who are unwilling to quit, personalized messages that are geared toward increasing motivation to quit are recommended.

TABLE 14–5 ■ The Four A's of Smoking Cessation

Ask every patient at every health care encounter if they smoke.
Advise all smokers to quit smoking in a clear, direct, and personalized message.
Assist patients who are willing to make a quit attempt:

- Set a quit date.
- Provide self-help materials with practical information about preparing to quit and staying quit.
- Provide pharmacologic cessation aides (e.g., nicotine replacement therapy, bupropion).

Arrange a follow-up visit or telephone call 2 weeks after the quit date attempt.

Patient Education During Treatment

Lung cancer surgery is a major procedure with the potential for significant morbidity and pain. Before surgery, patient teaching is important to help with the postoperative recovery course. This includes turning, coughing, deep breathing, and use of the incentive spirometry. After surgery, nurses play an important role in monitoring the patient for airway disorders, bleeding, pain management, and coping with major surgery. Key nursing interventions include monitoring vital signs and laboratory values. Patients undergoing major surgery may exhibit fear and anxiety. It is important for nurses to impart realistic and reassuring information to patients experiencing major surgery.

Nurses play an instrumental role in patient education and symptom management (see Unit V for specific symptoms) for the patient receiving chemotherapy. Patient education includes teaching patients and their families about the potential side effects of the specific chemotherapy agents used to treat lung cancer (see Chapter 7, Chemotherapy). The nurses often evaluate blood counts and are the first to recognize when a patient is neutropenic (absolute neutrophil count below 1000), which places the patient at risk for infection.

Patients undergoing radiation therapy often experience skin changes, fatigue, nausea, and esophagitis. The patient's weight and vital signs should be monitored during treatment to evaluate for dehydration. Patient education includes skin care and proper nutrition. If esophagitis occurs, viscous lidocaine can help decrease odynophagia. Soft foods and liquid dietary supplements can help provide calories and proteins. Radiation therapy has cumulative effects (see Chapter 8, Radiation Therapy); therefore, adverse reactions generally begin within

2 weeks and then increase in intensity until about 1–2 weeks after the end of treatment. Acute symptoms usually subside after 3–4 weeks; however, large doses of radiation can result in permanent damage, with some long-term side effects occurring greater than a year after the patient has ended treatment. These complications include radiation pneumonitis, signaled by dry cough, dyspnea on exertion, and fever. A possible side effect from radiation therapy to left-sided chest tumors is pericarditis with symptoms of chest pain, electrocardiographic abnormalities, and pericardial friction rub.

Symptom Management

Adults with lung cancer often experience multiple symptoms that change throughout the illness trajectory. Clinical research shows that patients undergoing all treatment modalities most frequently complained of pain, fatigue, changes in appetite, and respiratory symptoms and that these symptoms frequently cluster together. Because uncontrolled symptoms are associated with increased emotional distress and decreased quality of life, prompt recognition and intervention for distressing symptoms are essential. Management of these symptoms is discussed in Unit V.

■ Conclusion

Providing nursing care to adults with lung cancer and their family members is a challenging yet rewarding opportunity. Nurses can play a significant role in maintaining a patient's quality of life and decreasing patients' distress through patient education, symptom management, and psychosocial support. Because of the strong association between smoking and lung cancers, nurses can significantly affect the number of people with lung cancer through leadership, community education, and political activism to decrease the initiation of smoking and encourage smoking cessation.

■ Resources

Alliance for Lung Cancer Advocacy, Support, and Education (ALCASE): peer-to-peer telephone support network; hotline for people with lung cancer and their families; referral to lung cancer support groups. 800-298-2436 or *www.alcase.org*

American Cancer Society: *www.cancer.org.docroot/home/index/asp*

- "Double your chances of quitting": call 800-ACS-2345
- American Cancer Society. (2003). *Kicking butts: Quit smoking and take charge of your health*. Atlanta, GA: Author.
- NCCN Lung Cancer Treatment Guidelines for Patients: call 800-ACS-2345
- Smart Move: A Stop Smoking Guide: call 800-ACS-2345

American Lung Association: Tobacco control information and smoking cessation. *www.lungusa.org/tobacco*

It's Time to Focus on Lung Cancer: Sponsored by Cancer Care, Inc. and Oncology Nursing Society *www.lungcancer.org*

National Center for Chronic Disease Prevention and Health Promotion: Tobacco Information and Prevention Source (TIPS). *www.cdc.gov/tobacco/index.htm*

National Center for Chronic Disease Prevention and Health Promotion: Tobacco Information and Prevention Source (TIPS), Materiales y publicaciones en Espaniol. *www.cdc.gov/tobacco/SpanishSplash.htm*

National Comprehensive Cancer Network: Lung Cancer Treatment Guidelines for Patients.Version 1/December 2001. *www.nccn.org/patient_gls/_english/_lung/index.htm*

Bibliography

Cooley, M. E. (2000). Symptoms in adults with lung cancer: A systematic research review. *Journal of Pain and Symptom Management, 19,* 137–153.

Ingle, R. J. (2000). Lung cancer. In: S. L. Groenwald, M. H. Frogge, M. Goodman, & C. H. Yarbro (Eds.), *Cancer nursing: Principles and practice* (5th ed., pp. 1298–1328). Sudbury, MA: Jones & Bartlett.

Sarna, L., Padilla, G., Holmes, C., Tashkin, D., Brecht, M.L., & Evangelista, L. (2002). Quality of life of long-term survivors of non-small cell lung cancer. *Journal of Clinical Oncology, 20,* 2920–2929.

US Department of Health and Human Services. (2000). Reducing tobacco use: A report of the Surgeon General. Atlanta: US Department of Health and Human Services, Public Health Service, Centers for Disease Control, Center for Chronic Disease Prevention and Health Promotion, Office on Smoking and Health.

CHAPTER

15

Cancer in Children and Adolescents

Lona Roll

■ Incidence

About 9,000 new cases of cancer are diagnosed each year in children aged 0–14 years, and about 1,500 deaths occur each year in this age group. Although most statistics about childhood cancer focus on the age group of 0-14 years, recent data from the National Cancer Institute's Surveillance, Epidemiology and End Results program indicate that the incidence rate of cancer in adolescents 15–19 years of age in the United States is twice the incidence rate of cancer in younger age groups. From 1975–2000, the overall rate of cancer in the 15- to 19-year age group was 198.2 cases per million, compared with 138.4 cases per million for the 0- to 14-year age group.

Types of cancer occurring in children and adolescents differ from those occurring in adults. Childhood cancers include leukemia (30%), brain and spinal cord tumors (21%), neuroblastoma (7.3%), Wilms' tumor (5.9%), lymphoma (8.4%), rhabdomyosarcoma (3.4%), retinoblastoma (2.8%), osteosarcoma (2.7%), and Ewing's sarcoma (1.8%). The overall 5-year survival rate is 77%. This survival rate varies greatly, depending on the cancer site. The most common cancers among the 15- to 19-year ages are Hodgkin's disease (16%), germ cell tumors (15%), central nervous system (CNS) tumors (10%), non-Hodgkin lymphomas (8%), thyroid cancer (7%), malignant melanomas (7%), leukemia (15%), osteosarcomas (5%), and soft tissue sarcomas (7%) (see Chapter 2, Epidemiology of Cancer).

■ Risk Factors

For both children and older adolescents, the specific etiology of their most common cancers is unknown, but prenatal, in utero, and postnatal exposures have been identified as possible risk factors. Genetic inheritance has been limited to specific childhood cancers and accounts for only a small proportion of childhood and adolescent cancers. Exposures to environmental carcinogens (tobacco, sunlight, and diet) have not been shown to affect the development of the typical childhood/adolescent cancers (see Chapter 1, The Biology of Cancer).

■ Screening and Diagnosing

Cancers in children and adolescents are often difficult to recognize because initial symptoms can imitate common health problems in these populations. Also, the relatively small incidence of cancer in the 0–19 year olds when compared with the adult population makes cancer a low probability as a differential diagnosis. During any encounter with children and adolescents, health care providers need to be alert for an unusual mass or swelling; unexplained paleness and loss of energy; easy bruising; persistent pain or limping; prolonged fever or illness; frequent headaches, especially when accompanied by vomiting; vision changes; or rapid, unexplained weight loss.

Diagnosing cancer in children and adolescents includes a thorough history and physical examination, appropriate laboratory and imaging studies, evaluation of baseline organ function, and pathological confirmation of the diagnosis. Knowledge of the common sites and histologies of cancers in the 0- to 19-year age groups aids in directing the diagnostic and metastatic work-up. As the science of pediatric/adolescent cancers has developed, classification of tumors and leukemias/lymphomas has become more sophisticated. Precise diagnostic tools that aid in the planning of appropriate treatment are primarily located in pediatric cancer centers. A prompt referral from the primary health care provider to a pediatric cancer center provides the optimum opportunity for prompt confirmation of diagnosis and treatment planning. Care outcomes are better for children and adolescents treated at such centers.

Childhood and adolescent cancers are treated according to the type and stage of the tumor. Generally, management of cancer in children and adolescents differs from that in adults because of physiologic, psychological, and social differences in these populations. Progress in diagnosing and treating childhood and adolescent cancers has improved the outcome in the past 50 years from a once fatal prognosis to a treatable and potentially curable illness. This progression has been attributed to a cooperative effort by multidisciplinary specialists in pediatric cancer centers. This multidisciplinary team of experts includes pediatric oncologists/hematologists, pediatric pathologists, pediatric subspecialists, pediatric oncology nurses, social workers, psychologists, child life specialists, pharmacists, laboratory scientists, clinical research associates, and others who assist children and adolescents and their families. The goals of these teams are to cure children and adolescents with cancer, reduce long-term treatment effects, and improve quality of life for children and adolescents with cancer and their families. A pediatric cancer cooperative group, the Children's Oncology Group, is composed of pediatric cancer treatment centers and funded by the National Cancer Institute (NCI) to develop and implement clinical trials designed to cure pediatric cancers. For children and adolescents with cancer, participation in clinical trials significantly increases survival rates. Although approximately 90%–95% of children with cancer are treated at institutions that are participating in NCI-sponsored clinical trials, only about 20% of 15–19 year olds with cancer are treated in NCI-sponsored clinical trials.

■ Acute Leukemia

Incidence

Acute lymphocytic leukemia (ALL) is the most common childhood and adolescent cancer, occurring at an annual rate of 27.8 cases per million in the 0- to 19-year age group. Acute nonlymphocytic leukemia (ANLL) occurs at an annual rate of 6.7 per million in the 0- to 19-year age group. The exact cause of the acute leukemias is unknown, although certain factors are known to increase the risk of developing the disease. Among these are acquired genetic abnormalities; inherited genetic syndromes, such as Down syndrome; exposure to ionizing radiation; and exposure to mutagenic chemicals.

Clinical Presentation and Diagnosis

Children and adolescents with acute leukemia present with symptoms related to bone marrow failure. The most common symptoms are fever, fatigue, bone pain, bleeding, anorexia, petechiae, pallor, lymphadenopathy, and hepatosplenomegaly. The definitive diagnosis is confirmed by bone marrow examination. A diagnostic lumbar puncture determines the presence or absence of CNS involvement. The morphologic, immunophenotypic, and cytogenetic characteristics of the abnormal cells determine the diagnostic and treatment stratification of the disease.

Treatment

Treatment for ALL and ANLL has improved significantly since the 1970s. With the use of multidrug regimens in clinical trials, the cure rate for ALL has improved from 40% to 80%–85%. ANLL survival rates have improved from 5% to 40%–45%. Treatment of ALL involves chemotherapy regimens in four stages: remission induction, consolidation, maintenance therapy, and CNS sanctuary therapy with intrathecal chemotherapy with or without craniospinal irradiation. Therapy generally lasts 2.5–3 years. Therapy for ANLL includes intense induction therapy followed by intense short-term treatment that lasts about 6 months. An allogeneic hematopoietic stem cell transplantation after remission induction is recommended for children and adolescents with a matched sibling donor. CNS prophylaxis with intrathecal chemotherapy is also used. Commonly used agents for the induction phase of ALL are vincristine, prednisone or dexamethasone, and asparaginase with or without daunorubicin. This is followed by methotrexate, 6-mercaptopurine, vincristine, prednisone, asparaginase, daunorubicin, cyclophosphamide, and cytarabine for consolidation. Maintenance therapy includes methotrexate, 6-mercaptopurine, vincristine, and prednisone. ANLL remission therapy includes cytarabine and daunorubicin, with the addition of other agents, such as etoposide, dexamethasone, or thioguanine. New agents are regularly being tried to improve the survival rate in ANLL. The bone marrow is the most common site of relapse in the leukemias. Relapses are treated with reinduction of remission followed by allogeneic hematopoietic stem cell transplantation or intense consolidation chemotherapy.

■ Lymphomas

Incidence

Hodgkin's and non-Hodgkin's lymphomas occur at a rate of 24 per million in the 0- to 19-year age population. The diagnosis and treatment for these conditions are covered in Chapter 18 (Lymphomas).

Central Nervous System Tumors

Incidence

CNS tumors occur at a rate of 26.5 cases per million in the 0- to 19-year age group, and the incidence of CNS tumors in children and adolescents has increased over the past 20 years. The reason for this increase is not known, but it is speculated to be related to improvements in diagnostic imaging capabilities. There is an increased incidence in children with specific hereditary and familial syndromes, such as neurofibromatosis types I and II and bilateral retinoblastoma. The cause of CNS tumors is unknown. Risk factors include exposure to ionizing radiation and exposure to industrial and chemical toxins (see Chapter 1, The Biology of Cancer).

Clinical Presentation and Diagnosis

Children and adolescents with CNS tumors present with symptoms related to the location, histology, and size of the tumor. General signs and symptoms include headaches, seizures, changes in mental status, and signs of increased intracranial pressure (nausea, vomiting, drowsiness, vision problems, papilledema, and decreased level of consciousness). Additional signs and symptoms directed by the location of the tumor may include altered gait, paresis, nystagmus, double vision, communication difficulties, and emotional lability. Age and developmental stage are important factors in assessing for potential CNS malignancies. Primary health care providers need to be alert to delays in achieving normal developmental milestones in infancy, a history of personality changes, or altered school performance in school-aged children and adolescents. Diagnostic evaluation of CNS tumors begins with a thorough history and neurologic examination. Once a CNS tumor is suspected, the remainder of the work-up includes a combination of neuroimaging (magnetic resonance imaging [MRI], computed tomography [CT]), cerebrospinal fluid evaluation, and biopsy.

Treatment

Children and adolescents with CNS tumors are treated with a combination of surgery, radiation therapy, and chemotherapy. The therapeutic plan is determined by the tumor size, location, and histology, as well as by the age of the child. Although the overall survival rate has improved in the past 20 years from 55% to 64%, long-term survival rates vary greatly. The treatment regimen requires a multidisciplinary approach in a childhood cancer center. Members of this team include oncologists, neurologists, neurosurgeons, rehabilitation specialists, radiation oncologists, nurses, physical and occupational therapists, psychologists, and social workers. In addition to the treatment of the CNS tumors, children and adolescents with a CNS tumor frequently require support for the sequelae of the disease and its treatment (see Chapter 34, Pediatric Symptoms and Responses). Possible sequelae are neurocognitive deficits, altered mobility, sensory deficits, and seizure disorders. The support of community health care providers and educators may be required for the long-term management of these sequelae.

■ Neuroblastoma

Incidence

Neuroblastomas occur primarily in infants and young children. The incidence is 7.8 cases per million in the 0- to 19-year age group, with most cases presenting before the age of 2 years. There is no known cause for neuroblastoma.

Clinical Presentation and Diagnosis

Neuroblastomas arise at points along the sympathetic nervous system. Presenting signs and symptoms are directed by the site of the principle disease and the existence of metastases. Most primary neuroblastomas occur in the abdomen and present as an abdominal mass. Other common sites include the thorax, cervical area, and pelvis. Metastatic disease spreads via the blood and lymphatic system and results in signs and symptoms related to bone marrow, liver, skin, and lymph node involvement. Common signs and symptoms can include palpable masses, pain, low-grade fever, weight loss, fatigue, pallor, periorbital ecchymosis, lymphadenopathy, hepatosplenomegaly, and hypertension.

A diagnosis of neuroblastoma includes a thorough history and physical examination. Neuroblastoma is staged according to the International Neuroblastoma Staging System (INSS). The INSS staging system uses location and size of the tumor along with presence or absence of lymph node involvement to stage the disease from 1 to 4S. This tumor is further categorized as low, medium, or high risk through the use of a combination of INSS stage, child's age, and genetic markers. The diagnostic and staging work-up include bone marrow aspiration, measurement of urinary catecholamines, and a surgical procedure. Urinary catecholamines (homovanillic acid, vanillylmandelic acid) are increased in about 90% of neuroblastomas. Immunohistochemical, cytogenetic, and molecular studies are performed to assist in determining the risk group. The presence of a genetic mutation on chromosome 1 and the amplification of MYCN (a proto-oncogene) are strongly associated with a poorer prognosis. Additionally, diagnostic imaging studies are conducted to evaluate the extent of the primary disease and the presence of metastatic disease. Imaging studies can include: plain film studies, CT and bone scans, MRI, and an iodine 131—metaiodobenzylguanidine scan. The two most important factors in determining prognosis are age at diagnosis and stage of disease at diagnosis. The most favorable prognosis is for children < 1 year of age and for tumors located in the chest and pelvis. Survival rates are 80%–90% for those with low- and intermediate-risk disease and only 20%–30% for those with high-risk disease.

Treatment

Treatment of children with neuroblastoma is based on the identified risk group. Surgery is performed to obtain material for diagnosis, determine the stage of disease, and either debulk or completely resect the tumor. Low-risk patients are treated with complete tumor resection and careful follow-up. Intermediate-risk patients are treated with surgery, chemotherapy, and radiation therapy. High-risk patients require intense therapy using chemotherapy at myeloablative levels, followed by rescue with autologous peripheral blood stem cells. The Children's Oncology Group is currently using tandem autologous hematopoietic stem cell transplantation in this high-risk group. Localized radiation and use of a biologic modifier (13-*cis*-retinoic acid) contribute to survival for these children.

■ Wilms' Tumor

Incidence

Wilms' tumor is a malignant renal tumor occurring at an annual rate of 6.3 per million in the 0- to 19-year age group, with most cases appearing before the age of 5 years. The age at diagnosis peaks at 2-3 years. Wilms' tumors occur as a result of changes in one or more genes. These changes may be inherited or occur sporadically. The tumor is associated with certain congenital anomalies, including aniridia, genitourinary malformations, and Beckwith-Wiedemann syndrome.

Clinical Presentation and Diagnosis

Children with Wilms' tumor commonly present with the appearance of good health in the presence of a palpable abdominal mass. Additional signs may be abdominal pain, hematuria, anorexia, and hypertension. In addition to a detailed history and physical examination, abdominal ultrasound, CT, and MRI are used to determine the location, shape, and extent of the tumor. Laboratory studies include a complete blood count, liver and renal function tests, and urinalysis. A metastatic work-up includes CT of the chest because the most common metastatic site is the lung. Wilms' tumor is staged according to the degree of involvement as well as the histology of the tumor. The most important factor in determining prognosis is the histology, which is classified as either favorable or unfavorable. Prognosis is related to numerous factors but focuses on histology of the tumor and stage of the disease. Children with low-stage disease and favorable histology have survival rates of 90%. Children presenting with metastatic disease or unfavorable histology have survival rates of 80%. The presentation of tumor with diffuse anaplasia confers a much less favorable prognosis.

Treatment

Surgery is used for staging and initial treatment of children with Wilms' tumor. Preoperative chemotherapy is used in patients with unresectable disease or bilateral involvement. After surgery; children with low stage disease and favorable histology will receive no more therapy. Children with advanced stage or unfavorable histology will proceed to receive radiation and chemotherapy.

■ Retinoblastoma

Incidence

Retinoblastoma is a rare intraocular tumor, occurring in children at an annual rate of 3 per million in the 0- to 19-year age group. Most cases are diagnosed before the age of 5 years. Approximately 75% of children present with a unilateral retinoblastoma, and the remaining 25% present with bilateral disease. Retinoblastoma can be hereditary or nonhereditary, but most cases are nonhereditary. The inherited form of retinoblastoma is transmitted as an autosomal dominant trait, and the retinoblastoma gene is located on band 14 of chromosome 13.

Clinical Presentation and Diagnosis

The common presenting signs of retinoblastoma are leukocoria (a white spot in the pupil) and strabismus (the eye turning inward or outward). The clinical diagnosis of retinoblastoma is accomplished by ophthalmoscopic examination. This examination identifies the size and location of the tumor. Retinal imaging studies, which include CT, MRI, and plain film, aid in identifying the extent of the disease. The overall prognosis for retinoblastoma without extraocular disease is approximately 90%. The Reese-Ellsworth classification system is used for tumor staging and treatment decision making. The location and the size of the tumor determine the stage, which ranges from I to IV.

Treatment

Treatment for retinoblastoma centers on elimination of the tumor with preservation of vision. Treatment modalities include surgery, radiation therapy, and chemotherapy. Surgical options involve enucleation, cryotherapy, or photocoagulation. Patients with intraocular disease receive chemotherapy followed by local therapy, such as cryotherapy or photocoagulation, to preserve vision. Enucleation is the treatment of choice if there is no chance for preservation of vision.

■ Rhabdomyosarcoma

Incidence

Rhabdomyosarcoma is the most common soft tissue sarcoma in childhood and adolescence. Rhabdomyosarcoma occurs at an annual rate of 4.4 per million in the 0- to 19-year age group. There are two peaks of occurrence: between the ages of 2 and 5 years and between the ages of 15 and 19 years. The cause of rhabdomyosarcoma is unknown. It has been associated with familial syndromes, such as neurofibromatosis and the Li-Fraumeni syndrome.

Clinical Presentation and Diagnosis

Presenting symptoms vary according to the location of the tumor. The most common site is the head and neck (35%). Other sites are the genitourinary tract (20%) and the extremities (18%). Head, neck, and genitourinary rhabdomyosarcomas are most common in young children, and extremity rhabdomyosarcomas are most common in adolescents. Specific symptoms are related to the anatomic site of the tumor. The range of symptoms includes nosebleeds, sinus congestion, facial palsies, hematuria, urinary obstruction, and anatomic deformities of the extremities. Diagnosis begins with a history and physical examination, with particular attention being given to adjoining lymphatic structures. Tumor size and involvement are determined by MRI. Regional lymph node areas are thoroughly examined. Imaging studies of the chest and bone assist in determining metastatic spread. Bone marrow aspiration and biopsy are performed to assess for marrow involvement. Biopsy of the tumor and adjacent lymph nodes is necessary for histologic diagnosis.

Treatment

After the diagnostic work-up and biopsy, staging is performed to determine the choice of therapy. The clinical and histologic staging of rhabdomyosarcoma is complex and is best accomplished at a pediatric cancer center. The most current staging system uses size, invasiveness of the tumor, lymph node involvement, and primary site as criteria. The treatment plan for rhabdomyosarcoma includes a combination of surgery, chemotherapy, and radiation therapy. With multimodal therapy, 70% of patients with nonmetastatic rhabdomyosarcoma are long-term survivors.

■ Osteosarcoma

Incidence

Osteosarcoma is a malignant tumor of the bone, the exact cause of which is unknown. Bone tumors occur at an annual incidence of 8.5 cases per million in the 0- to 19-year age group and the incidence is highest in the 10- to 19-year age group. The incidence of bone tumors seems to occur with more frequency during periods of rapid growth and develops most often in the distal femur, proximal tibia, and proximal humerus.

Clinical Presentation and Diagnosis

Pain is the common presentation of osteosarcoma with or without a palpable mass. The child or adolescent may also experience difficulty with weight bearing. Once a bone tumor is suspected, imaging studies are performed to evaluate the tumor and the extent of the disease. A total-body bone scan and chest CT evaluate the presence of distant bone involvement and pulmonary metastases. An open biopsy is necessary to confirm the diagnosis and identify the tumor histology.

Treatment

Surgery is the primary treatment for bone tumors, with the addition of intensive chemotherapy to increase the possibility of long-term survival. The common surgical options used in the treatment of bone tumors are amputation and limb salvage. The surgical selection is influenced by the tumor location, the ability to preserve function of the affected limb, and the possibility of achieving a margin of healthy tissue after removal of the tumor. Osteosarcoma is resistant to radiation.

Prognosis for children and adolescents with osteosarcoma is greatly influenced by the presence of lung metastases at diagnosis and the ability to completely resect the tumor. Overall, the long-term survival for children and adolescents with osteosarcoma is 65%. The challenge for children and adolescents with osteosarcoma is the need for intense chemotherapy coupled with the need for rehabilitation. A multidisciplinary team is needed to address the multiple therapeutic and rehabilitation needs of this population.

■ Supportive Care and the Role of the Nurse

The physical side effects and toxicities of the treatment of cancer in the child and adolescent are covered in Chapter 34 (Pediatric Symptoms and Responses). Health providers caring for these patients must be aware of age-related physical needs and abilities in order to accurately assess and meet those needs.

Cancer in children and adolescents affects the entire family. A multidisciplinary approach is recommended to address the psychosocial needs of the child or adolescent with cancer, as well as the parents, the siblings, and the extended social network of this group. At each stage of the treatment process, care must be taken to identify psychosocial issues and to promote attainment of developmental milestones. Threats to development are unique to each child and can change as the child moves from diagnosis to treatment and long-term survivorship.

Infants, toddlers, and preschool children are learning trust and independence. Attention must be directed at supporting these developmental tasks while providing the care necessary to treat the illness. Opportunities are provided for the child and family to anticipate and understand each procedure, test, and treatment. The use of age-appropriate books, videotapes, and toys can assist in preparing young children for each experience. The use of play therapy, music and art therapy, relaxation, and imagery implemented by a child health professional can assist the young child in coping.

School-aged children are developing and refining their social and intellectual skills. Age-appropriate information should be provided to the child with ample opportunity to have his or her questions answered. The health care team blends the child's physical needs with the child's need to continue being a part of his expanding social environment.

School issues are addressed by supporting school reentry. Communication with teachers and classmates and prompt return to school and extracurricular activities provide the child with the opportunity to pursue academic and social goals available in the school experience. Parents and teachers should be encouraged to continue to expect age-appropriate behavior and to maintain discipline.

Adolescents with cancer present with multiple psychosocial needs and challenges. Their challenges include autonomy and independence, education, sexual maturation, social development, intimacy, and development of life skills. Health care providers working with adolescents need to establish a relationship with the adolescent that facilitates communication and promotes adaptation within the context of the family. Collaborating with the family, the health care provider establishes boundaries to support the adolescent as an integral part of the treatment and decision-making team. Adaptation to the experience can be facilitated by providing guidance and information about all treatments and side effects and by encouraging the adolescent to express concerns. The adolescent's need to continue to be part of the school and the community should also be addressed from diagnosis forward. Group activities with peers can provide opportunities for adolescents to share feelings, build social skills, and develop their abilities to cope with the cancer experience. The health care team must be open to assessing and interacting with the adolescent to provide the necessary emotional support and maximize independence.

■ Family-Centered Care

The diagnosis of cancer affects all members of the family. Parents are required to support their child through the cancer experience, continue in their established role within the family, and cope with their own intense fears and feelings. The health care team must address the needs of the patient's family with the same level of intensity used with the ill child or adolescent. Parents need to be informed of all aspects of care, be supported in their decisions, and have guidance in supporting their child. Assessing the family's available social support network and coping skills in an ongoing manner enables the health care team to develop a comprehensive plan for meeting family needs.

During the cancer experience, siblings have information and support needs coupled with their own need to continue to develop normally. It is important to acknowledge the impact of the cancer experience on the healthy sibling. Siblings can experience a sense of loss and disruption to their normal routines. Assisting parents to recognize the impact of this experience on the healthy sibling and to encourage frank communication regarding fears, needs, and expectations to help facilitate the adjustment of the healthy sibling. Siblings also benefit from participation in sibling support groups. Psychosocial care of the entire family requires careful assessment of the needs of each and every member of the family.

■ Cancer Survivorship Issues

With cancer survivorship comes the need for comprehensive long-term follow-up care to address the physiologic and psychological needs of survivors of childhood cancer. Programs have been developed to assess existing and potential health risks related to treatment, explore psychosocial issues that accompany cancer survivorship, and teach lifelong health promotion and disease prevention skills.

Physical effects of cancer treatment may appear immediately or months to years after the completion of therapy, and these effects can range from minor to life-threatening. Late effects of treatment could affect every organ system. The cancer survivor should be evaluated for these late effects on a regular basis by a team of experts who are knowledgeable about specific health risks associated with treatment for cancer during childhood and adolescence.

The cancer experience during childhood and adolescence also has potential for contributing to psychosocial difficulties. Survivors may fear recurrence and may experience developmental disruptions, neurocognitive challenges, survival guilt, physical deformity, and economic difficulties. Survivors and their families need to receive guidance regarding risk for late effects and the recommended monitoring after treatment. As survivors make the transition to long-term follow-up care, they can benefit from survivorship resources that put them in touch with other cancer survivors, such as the American Cancer Society's Cancer Survivors' Network (*www.cancer.org*).

■ Conclusion

Advances in treatment, supportive care, and comprehensive family-centered care have positively influenced the physical and emotional survival in children and adolescents with cancer. The result is an increasing number of cancer survivors who will interact with primary and specialty health care providers for years to come. Health care professionals will need to become knowledgeable about the special needs of this sizeable group in order to optimize their quality of life.

■ Resources

- The Children's Oncology Group: provides information on clinical trials for children, long-term follow-up guidelines, and help locating a treatment center. *www.childrensoncologygroup.org*
- Teens Living with Cancer: provides resources to support teens, their families, and friends. *www.teenslivingwithcancer.org*

Bibliography

American Academy of Pediatrics, Section on Hematology, Oncology. (1997). Guidelines for the pediatric cancer center: Role of such centers in diagnosis and treatment. *Pediatrics, 99,* 139–141.

Baggott, C. R., Kelly, K. P., Fochtman, D., & Foley, G. F. (Eds.) (2002). *Nursing care of children and adolescents with cancer* (3rd ed.). St. Louis: W. B. Saunders Company.

Bleyer, A. W. (2002). Cancer in older adolescents and young adults: Epidemiology, diagnosis, treatment, survival, and importance of clinical trials. *Medical and Pediatric Oncology, 38,* 1–10.

Murry, J. S. (1999). Siblings of children with cancer: A review of the literature. *Journal of Pediatric Oncology Nursing, 16,* 25–34.

CHAPTER

16

Cancer of Unknown Primary Sites

Jamie S. Myers

■ Incidence

Cancers of unknown primary sites (CUPs) are malignancies that present as metastatic lesions with no corresponding primary site. It is estimated that the incidence of CUPs ranges from 2%–10% of cancer diagnoses. The primary site may become obvious during the patient's lifetime in 15%–20% of certain categories of CUPs. However, 20%–30% cannot be identified at the time of autopsy. In most malignancies, the incidence increases in direct proportion to diagnostic skill and advanced technologies. The incidence of CUPs is decreasing because of our ability to differentiate between tumor types. In the future, DNA microarray technology may be extremely useful in determining the site of origin from gene expression.

■ Risk Factors and Detection

Because CUPs encompass a variety of different tumor types, there are no known specific risk factors. For the same reason, there are no specific screening procedures.

Diagnosis

CUPs are diagnosed only after an exhaustive evaluation for the primary site of cancer. A careful history and physical examination are performed. The site of presentation is biopsied. Based on the histologic category that is assigned and the location of the metastatic lesion, the patient undergoes further evaluation for the most likely primary site.

CUPs are currently grouped into the following categories:

- Poorly differentiated neoplasm
- Well-differentiated and moderately well-differentiated adenocarcinoma
- Squamous cell carcinoma
- Poorly differentiated carcinoma (with or without features of adenocarcinoma)

These categories are useful for conducting the clinical evaluation, planning the treatment, and predicting the response to treatment. The diagnostic work-up for each category of CUP is described in the following sections.

Poorly Differentiated Neoplasm

Approximately 5% of CUPs fall into this category. On further evaluation with immunoperoxidase staining and electron microscopy, most cases can be further defined as lymphoma, carcinoma, melanoma, or sarcoma. This process is most successful when a generous amount of tissue is available for analysis. Fine-needle aspirations do not preserve the histologic pattern and limit the ability to perform special studies. Genetic analysis may be used to identify chromosomal abnormalities and abnormal expression of specific genes. DNA microarray technology is being developed to classify neoplasms on the basis of gene expression and has the potential to identify the primary site of origin.

Well-Differentiated and Moderately Well-Differentiated Adenocarcinoma

Adenocarcinomas of unknown primary are also referred to as ACUPs. These represent about 60% of CUPs. The actual primary site is revealed in 15%–20% of patients before death, whereas 70%–80% are determined at autopsy. Lung and pancreas are the most common primary sites (40%), followed by stomach, colon, and liver. Breast, prostate, and ovary are more rare. Adenocarcinomas of unknown primary may demonstrate metastatic patterns of spread that are different than what is expected from a standard primary site presentation.

TABLE 16–1 ■ Clinical Evaluation for ACUPs

History and physical	Include family history of breast or ovarian cancer; history of tobacco use; prior exposure to asbestos, radiation, chemotherapy or other chemicals
Lab	Complete blood count (CBC) Liver function tests (LFTs) Serum Creatinine Prostatic specific antigen (PSA) Urinalysis
Radiology	Chest x-ray Computerized Tomography (CT) of abdomen and pelvis Mammogram Positron emission tomography (PET scan)

Patients in this category tend to be older adults. Metastatic tumors are commonly seen at multiple sites (e.g., lymph nodes, liver, lung, and bone). Most patients in this category have a poor prognosis, with a 3- to 4-month median survival. However, subsets of patients with primary breast, prostate, or ovarian cancers may respond to treatment. The clinical evaluation for ACUPs is listed in Table 16–1.

Axillary lymph node presentation in women may indicate a primary breast cancer. The node should be biopsied and tested for estrogen/progesterone receptor status as well as overexpression of the HER-2/*neu* oncogene.

Elevated prostate-specific antigen levels and/or osteoblastic bone metastases in men may be indicative of a primary prostate cancer (about 3% of cases). Specific proteins on prostate cancer cells may be detected by radiolabeled imaging, such as the ProstaScint scan (indium 111—labeled capromab pendetide).

Squamous Cell Carcinoma

Squamous cell carcinomas represent about 5% of CUPs. The diagnostic work-up differs, depending on the site of presentation. Cervical lymph node presentation occurs the most frequently. Positive upper or middle cervical nodes may indicate a primary head and neck cancer. Positive lower cervical or supraclavicular nodes more likely indicate a primary lung cancer. Inguinal nodes are most commonly associated with genital or anal cancers. Other sites of presentation most typically represent primary lung cancer.

TABLE 16–2 ■ Clinical Evaluation of Poorly Differentiated CUPs

History and Physical	
Lab	CBC
	LFTs
	Serum Cratinine
	Serum human chorionic gonadotropin (HCG)
	Serum alpha fetal protein (AFP)
	Serum Lactic Dehydrogenase (LDH)
Radiology	Chest x-ray
	CT of chest and abdomen

Poorly Differentiated Carcinoma (With or Without Features of Adenocarcinoma)

This category represents about 30% of CUPs. Approximately one third of patients have features of adenocarcinoma. These patients tend to be younger than patients with well- and moderately differentiated adenocarcinoma. History may reveal a rapid progression of symptoms and tumor growth. As in the poorly differentiated neoplasm category, histologic examination with light microscopy, immunoperoxidase staining, and genetic analysis is of value. Electron microscopy may also be used to determine subsets of lymphoma, sarcoma, melanoma, mesothelioma, and neuroendocrine tumors. The clinical evaluation of poorly differentiated CUPs is listed in Table 16–2.

Positron emission tomography may also be of value in determining other metastatic lesions and the primary site of origin. Patients with elevated human chorionic gonadotropin and alpha-fetoprotein levels, with or without enlargement of the mediastinal and/or retroperitoneal lymph nodes, may actually have an extragonadal germ cell tumor. These patients are potentially curable. Patients that fall into the poorly differentiated category may exhibit the presence of neurosecretory granules (by electron microscopy) in about 10% of cases. These granules are diagnostic for neuroendocrine carcinoma, a subgroup that is very responsive to treatment.

Staging

Due to the nature of CUPs' presentation as a metastatic lesion, it is not possible to use the tumor, node, metastasis staging system. The diagnostic work-up described earlier is important for revealing clues about the most likely primary site and for revealing other metastatic sites. Pa-

TABLE 16–3 ▪ Favorable Prognostic Indicators for CUPs

Younger age (≤ 35)
Performance status < 2 (ECOG scale)
Nonsmoker
< 2 sites of metastases
Normal serum lactic dehydrogenase (LDH)
Normal serum carcinoembryonic antigen (CEA)
Poorly differentiated carcinoma vs adenocarcinoma features
Single site of metastasis
Neuroendocrine features

Key: CUP = cancers of unknown primary sites; ECOG, Eastern Cooperative Oncology Group.

tients who present with a single site of metastasis may fall into a more favorable prognostic category. An example of this would be the woman who presents with CUP diagnosed on the basis of involved axillary lymph nodes. If there are no other signs of disease, she may have a stage II breast cancer with an occult primary site. Certain favorable prognostic indicators for CUPs have been identified (Table 16–3).

▪ Treatment

Like the diagnostic work-up, the treatment of CUPs varies, depending on the category and some specific subgroups of patients.

Poorly Differentiated Neoplasm

Unless the diagnosis can be further defined into a general category of neoplasm (e.g., carcinoma, adenocarcinoma), it is difficult to choose a treatment that may benefit the patient. Eligibility for a clinical trial should be explored.

Well-Differentiated and Moderately Well-Differentiated Adenocarcinoma

Women with peritoneal carcinomatosis are typically treated as if they have a peritoneal primary (see Chapter 19, Genitourinary Cancers). Treatment includes aggressive surgery to remove as much disease as possible. Surgery is followed with a platinum-based chemotherapy regimen. Chemotherapy may also be given before surgery.

Women who present with axillary lymph nodes and no known primary tumor are often treated as if they have a primary breast cancer (see Chapter 11, Breast Cancer). Positive estrogen/progesterone receptor assays support this diagnosis. Treatment choices include surgery or radiation therapy after lymph node dissection, followed by systemic chemotherapy. Hormonal therapy is dependent on the results of the estrogen/progesterone receptor assays and the woman's menopausal status. Women with additional sites of metastases should be treated as if they have a primary metastatic breast cancer. Overexpression of the HER-2/*neu* oncogene would make the woman an eligible candidate for monoclonal antibody therapy.

Men with osteoblastic bone metastases and/or elevated prostate-specific antigen levels may be treated for metastatic prostate cancer (see Chapter 13, Prostate Cancer). Hormonal therapy (ablation) would be a reasonable treatment option.

Approximately 90% of cases do not fall into one of the preceding groups. Various chemotherapy regimens have been tried in this patient population.

Squamous Cell Carcinoma

CUPs in the squamous cell carcinoma category are primarily treated based on anatomic presentation. Local treatment of the involved lymph nodes may include neck dissection and/or radiation therapy. Radical neck dissection identifies the primary tumor in 20%–40% of cases, but it has significant cosmetic impact and may negatively affect the patient's quality of life. Aggressive local therapy for patients with only supraclavicular disease yields long-term survival in 10%–15% of patients. Platinum- or paclitaxel-based chemotherapy regimens may also be beneficial (see Chapter 7, Chemotherapy). The use of neoadjuvant chemotherapy before radiation therapy is gaining acceptance for locally advanced head and neck cancers.

For disease spread to the inguinal lymph nodes, long-term survival can sometimes be achieved with surgical resection with or without inguinal radiation therapy.

Poorly Differentiated Carcinoma (With or Without Features of Adenocarcinoma)

Patients in this category may benefit from platinum-based chemotherapy regimens (see Chapter 7, Chemotherapy). Various combinations are under evaluation.

Rehabilitation

Rehabilitation for patients diagnosed with CUP depends on the type of treatment that is chosen, the patient's response to treatment, and the likelihood of long-term survival.

The Role of the Nurse

The diagnosis of cancer carries a profound psychosocial and emotional impact for the patient and his or her loved ones. That impact may be significantly magnified when there is no known primary site of origin for the disease. Fear of the unknown can be a more formidable enemy than facing a known entity. It is not uncommon for people diagnosed with cancer to seek a reason or a cause for their illness (see Chapter 27, Anxiety and Depression in the Oncology Setting). Many cancers have known risk factors, but CUPs are in many ways indefinable. Without knowing where the cancer started, there is no way to speculate on how or why the disease occurred.

The role of the nurse is essential to supporting the patient and family through the diagnostic process. It is important for the nurse to be present as the test results are discussed and the diagnosis of CUP is described. Familiarity with the treatment options is necessary to reinforce the information provided to the patient and family. Educating the patient and family about the identification and management of potential side effects and toxicities of the planned treatment is also a vital nursing function (see Unit V for specific symptoms).

Conclusion

Further investigation through clinical trials is necessary to determine the ideal treatment strategies for the various categories of CUPs. As we learn more about tumor types and molecular biology, targeted therapies will continue to evolve. The incidence of CUPs will continue to decline, as we are able to determine primary sites with increasing accuracy.

Resources

- OncoLink (*www.oncolink.com*), web site sponsored by the University of Pennsylvania Cancer Center

  To read about CUPs, click on the following:

  - Types of cancer
  - Miscellaneous/other diseases
  - Cancers of unknown primary
  - NCI/PDQ Patients: cancers of unknown primary

  To search for information on a clinical trial

  - Click on cancer.gov at the end of the PDQ information

  To join an on-line support group (list server) sponsored by the Associates of Cancer On-line Resources (ACOR)

  - Click on Support (in the left hand column of the PDQ page)
  - Choose group for Rare Cancer, or ACUP (adenocarcinoma of unknown primary)

Bibliography

Culine, S., Kramar, A., Saghatchian, M., Bugat, R., Lesimple, T., Lortholary, A., Merrouche, Y., Laplanche, A., & Fizazi, K. (2002). French Study Group on Carcinomas of Unknown Primary. Development and validation of a prognostic model to predict the length of survival in patients with carcinomas of an unknown primary site. *Journal of Clinical Oncology, 20*:4679–4683.

Greco, A. F., & Hainsworth, J. D. (2001). Cancer of unknown primary site. In V. T. Devita, S. Hellman, & S. A. Rosenberg (Eds.), *Cancer: Principles & practice of oncology* (5th ed., pp. 2537–2560). Philadelphia: Lippincott-Raven.

Kramar, A. K., Culine, S., Laplanche, A., et al. (2002). Prognostic factors for survival in patients with carcinomas of unknown primary: construction and validation of a simple prognostic model for the design of clinical trials. From the French Study Group of Carcinomas of Unknown Primary (GEFCAPI), abstract no. 1747. Retrieved April 3, 2003, from *http://www.asco.org/asco/publications/abstract_print_view/0,1148,_12-002324_18-002002*

NCI/PDQ Physician statement: carcinoma of unknown primary. Posted January 16, 2003. *http://oncolink.upenn.edu/pdq_html/1/enl/103331-1.html*

CHAPTER

17

Leukemia

Belinda Mandrell

Leukemia is the uncontrolled replication of the hematologic progenitor cells involved in the development of white blood cells, red blood cells, and platelets. This malignancy may originate in any of the blood-forming organs, including the bone marrow, lymphatic system, and spleen. Leukemia is a heterogeneous disease with various biologic and clinical presentations that influence a person's response to therapy.

■ Classification

Leukemia originates from either the lymphoid or myeloid progenitor cells infiltrating the bone marrow, lymphatic system, and organs. The leukemia is further classified as being acute or chronic on the basis of its clinical presentation and cell maturity (see Chapter 1, The Biology of Cancer). In the acute phase, the malignancy occurs during early cell differentiation, resulting in rapid replication with blasts; in the chronic phase, unregulated replication of differentiated cells occurs. Thus, there are four major classifications of leukemia: acute lymphocytic leukemia (ALL), chronic lymphocytic leukemia (CLL), acute myelogenous leukemia (AML), and chronic myelogenous leukemia (CML).

■ Incidence

It is estimated that 33,440 new cases of leukemia will be diagnosed in 2004, with an equal distribution of the acute and chronic forms.

TABLE 17–1 ■ Total Estimated Number of Leukemia Cases in 2003

Type of Leukemia	Number of Individuals
Acute lymphocytic leukemia (ALL)	3,600
Chronic lymphocytic leukemia (CLL)	7,300
Acute myelogenous leukemia (AML)	10,500
Chronic myelogenous leukemia (CML)	4,300
Other, unclassified leukemia	4,900
Total	30,600

Source: Surveillance, Epidemiology and End Results (SEER) Program 1079-1998. National Cancer Institute. Courtesy of the American Cancer Society.

Leukemia is 10 times likelier to occur in adulthood than in childhood. The overall incidence of leukemia is slightly higher in males than in females and is higher in Americans of European descent (see Chapter 2, Epidemiology of Cancer).

Leukemia occurs more often in the older adult, with more than half the cases occurring in the sixth decade. The most common leukemias among adults are AML and CLL. CML is one of a group of diseases called the myeloproliferative disorders, seen more frequently in adults and accounting for a small proportion of the overall leukemias. Although ALL makes up the smallest proportion of leukemias, it is most frequently seen in the pediatric leukemia patient (see Chapter 15, Cancer in Children and Adolescents). The total estimated numbers of adult and pediatric leukemia cases in 2003 are listed in Table 17–1.

■ Risk Factors

Although most cases of leukemia have no identifiable etiology, several risk factors have been proposed. The most commonly associated factors include genetics, environmental exposures, viral infections, and immunodeficiency. The genetic and immunologic predispositions for the development of leukemia are well known, especially in childhood leukemia. Children with Down syndrome, trisomy 21, are approximately 20 times likelier to develop leukemia than the general population, with children younger than 3 years of age likeliest to develop the megakaryoblastic subset of AML and older children likeliest to develop ALL. Fanconi's anemia, a constitutional aplasia of the bone marrow, is frequently associated with the development of AML. Bloom's syndrome, a recessive chromosomal fragility disorder, is associated with AML and, less frequently, ALL. Patients with ataxia-telangiectasia, an autosomal recessive syndrome, have a 100-fold greater incidence of developing T-cell leukemia/lymphoma. Other syndromes associated with leukemia include Klinefelter's syndrome, trisomy G syndrome, Rubinstein-Taybi syndrome, Schwachman-Diamond syndrome, Poland syndrome, and neurofibromatosis.

A genetic predisposition to leukemia has been observed in some families. Siblings of children with leukemia are at a two- to fourfold greater risk of developing the disease, and family members have a fivefold greater risk of AML if another family member is diagnosed with the leukemia. There is also a high correlation for leukemia among identical twins, especially if the disease is diagnosed within the first year of life. This may be the result of a prepregnancy/intrauterine event or may be spread through the shared placenta.

Certain environmental factors have also been associated with the development of leukemia. This relationship was well documented through long-term follow-up of persons exposed to the atomic bomb radiation in World War II. This finding promoted investigation into other environmental agents, including diagnostic and ionizing radiation, cigarette smoke, and electromagnetic fields or high power lines. Although ionizing radiation and smoking have been linked with leukemia, the electromagnetic field factor is unproved.

Occupational and therapeutic chemical exposures are also considered a risk factor for the development of leukemia (see Chapter 3, Cancer Screening, Early Detection, Risk Reduction, and Genetic Counseling). Exposures to benzene and solvents, such as toluene and butadiene, are linked to acute leukemia. However, hair dyes have not been conclusively shown to be a risk factor. Exposure to epipodophyllotoxins and alkylating chemotherapeutic agents is associated with secondary AML.

Viruses can be a causative factor in the development of leukemia. Epstein-Barr virus has been associated with B-cell leukemia and lymphoma, and retrovirus human T-cell lymphotropic virus type 1 has been associated with T-cell and hairy-cell leukemia.

Immunodeficiency disorders have also been associated with the development of leukemia and lymphoma. Patients with the human immunodeficiency virus have a higher risk of developing lymphoma and B-lineage leukemia. Patients with Wiskott-Aldrich, congenital hypogammaglobulinemia, or severe combined immunodeficiency disease have an increased risk of lymphoid malignancies. Long-term immunosuppressive therapy has also been associated with the development of leukemia-lymphoma.

■ Detection

The clinical presentation of leukemia results from the malignant replication of abnormal blood cells and is dependent upon the involved leukemia subset. During replication of rapidly dividing malignant cells, there is a crowding and inhibition of normal cells, resulting in hypermetabolism and cellular starvation. The patient experiences symptoms within weeks to months of the beginning of the acute malignant process. The most common symptoms and physical findings at diagnosis are anemia, fever, thrombocytopenia, neutropenia, pallor, fatigue, anorexia, petechiae, bleeding, and infection. In addition, the patient may have extramedullary disease and present with generalized or local lymphadenopathy, hepatomegaly, splenomegaly, bone pain, bone fracture, and parotid gland and testicular infiltration. A mediastinal mass may also be present and is most commonly associated with T-cell involvement. Extramedullary disease may involve the central nervous system, with presenting symptoms resulting from increased intracranial pressure that include vertigo, nausea, vomiting, papilledema, and blurred vision. An algorithm of acute leukemia symptomology is outlined in Figure 17-1.

Clinical manifestations of chronic leukemia are similar to those of acute leukemia but have an insidious onset. The first symptoms may include fatigue, exercise intolerance, night sweats, or abdominal fullness secondary to splenomegaly. Infection may also be a presenting symptom for leukemia and is common with CLL as a result of the associated hypogammaglobulinemia. Most chronic leukemias are diagnosed on routine examination or during an unrelated visit.

■ Diagnosis

A complete history and physical examination, blood count, and chemistry panel can indicate leukemia. If a diagnosis of leukemia is suspected, the patient should be referred to a hematology-oncology practice to confirm diagnosis and staging. After referral, the initial interview should include a history and physical examination, with interpretation of the complete blood count and chemistry panel. A bone marrow aspirate/biopsy is performed to confirm the diagnosis. The bone marrow sample is then processed for morphology/cytochemistry, immunophenotype, and cytogenetic/molecular features. A lumbar puncture is performed in children with ALL and AML, and in most adults with ALL. In adults with AML, a lumbar puncture is performed only if there are symptoms such as headaches or nerve damage.

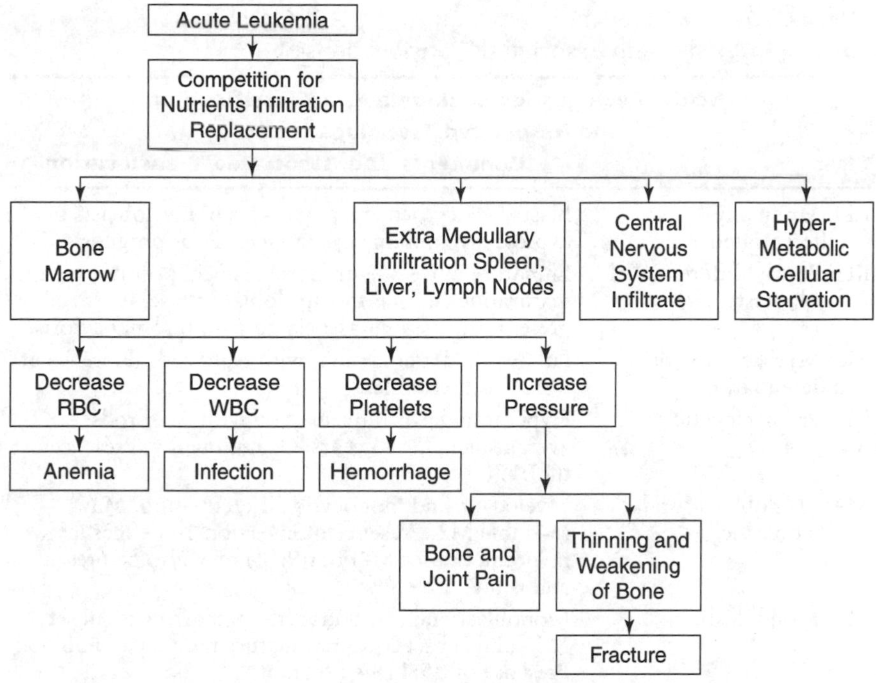

FIGURE 17–1 ■ An Algorithm of Acute Leukemia. Key: RBC = red blood cell; WBC = white blood cell.

Source: Reprinted from Crom, D. B., Boggs, T. B., Mandrell, B. N., & Norvill, R. (1999). Pediatric cancers. In C. Miaskowski, & P. Buchsel. (Eds.), Oncology nursing: Assessment and clinical care. St. Louis: Mosby. Copyright (1999) with permission from Elsevier.

Leukemia Classification

Once the bone marrow aspirate and spinal fluid have been obtained, the leukemia is classified according to the French-American-British classification system. Acute lymphocytic leukemia has three subsets (L1, L2, and L3) according to morphologic feature. Knowing the subtype will further classify the leukemia and helps predict which treatment will work best. For example, the three subtypes of ALL have a better prognosis when they are treated with intensive chemotherapy. The acute myeloid leukemias are also classified by the French-American-British system and are placed into morphologic subsets M0-M7 (Table 17–2).

The classification for CML begins with evidence of hyperleukocytosis and increased peripheral granulocytes. The phases of CML

TABLE 17–2 ■ French-American-British (FAB) Classification and Associated Translocations

Acute Myelogenous Leukemia FAB Classification and Associated Translocations

Class	Comments and Associated Translocation
M0: Minimally differentiated	Blasts lack cytochemical markers of myeloblasts but express myeloid lineage antigens. Poor prognosis.
M1: Poorly differentiated myeloblast	Immature but > 3% are cytochemical positive, little maturation beyond the myeloblast phase. Auer rods present. Inversion 3 associated with thrombocytosis.
M2: Myeloblast with differentiation	Full myeloid maturation, with Auer rods. Presence of t(8:21) is favorable.
M3: Promyelocytic	Hypergranular promyelocytes, with Auer rods; average age, 35–40 years. Coagulopathy. Presence of t(15:17).
M4: Myeloblastic and monoblastic	Myelocytic and monocytic differentiation. May resemble M2. Presence of inversion 16 defines a favorable subset M4Eo. t(9:11) may also be present and is favorable.
M5: Monoblastic	Monoblast and promonocytes in marrow is subset M5a and subset M5b has mature monocytes in blood. Presence of t(9:11) is favorable.
M6: Erythroleukemic	Dysplastic erythroid precursors and some myeloblast, seen in advanced age, poor outcome.
M7: Megakaryoblastic	Megakaryocytic blasts. Presence of t(1:22) may be present in infants. Poor prognosis; however, children with Down syndrome do well.

disease progression are outlined in Table 17–3. The hallmark of CML is the Philadelphia (Ph-1) translocation of chromosome 9 and 22, but this translocation can be seen in a subset of pediatric and adult ALL. Although Ph-1 in ALL is an unfavorable translocation, patients without Ph-1 translocation in CML have a poorer response than those with the Ph-1 translocation.

CLL presents with immature lymphocytes that accumulate in the marrow, blood, and lymph nodes. Patients with CLL have an average survival of 4–6 years; however, the leukemia may progress to a more aggressive lymphoid malignancy.

Staging for CLL has been confusing because two different systems, the Rai and the Binet, are currently used. The International Workshop on Chronic Lymphocytic Leukemia has recommended integration of the two systems. These classification criteria are outlined in Tables 17–4 and 17–5.

TABLE 17-3 ■ Phases of Chronic Myelogenous Leukemia Disease Progression

Chronic phase:	Bone marrow and cytogenetic findings of chronic myelogenous leukemia with 5% or fewer blast and promyelocytes in the peripheral blood and bone marrow
Accelerated phase:	Greater than 10%–15% blast in either the peripheral blood or bone marrow but with 30% or fewer blasts in both the peripheral blood and bone marrow
Blastic phase:	Greater than 30% blast in the peripheral blood or bone marrow

TABLE 17-4 ■ The Rai Staging System for Chronic Lymphocytic Leukemia

Stage O CLL:	White count > 15,000 cu/ml, without adenopathy, hepatosplenomegaly, anemia or thrombocytopenia
Stage I CLL:	White count > 15,000 cu/ml, with lymphadenopathy, without hepatosplenomegaly, anemia, or thrombocytopenia
Stage II CLL:	White count > 15,000 cu/ml, with either hepatomegaly or splenomegaly, with or without lymphadenopathy
Stage III CLL:	White count > 15,000 cu/ml, anemia, with or without hepatomegaly, splenomegaly, or lymphadenopathy
Stage IV CLL:	White count > 15,000 cu/ml, thrombocytopenia, with or without hepatomegaly, splenomegaly, lymphadenopathy, or anemia

TABLE 17-5 ■ The Binet Classification for Chronic Lymphocytic Leukemia[a]

Clinical stage A:	No anemia or thrombocytopenia and < 3 areas of nodal involvement. Rai stages 0, I, and II
Clinical stage B:	No anemia or thrombocytopenia and > 3 areas of nodal involvement. Rai stages I and II
Clinical stage C:	Anemia and/or thrombocytopenia regardless of nodal involvement. Rai stages II and IV

[a]The International Workshop on chronic lymphocytic leukemia has recommended integration of both the Rai and Binet system as follows: A(0), A(I), A(II); B(1), B(II); and C(III), C(IV).

Hairy cell leukemia is also a chronic lymphoproliferative disorder that may be confused at diagnosis with CLL. Hairy cell presents with splenomegaly, pancytopenia, and bone marrow infiltration by atypical cells that have prominent cytoplasmic projections that resemble hair. Treatment with cladribine has greatly improved outcome, with 85% survival at 5 years.

■ Treatment

The goal of leukemia therapy is to eradicate the malignant clone, allowing growth of normal hematopoietic cells. Once the diagnosis, immunophenotype, and cytogenetic/molecular classification are complete, the treatment plan is prescribed accordingly. Therapy for ALL is divided into stages: induction, consolidation, and maintenance. Based on the patient's prognostic factors, the remission induction chemotherapy program generally includes some if not all of the following drugs: cyclophosphamide, vincristine, dexamethasone or prednisone, L-asparaginase, and doxorubicin. Some programs include high doses of methotrexate and cytosine arabinoside as part of the induction scheme. Others use a drug called etoposide.

The patient is monitored closely for the disappearance of peripheral blasts and treatment-related side effects. At the end of induction, the marrow is examined for morphologic and molecular presence of disease. Many treatment regimens have a month of reintensive induction within the first year of therapy. Consolidation is several weeks long and includes courses of methotrexate or cytarabine. At the conclusion of consolidation, maintenance therapy begins with drugs used in a combination, rotational schedule. Maintenance therapy may include cytarabine, thioguanine, methotrexate, cyclophosphamide, vincristine, prednisone/dexamethasone, doxorubicin, L-asparaginase, mitoxantrone, and 6-mercaptopurine. This rotational therapy is administered over a 2- to 3-year course. Additionally, patients with ALL receive intrathecal chemotherapy with methotrexate or cytarabine for prophylaxis or treatment of central nervous system involvement. If the initial lumbar puncture finds leukemia in the spinal fluid, radiation therapy may also be given to the brain. Bone marrow/stem cell transplantation may be a treatment option for patients who have an early relapse, have disease that is unresponsive to therapy, or have unfavorable cytogenetics.

Patients with ALL, L3 morphology have a mature B-cell leukemia that is treated with the same drugs; however, this leukemia is treated with high-dose combination therapy given every 3–4 weeks over 6–9 months. Although most patients have an excellent outcome, poor prognosis is associated with central nervous system involvement.

Approximately 60%–80% of adults with ALL attain complete remission after induction therapy. However, the mean duration of remission is 15 months, with only a 40% survival at 2 years with aggressive therapy.

AML, like ALL, is a very heterogeneous disease with the choice of treatment being dependent on subset, translocation, and response to initial therapy. Approximately 60%–70% of adults with AML achieve remission; however, only 25% of those in remission survive greater than 3 years. Higher age at diagnosis correlates with a higher morbidity and mortality rate. Prognosis is especially dismal for those who develop AML secondary to myelodysplastic syndromes, have a deletion or monosomy of chromosome 5 and 7, and have chemotherapy-related disease. Treatment for AML is in two phases: (a) induction and (b) postremission or consolidation to maintain remission. Induction usually involves treatment with two chemotherapy drugs, cytarabine and an anthracycline, such as daunorubicin or idarubicin. This intensive therapy, which usually takes place in the hospital, typically lasts 1 week. The options for AML postremission therapy are (a) several courses of high-dose cytarabine chemotherapy, (b) allogeneic (donor) stem cell transplantation, or (c) autologous stem cell transplantation. Because of the high recurrence rate of AML and the reduced cure rate, bone marrow/stem cell transplantation is recommended for patients with an unfavorable response to therapy or unfavorable subset/cytogenetics.

An exception to these recommendations is AML M3, which is a malignancy of the promyelocyte. Treatment of this subtype of AML differs from the usual AML treatment because a nonchemotherapy drug, all-*trans* retinoic acid (ATRA), a drug related to vitamin A, is also used. Although remission induction is usually possible with ATRA alone, combining the ATRA with chemotherapy produces the best results. During treatment, some people experience coagulopathies and treatment may be needed to prevent this. Patients are usually given an anticoagulant or fresh frozen plasma to prevent or treat clotting problems.

Remission is usually induced by treatment with ATRA and the chemotherapy used for AML. The side effects of this treatment differ from those of standard AML induction chemotherapy because retinoic acid syndrome may occur. This syndrome involves rash, respiratory distress, edema, pleural or pericardial effusions, renal dysfunction, hyperleukocytosis, and pseudotumor cerebri.

Consolidation therapy usually consists of two or more courses of chemotherapy, followed by maintenance therapy with ATRA for at least 1 year. About 70% of patients are cured with this treatment.

For patients experiencing relapse, arsenic therapy is used to induce remission, followed in some cases by bone marrow transplantation.

CML is a chronic leukemia with chronic, accelerated, and blast phases. Although the disease may remain stable for many years, a blast crisis is inevitable and usually occurs within 3 years of diagnosis. With an indolent course, immediate intensive therapy is not required, unless the patient presents with a high white blood cell count. Hydroxyurea is then required for rapid count reduction and prevention of leukostasis, which could result in cerebrovascular events or death.

For newly diagnosed CML, the only curative therapy is allogeneic bone marrow or stem cell transplantation (see Chapter 9, Hematopoietic Stem Cell Transplantation). For those who are ineligible, unwilling, or waiting to undergo transplantation, interferon alfa and imatinib mesylate (Gleevec) are treatment options. Approximately 80% of patients treated with interferon experience a hematologic remission, whereas 10%–20% of patients treated with interferon have a complete cytogenetic response (loss of Ph-1 translocation) and remain disease free beyond 10 years. However, 90% of patients experience side effects that may preclude the continuation of therapy. A specific inhibitor of the Ph-1 translocation, Gleevec has now become front-line therapy. For untreated patients, approximately 60% have a complete response with few side effects. However, long-term response rates are yet unknown. Patients receiving Gleevec should avoid grapefruit juice, which is known to increase the Gleevec level.

CLL is the most common chronic leukemia, with variable treatment options, depending on the progression of the leukocytosis. Because CLL is a slowly progressing leukemia occurring within the elderly population, most are conservatively observed. Therefore, treatment options depend on the stage of disease progression. Treatment options may include observation, chemotherapy (see Chapter 7, Chemotherapy), and monoclonal antibiotics, which target the surface antigen. Chemotherapy agents include oral alkylating agents, such as chlorambucil or cyclophosphamide with prednisone; fludarabine; cladribine; pentostatin; and vincristine or the monoclonal antibiotics alemtuzumab (Campath) or rituximab. Low-dose radiation therapy may also be used to symptomatically treat enlarged nodal sites. Lastly, bone marrow transplantation may be a treatment option for the younger patient (see Chapter 9, Hematopoietic Stem Cell Transplantation).

■ Rehabilitation

Once leukemia is diagnosed, the patient and family must balance the treatment regimen and uncertainty of the future, while attempting to maintain a sense of control and normalcy. This may be further compounded by the emotional, mental, and physical responses to therapy. During and after the completion of therapy, the patient should be closely monitored for such responses. Fatigue is a common complaint (see Chapter 25, Fatigue) expressed by both children and adults, and it contributes to psychological, physical, spiritual, and social despair. The patient should be closely assessed for symptoms of fatigue, which include feelings of sadness, sleepiness, dizziness, nausea, as well as feeling heavy, mentally tired, not one's self, and sorry for one's self (see Unit V for specific symptoms).

Patients may not resume their life as it was before leukemia. The experience could have a positive effect, resulting in personal growth, assessment of life priorities, and an increased appreciation of life and family. However, other patients experience lower self-esteem, isolation, and educational or occupational difficulties. These patients should be monitored closely for psychological distress, which may require medical and psychological intervention (see Chapters 34 [Pediatric Symptoms and Responses] and 35 [Psychosocial-Spiritual Responses to Cancer and Treatment: Living with Cancer]).

■ The Role of the Nurse

Five categories of nursing care strategies exist for the leukemia patient (Table 17–6). The first category is patient and family education. The nurse has a responsibility to be knowledgeable about the disease, its treatment, and side effects of therapy. For example, patients undergoing leukemia treatment are at greater risk for infection. Therefore, the patient and family should be educated on signs and symptoms of infection and ways to prevent infection (e.g., avoidance of crowds). The second category for nursing care is a supportive presence, and this support may be demonstrated through the nurse's availability to answer questions, address concerns, and be present during discussion of treatment. The third category is active monitoring and anticipation on the part of

TABLE 17–6 ■ Nursing Care Requirements for Patients with Leukemia

- Patient and family education
- A supportive presence by the caregiver
- Actively monitoring and anticipating events
- Technical competence
- Advocacy

the nurse. At all times, the nurse should be monitoring the disease response of the patient, with anticipation of the upcoming needs of the patient and the family. For example, this becomes very important when the patient fails to respond to therapy and the nurse must meet the palliative needs of the patient and family. If the nurse fails to anticipate these needs, it becomes an even more distressing situation for the nurse and may result in an inability to care for the patient. The fourth category is that the nurse be technically competent. This is especially true in caring for the leukemia patient, who has a central access device, receives blood/platelet transfusions (see Chapter 22, Myelosuppression), and is given drugs with multiple side effects. The nurse should also be competent in assessing the patient for problems that should be brought to the attention of the health care team. Last, the nurse should serve as an advocate for the patient and the family. The leukemia patient experiences a loss of control because of the intensive therapy and prolonged hospitalizations. It becomes the nurses' responsibility to ensure that the patient and family are involved to the extent that they prefer in treatment decision making.

When developing a care plan for the patient with leukemia, the nurse should incorporate these strategies throughout the continuum of care while taking into consideration the environmental influences of the patient, family, health care team/system, and society. Therefore, the nurse can tailor care according to the circumstances of the patient, family, and treatment plan.

■ Conclusion

Nurses should care for patients with leukemia with an analytical approach. Such an approach involves analyzing the care outcomes of previously treated patients to deduce ideas that can improve care and long-term outcomes of future patients. In giving care to adults or children with leukemia, nurses need to convey hope, as well as their commitment to optimal care outcomes and quality of life for patients and their family members whose lives are affected by leukemia.

■ Resources

- American Cancer Society Leukemia Resources:
  - Adult chronic: *www.cancer.org/docroot/CRI/CRI_2x.asp?sitearea=&dt=62*

  - Adult acute:
    www.cancer.org/docroot/CRI/CRI_2x.asp?sitearea=&dt=57
  - Children's:
    www.cancer.org/docroot/CRI/CRI_2x.asp?sitearea=&dt=24
- The Leukemia and Lymphoma Society: *www.leukemia.org*
- National Cancer Institute Leukemia home page: *www.nci.nih.gov/cancerinfo/types/leukemia*

Bibliography

Breed, C. D. (2003). Diagnosis, treatment, and nursing care of the patient with chronic leukemia. *Seminars in Oncology Nursing, 19,* 109–117.

Hinds, P. S. & Gattuso, J. S. (1999). Nursing care. In C-H. Pui (ed.), *Childhood Leukemia* (pp. 542–552). New York, NY: Cambridge University Press.

National Cancer Institute. Leukemia treatment. Retrieved June 1, 2003, from *www.cancer.gov/pdq/treatment/healthprofessionals*

Viele, C. S. (2003). Diagnosis, treatment, and nursing care of the patient with acute leukemia. *Seminars in Oncology Nursing, 19,* 98–108.

CHAPTER

18

Lymphomas

Adonica L. Jones

Lymphomas are one of a group of malignancies that originate from the lymphatic system. Depending on the histology and the pattern of behavior, lymphomas can be divided into two groups: Hodgkin's lymphoma or Hodgkin's disease and non-Hodgkin's lymphoma (NHL). Leukemias and myelomas are also malignancies that arise from the lymphoid cell line. These are discussed in separate chapters.

Hodgkin's Disease

Incidence

An estimated 7,880 new cases of Hodgkin's disease are diagnosed annually, and approximately 1,300 deaths occur as a result of the disease. There is an age-related bimodal incidence distribution, with the incidence peaking in the mid 20s, declining until the mid 40s, and then increasing after age 60. Hodgkin's disease is rare before the age of 10, and it is more common in males than in females. In adults, the annual incidence is 4,000 in males and 3,600 in females. Since the introduction of combination chemotherapy, adult Hodgkin's disease has become one of the most curable malignancies.

Risk Factors

Although the exact etiology of Hodgkin's disease is not known, it has been suggested that the Epstein-Barr virus plays a role in its development. A greater incidence of Hodgkin's disease has been observed in young individuals who previously had infectious mononucleosis, and this virus is found in the lymph nodes of many young patients with Hodgkin's disease. The presence of large, multinucleated Reed-Sternberg cells, an abnormal B cell with two or more identical nuclei, in the tumor is characteristic of the disease. Hodgkin's disease is thought to originate from a single focus, usually a lymph node. Patients with Hodgkin's disease exhibit defects in immune system function throughout the course of the disease but to a lesser degree after remission is obtained. An increased incidence of Hodgkin's disease among siblings suggests a possible genetic risk, but this has not been proved.

Clinical Presentation

Patients are often asymptomatic and may present with lymphadenopathy that is painless. Lymphadenopathy is most commonly found in the supraclavicular, cervical, and mediastinal lymph node regions. The spread of disease is contiguous and predictable, first involving adjacent lymph nodes before spreading to other organs. The spleen, liver, and retroperitoneal lymph nodes may be involved, although patients may not exhibit clinical signs of involvement at diagnosis. Associated symptoms of unexplained weight loss of more than 10% of body weight in the 6 months before diagnosis; frequent, drenching night sweats; fever with temperatures above 38° C; and pain with alcohol ingestion may be present. Pruritis, an additional systemic symptom, is associated with more advanced disease. These symptoms, defined as "B" symptoms for staging purposes, occur with greater frequency in older patients and are associated with a poorer prognosis.

Diagnosis and Staging

The diagnostic process for Hodgkin's disease includes a thorough history and physical examination, plus hematology and chemistry profiles. Diagnosis is made by histologic examination of the excised lymph node. A chest x-ray study may demonstrate mediastinal involvement. The extent of disease is best determined by computed tomography of the thoracic, abdominal, and pelvic areas, and positron emission tomography to better characterize lymph nodes. In the past, a staging laparotomy was usually performed if the extent of disease could not be determined by other diagnostic tests and if confirmation of abdominal disease would alter the choice of therapy. With the advent of combination chemotherapy and radiation therapy for early-stage disease, the need for surgery has diminished. The overall treatment plan or outcome is not changed by surgical staging. Current staging practices are to assign a clinical stage based on the findings of the diagnostic studies previously indicated and a pathological stage based on the biopsy specimen. The widely used Ann Arbor–Cotswold Staging Classification shown in Table 18–1 allows for both clinical and pathological staging. It is used to determine treatment and prognosis and to enable the clinician to compare patients enrolled in various treatment protocols.

Treatment

Therapy for Hodgkin's disease has improved over the past 30 years, resulting in a long-term survival rate of nearly 80% today. The role of surgery in Hodgkin's disease is limited to diagnostic biopsy, staging procedures, or splenectomy in selected cases.

Radiation Therapy Radiation therapy alone is curative in most patients with stage I or stage II disease (see Chapter 8, Radiation Therapy). The

TABLE 18–1 ■ Ann Arbor–Cotswold Staging Classification Indicated for Both Hodgkin's and Non-Hodgkin's Lymphoma

Clinical Staging	
Stage I	Involvement of a single lymph node region. Extension into an extralymphatic organ or site (I_E)
Stage II	Involvement of two or more lymph node regions on the same side of the diaphragm. Extension into an extralymphatic site (II_E)
Stage III	Involvement of lymph node regions or structures on both sides of the diaphragm. May be divided into disease of the upper (III_1) or lower (III_2) abdomen, if spleen is involved (III_S); if extralymphatic extension, (III_E)
Stage IV	Diffuse involvement of liver, bone marrow, lung, or diffuse extralymphatic disease
For all stages	A: No symptoms B. Presence of symptoms (fever, sweats, weight loss of >10% of body weight

Pathological Staging

E: Well-localized extranodal lymphoid malignancies arise in or extend to tissues beyond but near the major lymphatic aggregates.

Sites of involvement are identified by initial notations and a plus (+) sign.

N=nodes H=liver L=lung M=bone S=spleen P=Pleura O=bone D=skin

Source: Yarbro, C. H. (2000). Malignant lymphomas. In C. H. Yarbro, M. H. Frogg, M. Goodman, & S. L. Groenwald (Eds.), *Cancer nursing principles and practice* (5th ed., pp. 1329–1353). Sudbury, MA: Jones & Bartlett.

addition of chemotherapy to the treatment plan may be indicated in patients with poor prognostic factors, such as "B" symptoms, or in those with very large mediastinal lymph nodes or stage III or stage IV disease. Radiation therapy fields designed to treat all involved lymph nodes with the same radiation dose are illustrated in Figure 18-1. Radiotherapy may also be given prophylactically to chains of clinically uninvolved nodes to limit the spread of disease along its predictable routes. When radiation therapy is used in combination with chemotherapy, the total dose of radiation may be decreased. Therapy is usually administered over a period of 3–4 weeks. Figure 18-1 shows standard radiation ports used for the treatment of Hodgkin's disease.

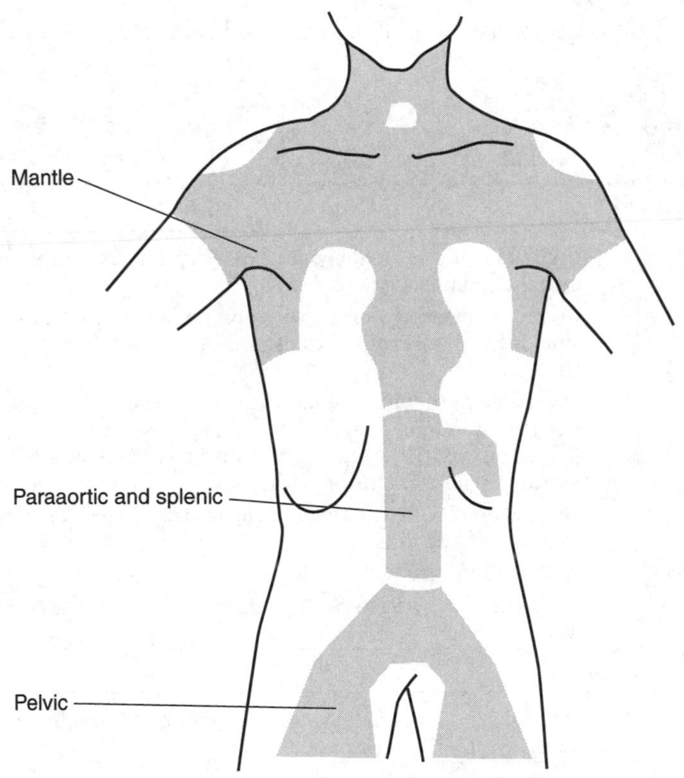

FIGURE 18–1 ■ Standard Radiation Ports Used for the Treatment of Hodgkin's Disease.

Source: Adapted with permission from Salzman, J. R., & Kaplan, H. S. (1972). Effect of prior splenectomy on hematologic tolerance during total lymphoid radiotherapy of patients with Hodgkin's disease. *Cancer 27,* 472.

For disease presenting above the diaphragm, the mantel plus the paraaortic and splenic ports are regarded as extended-field radiation therapy. Use of all three ports is considered total nodal irradiation. This is rarely performed, and most oncologists use chemotherapy added to limited radiation therapy for extensive disease.

Chemotherapy Intensive chemotherapy is used in most patients with stage III and stage IV disease and in some patients with earlier-stage disease. Combinations of at least four chemotherapeutic drugs are used to achieve a cure (see Chapter 7, Chemotherapy). The most commonly used combination is ABVD (doxorubicin, bleomycin, vinblastine, and dacarbazine). This regimen induces a complete remission in more than 80% of patients. In the past, MOPP (nitrogen mustard, vincristine, procarbazine, and prednisone) was the standard chemotherapy, but it is no longer used because of the risk of late effects from therapy, such as secondary leukemia.

The risk of acute leukemia 10 years after therapy with MOPP is about 3%. For those treated with ABVD, the risk for the same period is about 1%. The most frequently observed acute side effects of chemotherapy include nausea and vomiting, myelosuppression, alopecia, fatigue, and mood changes associated with steroid therapy. Neurotoxicity related to treatment with vincristine is also seen.

Hematopoietic Cell Transplantation (see Chapter 9) The use of high-dose chemotherapy and autologous bone marrow and/or peripheral stem cell rescue may be considered for refractory and relapsed stage III and stage IV Hodgkin's disease. Clinical trials are ongoing for this treatment option.

Symptom Management, Long-Term Sequelae, and the Role of the Nurse

Treatment approaches for Hodgkin's disease are frequently complex, and nurses have an essential role in teaching patients and families about the treatment and its impact. Nurses also play a crucial role in managing the symptoms of patients receiving chemotherapy and radiation therapy (see Unit V for specific symptoms) and in explaining the importance of long-term surveillance.

Issues related to the long-term effects of radiation therapy and chemotherapy are particularly relevant to the large proportion of patients who are young adults. Risks of a second malignancy and reproductive ability are also a concern (see Chapter 33, Sexuality).

The occurrence of infertility is age dependent in females. Forty percent to 50% of women older than 35 years experience ovarian dysfunction after MOPP therapy. Males in the same age group who receive MOPP have a greater than 80% chance of irreversible sterility. Because fertility cannot be ensured after treatment, patients should be encouraged to discuss their concerns before therapy begins. These patients may wish to consider egg harvesting or sperm storage through a banking program before treatment if time and urgency of treatment permit. Because patients may still be able to conceive during therapy, all sexually active patients undergoing treatment should be advised to use contraceptives during and for 6 months after treatment. Patients need to be informed of the risk and assisted in balancing the long-term risks for therapy with the benefits of treating a life-threatening disease. Long-term follow-up after treatment is essential (see Chapter 36, Cancer Survivorship).

■ Non-Hodgkin's Lymphoma

NHL is seven times more common than Hodgkin's disease. Of the estimated 54,370 new cases of NHL diagnosed annually, as many as 19,410 will die of the disease. Overall survival at 5 years with optimum treatment for all patients with NHL is approximately 50%–60%. Males are more often affected than females. Individuals with congenital or acquired immunodeficiencies, including individuals with acquired immunodeficiency syndrome (AIDS), those undergoing organ transplantation, and those with autoimmune diseases, are at increased risk for developing NHL (see Chapter 2, Epidemiology of Cancer).

Etiology

NHL is a malignancy of the B or T lymphocytes. Clones of the malignant cells may infiltrate the lymph nodes, bone marrow, peripheral blood, or other organs (see Chapter 1, The Biology of Cancer). Most NHLs fall into two broad categories related to their clinical behavior: indolent type and aggressive lymphomas. The pattern of spread is less predictable in NHL than in Hodgkin's disease. The disease is frequently disseminated at the time of diagnosis.

Clinical Manifestations

Patients with NHL present with localized or generalized lymphadenopathy, which they may identify as having waxed and waned over a period of several months. Early involvement of the oropharyngeal lymphoid tissue or infiltration of the bone marrow is common. Abdominal mass may be detected with gastrointestinal involvement, or the patient may describe vague symptoms of back or abdominal discomfort. Patients may also exhibit systemic "B" symptoms, including night sweats, fever, and/or weight loss. Approximately one third of patients have splenomegaly or hepatomegaly.

Diagnosis and Staging

In addition to careful examination of all lymph node regions, a complete blood count, chemistry, bone marrow, and lymph node biopsy are used to diagnose NHL. The Ann Arbor–Cotswold Staging Classification is used but is of less value with NHL because it does not account for the histology or type of tumor. Having the clinical stage within each histologic subtype appears to help identify tumor activity for each subtype thus, carrying a reliable prognostic significance.

Treatment

Surgery The primary role of surgery is to establish diagnosis and to assist with staging. Surgery is rarely needed to prevent bowel obstruction or for splenectomy in patients exhibiting hypersplenism.

Radiation and Chemotherapy Unlike the contiguous node extension seen in Hodgkin's disease, NHL is disseminated via the vascular system. Consequently, radiation therapy is generally used as an adjuvant with chemotherapy as opposed to being the primary treatment. Radiation therapy may be used alone in stage I lymphoma, although it is more common to combine radiation therapy with chemotherapy. The patient's age and clinical condition may affect the choice of treatment. Therapy for low-grade lymphoma remains controversial because this disease is not curable with current therapies. These indolent lymphomas do have a long natural history, with a median survival approaching 10 years in untreated patients.

Patients with intermediate- and high-grade, aggressive lymphomas are routinely treated with combination chemotherapy with or without radiation therapy. Combination chemotherapy with a variety of regimens, such as MOPP or CHOP (cyclophosphamide, doxorubicin, vincristine, and prednisone) has led to high rates of remission, although the remission usually lasts for less than 5 years. After relapse, the remissions achieved are generally shorter. Unfortunately, only about 50% of patients with aggressive lymphomas are cured. Colony-stimulating factors are used to enable the delivery of more intensive chemotherapy, but research has not confirmed an overall decrease in drug toxicity (other than neutropenia) or increased survival rates with this approach. Hematopoietic cell transplantation (see Chapter 9, Hematopoietic Stem Cell Transplantation) after high-dose chemotherapy has resulted in long-term remissions for some patients with relapsing lymphomas.

Immunotherapy/Biotherapy Biotherapy, namely rituximab, a monoclonal antibody, was approved by the US Food and Drug Administration in 1997 for the treatment of relapsed or refractory low-grade or follicular CD20-positive B-cell NHL. It is also indicated as a first-line treatment with combination chemotherapy for aggressive lymphomas. Iodine I 131 tositumomab and yttrium Y 90 ibritumomab monoclonal-based radioimmunotherapeutic agents are approved by the US Food and Drug Administration for the treatment of CD20-positive follicular NHL that has relapsed after chemotherapy and is refractory to rituximab. Clinical trials are underway in this field.

Symptom Management, Long-Term Sequelae, and the Role of the Nurse

The nurse plays a very important role in education about treatment modalities, symptom management, and potential side effects and long-term effects. Many patients remain neutropenic for extended periods of time during treatment and must be able to protect themselves when they are vulnerable to infection (see Chapter 22, Myelosuppression). Bulky tumors may cause obstruction and pressure, resulting in complications such as spinal cord compression, superior vena cava syndrome, ascites, and gastrointestinal or ureteral obstruction. These oncology complications are discussed in Unit V.

Permanent sterility associated with radiation therapy and long-term treatment with cyclophosphamide is a risk. A risk of a second primary malignancy exists for up to 2 decades after diagnosis and treatment. As with Hodgkin's disease, the nurse can teach the patient about these risks.

■ AIDS-Related Lymphoma

Incidence

The prevalence of lymphoma in patients with human immunodeficiency virus (HIV) is 3%–6%. In approximately 30% of cases, the diagnosis of AIDS is made at the time of the diagnosis of NHL. As improved therapies called highly active antiretroviral therapy have boosted the immune status of patients, the incidence of lymphomas has decreased.

Etiology

The relationship between AIDS and NHL is not completely understood; however, nearly 95% of all HIV-associated malignancies are either NHL or Kaposi's sarcoma. Patients with central nervous system (CNS) lymphoma generally have advanced AIDS, are severely debilitated, and are usually considered to be in the terminal stages of their disease.

Clinical Manifestations

The patient with AIDS-related lymphoma often presents with advanced-stage disease. The CNS is the most common extranodal site, followed by the bone marrow and the bowel. Diagnosis of NHL outside the CNS is complicated by a history of fevers, night sweats, and significant weight loss, also common HIV symptoms.

Diagnosis and Staging

Diagnosing AIDS-related lymphoma is similar to diagnosing non-AIDS-related lymphoma. Cultures are required in order to rule out complicating opportunistic infections. Unfortunately, imaging cannot distinguish between CNS lymphoma and toxoplasmosis, which may occur simultaneously and is present in up to 43% of patients. The Ann Arbor–Cotswold Staging Classification is used. Most patients present with advanced disease with high-grade lymphoblastic histology. Prognosis and optimal treatment are related to many factors, including severity of the immune deficiency, bone marrow involvement, extranodal disease, antiretroviral therapy, prophylaxis for opportunistic infections, rapid recognition and treatment of infections, and performance status.

Treatment

Treatment of NHL in the presence of HIV/AIDS poses a challenge. The underlying immunodeficiency of AIDS limits the potential for dose-intensive regimens of chemotherapy. Dose reduction and CNS prophylaxis are often indicated. Response rates tend to be lower than for patients without HIV. Surgical intervention is typically limited to diagnostic biopsy or treatment of complications such as obstructions because of the diffuse nature of CNS lymphoma. Radiation therapy is limited to patients with primary CNS lymphoma. These patients are usually extremely debilitated and demonstrate focal neurologic symptoms, such as seizures and paralysis. Disease recurs in the brain in more than 92% of patients after high doses of radiation, and the median survival for this group of patients is generally less than 6 months.

Side Effects and the Role of the Nurse

Managing the complex side effects of radiation therapy and chemotherapy is further complicated by the fact that patients are often severely debilitated and have advanced-stage disease. The immunosuppressive nature of HIV infection and the incidence of coexisting opportunistic infection limit the treatment options available. The patient is often dealing with depression and loss, the financial burden imposed by illness, isolation, and at times, rejection by friends and family. Nursing care must include the often-overwhelming emotional consequences of AIDS (see Chapters 34 [Pediatric Symptoms and Responses] and 37 [End of Life]).

■ Conclusion

The lymphomas are a unique group of malignancies that present many challenges to nurses. Treatment and or symptom management is often complex, requiring highly skilled nursing care. Ongoing research leading to new treatment modalities is improving cure rates and quality of life for those living with the lymphoma and is providing much hope for the future.

■ Resources

- American Cancer Society: 800-ACS-2345 or *www.cancer.org*
  - Lymphoma, non-Hodgkin's type; *www.cancer.org/docroot/CRI/CRI_2x.asp?sitearea=&dt=32*
  - Hodgkin's disease: *www.cancer.org/docroot/CRI/CRI_2x.asp?sitearea=&dt=20*
- The Leukemia and Lymphoma Society
  - Information Resource Center: 800-955-4572 (free literature)
  - Website: *www.leukemia-lymphoma.org*
  - Publications: *The lymphomas: Hodgkin's and Non-Hodgkin's lymphoma.* Publication # P038.
- National Cancer Institute Website
  - AIDS-related lymphoma: *www.nci.nih.gov/cancerinfo/types/AIDS/*
  - Non-Hodgkin's lymphoma: *www.nci.nih.gov/cancerinfo/types/non-hodgkins-lymphoma/*
  - Hodgkin's lymphoma: *www.nci.nih.gov/cancerinfo/tyhpes/hodgkinslymphoma/*

- Physician Data Query
- Lymphomas Data Base for Healthcare Professionals and Patients

Bibliography

Adult Hodgkin's Lymphoma: Treatment (2003). *Physician data query* (*PDQ®*). Retrieved June 7, 2003 from National Cancer Institute Cancer.gov database. *http://www.nci.nih.gov/cancerinfo/pdq/treatment/adulthodgkins/health professional/*

Aids-related lymphoma (2003). *Physician data query* (*PDQ®*). Retrieved June 8, 2003 from National Cancer Institute Cancer.gov database. *http://www.nci.nih.gov/cancerinfo/pdq/treatment/AIDS-related-lymphoma/healthprofessional/*

Adult Non-Hodgkin's Lymphoma: Treatment (2003). *Physician data query (PDQ®).* Retrieved June 7, 2003 from National Cancer Institute Cancer.gov database. *http://www.nci. nih.gov/cancerinfo/pdq/treatment/adult-non-hodgkins/health professional/*

Trahan-Reiger, P. (Ed.). (2001). *Biotherapy: A comprehensive overview* (2nd ed.). Sudbury, MA: Jones & Bartlett.

Yarbro, C. H. (2000). Malignant lymphomas. In C. H. Yarbro, M. H. Frogg, M. Goodman, & S. L. Groenwald (Eds.), *Cancer nursing principles and practice* (5th ed., pp. 1329–1353). Sudbury, MA: Jones & Bartlett.

CHAPTER

19

Genitourinary Cancers

Jane Clark

Genitourinary (or urogenital) cancers are cancers of the organs concerned with reproduction and the production and excretion of urine. This chapter covers testicular cancer, penile cancer, urethral cancer, bladder cancer, and renal cancer.

■ Testicular Cancer

Incidence

Testicular cancer is a relatively uncommon malignancy, with approximately 8,960 new cases predicted to be diagnosed in 2004. However, the disease is the most common solid tumor malignancy in males between the ages of 15 and 35 years of age. The worldwide incidence of testicular cancer has doubled in the past 40 years. The highest incidence rates of testicular cancer occur in North America, Scandinavia, Germany, and New Zealand. Testicular cancer occurs four to five times more frequently in white males than in African American males (see Chapter 2, Epidemiology of Cancer).

More than 50% of testicular cancer cases are diagnosed at an early stage. Although more than 90% of individuals with testicular cancer achieve a 5-year survival, the American Cancer Society (ACS) estimates that 360 males will die from the disease in 2004.

Risk Factors

Risk factors for testicular cancer include cryptorchidism, genetics, and personal history of testicular cancer. The most significant risk factor is cryptorchidism (undescended testicle). Males with a history of cryptorchidism have a 30- to 40-fold increased risk for testicular cancer. Successful orchiopexy, performed before the patient is 6 years of age, reduces the risk of testicular cancer. However, data do not support a decreased risk for the disease when orchiopexy is performed in adults.

Scientists continue to study the role of genetics in the development of testicular cancer. The incidence of testicular cancer is greater in individuals with Klinefelter's syndrome, Down's syndrome, and testicular feminization, although the exact mechanisms of risk are unknown. In addition, sons of men with a history of testicular cancer have a four times greater risk of developing testicular cancer, and male siblings of individuals with testicular cancer have a 10 times greater risk of developing the disease (see Chapter 1, The Biology of Cancer).

The incidence of bilateral testicular cancer is 1%–2%. However, a personal history of unilateral testicular cancer results in a 500 times greater chance of development of the disease in the contralateral testicle.

Detection

Most cases of testicular cancer can be diagnosed at an early stage because early symptoms lead men to seek medical attention. Unfortunately, however, some testicular cancers may not cause symptoms until after reaching an advanced stage.

Most health care providers agree that examination of a man's testicles should be part of a general physical examination. The ACS recommends a testicular examination as part of a periodic checkup.

The ACS advises men to be aware of testicular cancer and to seek prompt medical evaluation if a mass is found. Because regular testicular self-examinations have not been studied enough to show a reduction in the death rate from this cancer, the ACS does not recommend regular testicular self-examinations for men without specific testicular cancer risk factors.

However, some health care professionals think that not noticing masses promptly is an important factor in delaying treatment, and they recommend that all men perform monthly testicular self-examinations after puberty.

The choice of whether a monthly self-examination is to be performed should be made by each man. Men with risk factors such as cryptorchidism, previous germ cell tumor in one testicle, or a positive family history should seriously consider monthly examinations and discuss this issue with their health care providers.

Signs and symptoms of testicular cancer include a lump, swelling, dull ache, heaviness, and pain in the scrotum. The most common presenting symptom is a mass in the scrotum that the individual or sexual partner discovers. In contrast to the findings on breast self-examination, 95% of all masses of the testicle are malignant. Less common symptoms of testicular cancer include oligospermia. Often diagnosed as a component of an infertility evaluation, breast tenderness may also be present.

Symptoms of chronic cough, shortness of breast, chest pain, and hemoptysis are characteristic of spread of the disease to the lungs. Other common sites of metastases include the liver, brain, and bone.

Diagnosis

The diagnosis of testicular cancer is based on a combination of physical examination findings, laboratory tests, radiographic tests, and orchiectomy for tissue diagnosis. Orchiectomy is the recommended surgical procedure for obtaining a tissue diagnosis because fine-needle biopsy increases the risk of metastases. Physical examination should include an evaluation of the testicles, lymph nodes, and breast (because hormonally active testicular cancers can cause breast enlargement). Laboratory tests include beta-human chorionic gonadotropin levels and alpha fetoprotein markers. Radiographic tests include chest x-ray study and computed tomography of the abdomen and chest to determine the presence of distant metastases.

Testicular cancer is staged using the tumor, node, metastasis (TNM) system created by the American Joint Committee on Cancer.

The staging system contains four key pieces of information:

T refers to the extent of spread of the primary tumor to tissues next to the testicle.

N describes the extent of spread to regional (nearby) lymph nodes.

M indicates whether the cancer has metastasized (spread to nonregional [distant] lymph nodes or other organs of the body).

S indicates the serum levels of certain proteins produced by some testicular cancers.

TABLE 19–1 ▪ Testicular Cancer Staging Simplified (TNM) Version

Stage 0 (carcinoma in situ):	Preinvasive germ cell cancer.
Stage I:	No spread to lymph nodes or distant organs, and blood tests are normal.
Stage II:	Cancer has spread to regional lymph nodes but not to lymph nodes in other parts of the body or to distant organs.
Nonbulky stage II:	Spread to retroperitoneal (behind the abdominal cavity) lymph nodes, and lymph nodes are not larger than 5 cm (2 inches).
Bulky stage II:	Cancer has spread to 1 or more retroperitoneal lymph nodes, and they are larger than 5 cm.
Stage III:	Cancer has spread to distant lymph nodes and/or to distant organs, e.g., the lungs or liver.
Nonbulky stage III:	Metastases are limited to lymph nodes and lungs, and no mass is larger than 2 cm (about 3/4 inch).
Bulky stage III:	There are large metastases and lymph node metastases are larger than 2 cm, and/or cancer has spread to other organs, e.g., the liver or brain.

For selecting treatment, staging of testicular cancer is sometimes simplified to that seen in Table 19–1.

Another application of the TNM system used for advanced disease takes into account the markers and classifies the cancer as conferring low, medium, or poor prognosis. Some doctors give more aggressive chemotherapy regimens to patients who are in a high-risk category (Table 19–2).

Treatment

Treatment of testicular cancer is based on the pathology (seminoma and nonseminoma), the extent to which the disease has spread beyond the testicle, and the serum tumor markers present. Researchers developed the International Germ Cell Tumor Prognostic Classification to determine good, intermediate, and poor prognosis for individuals with seminoma or nonseminoma malignancies (Table 19–2).

For individuals with early-stage disease, treatment involves surgical removal of the testicle through the groin and may include standard or nerve-sparing retroperitoneal lymphadenectomy and postoperative radiation therapy (see Chapter 6, Surgical Oncology). For individuals with regional disease, cytotoxic chemotherapy may be added to the standard treatment modalities mentioned previously (see Chapter 7, Chemotherapy). Agents that have demonstrated activity in testicular

TABLE 19-2 ■ Risk Status

Risk Status	Nonseminoma	Stages	Seminoma	Stages
Good prognosis	No nonlung spread	IS (S1)	No nonlung spread	IIC
	Good markers	IIA (S1)	AFP normal	IIIA
	AFP < 1,000	IIB (S1)	HCG and LDH can be any level	IIIB
	HCG <5,000	IIC (S1)		IIIC
	LDH < 1.5	IIIA		
Intermediate prognosis	No nonlung spread	IS (S2)	Nonlung spread	IIIC with Non lung spread
	Intermediate markers	IIC (S2)	AFP normal	
	AFP 1000–10,000	IIIB	HCG and LDH can be any level	
	HCG 5000—50,000			
	LDH 1.5–10			
Poor prognosis	Nonlung spread	IS (S3)	None	
	High markers	IIC (S3)		
	AFP >10,000	All IIIC		
	HCG > 50,000			
	LDH > 10			

Key: AFP = alpha-fetoprotein; HCG = human chorionic gonadotropin; LDH = lactate dehydrogenase.

cancer include bleomycin, etoposide, cisplatin, vinblastine, dactinomycin, ifosfamide, and cyclophosphamide. In individuals with disseminated disease, cytotoxic therapy is the treatment of choice with surgery or radiation therapy to remove or treat residual disease for selected patients. High-dose cytotoxic therapy with hematopoietic cell transplantation (see Chapter 9, Hematopoietic Stem Cell Transplantation) is indicated for selected patients.

Rehabilitation

Rehabilitation for patients with testicular cancer includes counseling regarding potential sexual health issues related to the disease or treatment (see Chapter 33, Sexuality). Sexual health encompasses how the individual sees himself as a male (body image, self-concept), his perceptions of how others see him, and how he expresses his sexuality (relationships with others, intimacy, sexual desire and function, and fertility). Availability of psychosexual counseling, prosthetic devices, hormone replacement therapy, and sperm banking offer potential rehabilitation interventions for individuals with testicular cancer and their partners.

Because many survivors of testicular cancer receive a combination of cytotoxic drug and radiation therapy, evaluation for the occurrence of late treatment-related effects is a critical component of long-term care. Potential late effects include infertility, secondary malignancies (leukemias and solid tumors of the stomach, bladder, colon, rectum, and pancreas), renal dysfunction, pulmonary dysfunction, and hearing loss (see Chapter 36, Cancer Survivorship).

The Role of the Nurse

Nurses have a comprehensive role to play in the care individuals at risk for, or with, a diagnosis of testicular cancer. Nurses can offer counseling about testicular cancer risks and potential risk reduction treatments to parents who have male children with cryptorchidism and selected genetic abnormalities. Nurses also have a role in education of the public, particularly adolescent and young adult males, about testicular self-examination and critical signs and symptoms to be reported to the health care team immediately.

Once diagnosed, nurses work with the health care team to discuss treatment options with the patient. Side effect management and potential participation in clinical trials for testicular cancer should also be discussed. Finally, the nurse participates in the evaluation of patients after the completion of treatment for changes in quality of life for the patient and partner, compliance with recommended follow-up examinations and tests, signs and symptoms of recurrent disease, and late effects of cancer treatments (see Chapter 36, Cancer Survivorship).

Conclusions

Testicular cancer is a disease that occurs primarily in young men. The disease is treatable and often curable, regardless of stage at the time of diagnosis. Advances in surgical, radiation, and cytotoxic therapies have resulted in dramatic improvements in survival as well as quality of life. Access to a multidisciplinary care team, diagnostic, treatment, and rehabilitative services, as well as well-designed clinical trials, is a key component to improvements in clinical outcomes for patients with testicular cancer.

■ Penile Cancer

Incidence

The incidence of penile cancer is rare in the United States, accounting for less than 1% of all male genital cancers. Penile cancer occurs most frequently in males in the sixth and seventh decades of life. The incidence of penile cancer has decreased over the past 50 years with improved socioeconomic status in the United States. In addition to a decrease in the incidence of penile cancer, a shift toward diagnosis at an earlier stage has been observed.

Risk Factors

Risk factors for penile cancer include a nonretractable prepuce, human papillomavirus infection, smoking, and history of treatment of psoriasis with methoxsalen and ultraviolet A photochemotherapy. Circumcision may provide protection against cancer of the penis. However, circumcision is a controversial issue. Although penile cancer risk overall is lower among circumcised men, penile cancer risk is low in some uncircumcised populations. Circumcision is strongly associated with other socioethnic practices that decrease risk. The consensus among studies that have taken these other factors into account is that circumcision alone is not the major factor preventing cancer of the penis. It is important that the issue of circumcision not distract the public's attention from avoiding known penile cancer risk factors—having unprotected sexual relations with multiple partners (increasing the likelihood of human papillomavirus infection), poor penile hygiene, and cigarette smoking. For males who are uncircumcised, retraction of the prepuce during penile hygiene is recommended.

Detection

The most common presenting symptom in males with penile cancer is a mass, nodule, or ulcerated lesion on the penis. Other symptoms include swelling, erythema, itching, or burning under the foreskin, and a foul-smelling, purulent discharge.

Diagnosis

Diagnosis of penile cancer is based on results of an excisional or incisional biopsy of the lesion. To evaluate for evidence of spread of the disease, a thorough physical examination with a careful assessment of the groin for evidence of lymphadenopathy, chest x-ray study, and bone scan may be indicated.

Staging

Penile cancer is staged using the TNM classification as designated by the American Joint Committee on Cancer. After determining the tumor size, lymph node status, and presence of metastasis, the patient is assigned a Stage from 0 to 4.

Treatment

The treatment choices for patients with penile cancer depend on the size, location, and invasiveness of the lesion and the stage of disease. Treatment for localized disease may include wide local surgical excision, microscopically guided excision using Mohs' techniques, application of fluorouracil cream to local/superficial lesions, partial or complete penile amputation, and radiation therapy. For patients with regional disease, partial, complete, or radical penile amputation is recommended, with or without inguinal lymph node dissection and postoperative radiation therapy. For patients with disseminated disease at diagnosis, palliative surgery for control of local disease and palliative radiation therapy to sites of metastases (regional lymph nodes, bone) may be warranted.

New treatments for penile cancer designed to preserve appearance and function are being evaluated. Examples include use of CO_2 and yttrium-aluminum-garnet laser for localized lesions, use of radiosensitizers, cytotoxic drugs (cisplatin, 5-fluorouracil, vincristine, bleomycin, methotrexate), and biologic therapies for invasive and regional and distant metastases.

Rehabilitation

Rehabilitation for individuals with penile cancer involves collaboration with care providers before and after primary treatment of the disease. Body image, intimacy, urinary voiding, and sexual function issues need to be addressed. Evaluation for a penile prosthesis may be appropriate for selected patients (see Chapter 33, Sexuality).

The Role of the Nurse

Nursing care for patients with penile cancer depends on the site of the lesion, the type of treatment, and the extent of treatment. Care focuses on the postoperative care of the surgical site (wound healing, skin care), teaching self-care skills (perineal care, lower-extremity care on the side of inguinal node dissection, voiding techniques), and management of side effects of cytotoxic therapy (oral hygiene, skin care, safety precautions for neurotoxicities, infection precautions, pulmonary hygiene, and perineal care).

Conclusions

Penile cancer is a relatively rare cancer in the United States. However, for individuals diagnosed with the disease, access to a multidisciplinary team of care providers that offer a full range of diagnostic, treatment, and rehabilitation services is critical to high-quality care.

■ Urethral Cancer

Incidence

Urethral cancer is a rare disease, with fewer than 2000 cases having been reported in the literature. The disease occurs more commonly in females than in males. The peak incidence for urethral cancer is between 50 and 70 years of age.

Risk Factors

Specific risk factors for urethral cancer are unknown. However, associations exist between urethral cancer and frequent infection, chronic irritation, venereal disease, and urethral strictures.

Detection

Common presenting symptoms of urethral cancer include a palpable urethral mass, urethral obstruction, discharge, bleeding, dysuria, and overflow incontinence. In males, penile, erosion, priapism, and impotence may be present. In females, hematuria and dyspareunia may be present.

Diagnosis

The diagnosis of urethral cancer is based on the findings on physical examination (external genitalia, perineum, palpation of inguinal lymph nodes, bimanual examination), radiologic examinations (computed tomography and/or magnetic resonance imaging of the abdomen and pelvis, chest x-ray study, intravenous pyelography, cystourethroscopy, and retrograde urography in males), urine cytology, and tissue biopsy.

Treatment

Treatment for urethral cancer is based on the gender of the patient, the site of the lesion, and the stage of the disease. For males, treatment may include partial or total penectomy, with or without inguinal lymphadenectomy, and with or without interstitial radiation or external radiation therapy. For advanced disease, patients may be evaluated for en bloc cystoprostatectomy. For females with limited invasion, laser ablation or partial urethrectomy are treatment options. For advanced disease, anterior pelvic exenteration may be considered. Researchers have not demonstrated benefit from the use of radiation therapy alone in the treatment of urethral cancer. Various cytotoxic agents, including 5-fluorouracil, methotrexate, vinblastine, doxorubicin, cisplatin, paclitaxel, carboplatin, and mitomycin C, have shown some activity in the treatment of urethral cancer.

Rehabilitation

Rehabilitation for the patient with urethral cancer encompasses psychosexual counseling, care of urinary or bowel diversions, and toileting techniques.

The Role of the Nurse

Nursing care for patients with urethral cancer is consistent with care described in the section for penile cancer.

Conclusions

Urethral cancer is an uncommon malignancy that threatens both quality and quantity of life for the individual. The care of patients with urethral cancer demands coordination of the expertise of multiple disciplines in evaluation, treatment, and rehabilitation of the patient.

■ Bladder Cancer

Incidence

The American Cancer Society estimates that 60,240 people in the United States will be diagnosed with bladder cancer in 2004, with approximately 12,710 people dying from the disease in 2004. The incidence of bladder cancer in males is three times greater than in females, and this disease occurs almost twice as frequently in white males than in African American males. Up to 90% of cancers of the bladder are localized at diagnosis and occur in the transitional epithelium of the bladder lining.

Risk Factors

Risk factors for bladder cancer include lifestyle choices, exposure to industrial and occupational carcinogens, and concurrent health problems. Lifestyle risk factors associated with an increased risk for bladder cancer are cigarette smoking, high dietary intake of nitrosamines, and phenacetin use. Industrial exposure to arylamines, toluidine, benzidine-based dyes, arsenic, leather dyestuff, and dry cleaner agents is associated with an increased risk for bladder cancer. Occupations at risk for bladder cancer include painters, truck drivers, drill press operators, leather workers, and dry cleaners. Individuals with spinal cord injuries or who have been exposed to *Schistosoma haematobium,* a parasite found primarily in Africa and the Middle East, are at increased risk for bladder cancer.

Detection

Individuals with bladder cancer often present to the health care system with one or more of the following signs and symptoms: gross hematuria, dysuria, frequency, urgency, and flank pain. Symptoms of advanced disease may include pelvic pain, lower-extremity edema, enlarged pelvic lymph nodes, and deep vein thrombosis.

Diagnosis

The diagnosis of bladder cancer is based on findings from physical examination, examination under anesthesia, urine cytology, intravenous pyelography or urography, cystoscopy, and biopsy of any suspicious lesions. More than 90% of cancers of the bladder are transitional cell carcinomas, 8% are squamous cell, and 2% are adenocarcinomas. In addition to histology, pathological grading of the tumor has a significant impact on treatment decisions and prognosis. Flow cytometry may be performed to evaluate the DNA content of the bladder tissue.

Staging

Staging of bladder cancer is based on clinical examination and depth of invasion of the bladder wall. The American Joint Committee on Cancer recommends the use of the TNM classification for bladder cancer.

Treatment

For individuals with superficial disease, transurethral resection and fulguration with or without intravesical cytotoxic therapy is the standard of care. Intravesical therapy is designed to concentrate the drug at the tumor sites in the bladder. Agents commonly used for intravesical therapy include thiotepa, mitomycin, gemcitabine, methotrexate, cisplatin, paclitaxel, and doxorubicin. A decrease in disease progression, conservation of the bladder, and decreased recurrence have been documented with immunotherapy with intravesical and subcutaneous bacillus Calmette-Guerin. Radical cystectomy with or without pelvic lymphadenectomy may be considered for patients with extensive superficial or refractory disease. In addition to surgery and cytotoxic drug

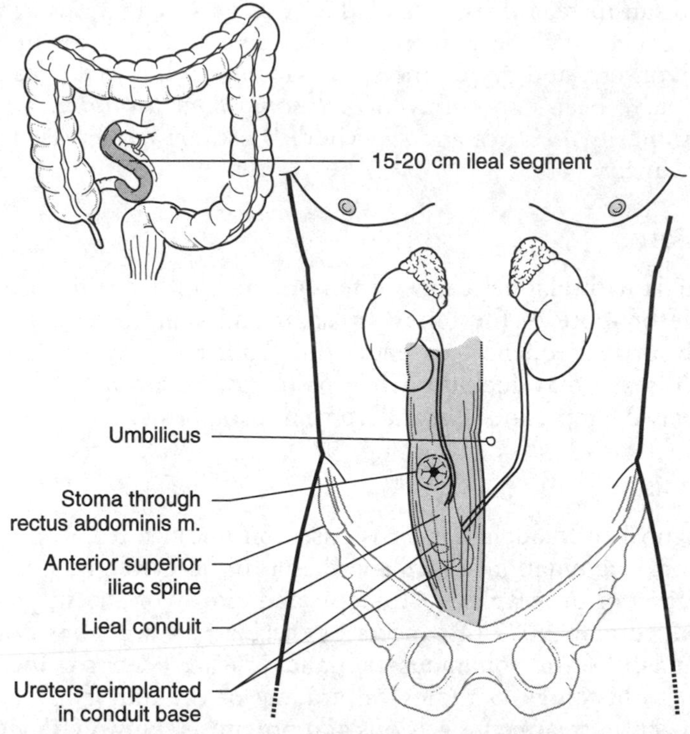

FIGURE 19–1 ■ Urinary Diversion Using a Segment of Ileum. As short a segment as possible is used, and it is usually positioned in the right lower quadrant of the abdomen in an isoperistaltic direction. *Source:* From Carroll, P. R. & Barbour, S. (1992). Urinary diversion & bladder substitution. In E. Tanagho & J. McAninch (Eds.), *Smith's general urology* (13th ed. p. 427). Norwalk, CT: Appleton & Lange.

therapy, some patients with local disease are candidates for interstitial radioisotopes with or without external radiation therapy.

For more advanced disease, radical cystectomy with urinary diversion is the treatment of choice. Urinary diversion is constructed using a piece of ileum to form a conduit (Figure 19–1) or with newer surgical techniques, a continent urinary reservoir (Figure 19–2). The advantage of the continent urinary reservoir is that there is no need to wear an external urine collection appliance and voiding can be achieved through self-catheterization of the reservoir. For individuals who are not good surgical candidates, external radiation therapy with or without interstitial radioisotopes or cytotoxic drug therapy may be considered.

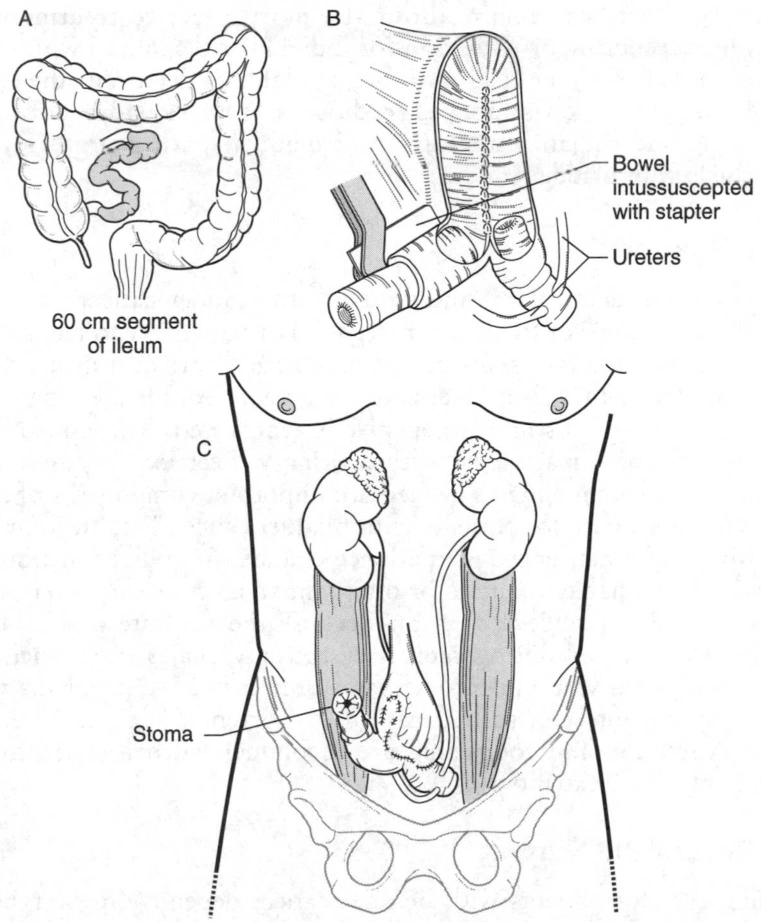

FIGURE 19–2 ■ Kock Pouch Urinary Reservoir.
(A) Shaded area indicates section of small intestine selected for reservoir construction. (B) Ureters implanted on afferent (nonrefluxing) limb and efferent limb (with nipple valve) for stoma created by using stapling devices. (C) Completed reservoir with the efferent limb drawn through the abdominal wll and stoma created.
Source: From Carroll, P. R. & Barbour, S. (1992). Urinary diversion & bladder substitution. In E. Tanagho & J. McAninch (Eds.), *Smith's general urology* (13th ed. p. 432). Norwalk, CT: Appleton & Lange.

Many questions remain about the most effective treatment to achieve cure, control, or palliation for individuals diagnosed with bladder cancer. Currently, clinical trials are available to determine the effectiveness of prevention strategies, radiosensitizers, neoadjuvant cytotoxic drug and radiation therapy, and bladder-sparing strategies for individuals with bladder cancer.

Rehabilitation

Rehabilitation needs of the individual with bladder cancer vary, depending on the type of treatment received. For patients who have a urinary diversion, self-care skills in application and care of a urinary collection appliance or self-catheterization are required; for these patients, referral to an enterostomal therapist is warranted. Threats to self-concept and body image exist with a urinary diversion. Psychological evaluation and counseling as needed are important components of a rehabilitation program for patients with bladder cancer. Finally, individuals with bladder cancer may experience changes in sexual functioning. Males may be unable to obtain or maintain an erection; however, some males are able to achieve orgasm. Because the prostate and seminal vesicles are removed during radical cystectomy, males experience dry orgasms. Women who undergo a cystectomy may have problems with penile-vaginal intercourse because of a shortened vagina. A sexual health evaluation and counseling are recommended before treatment (see Chapter 33, Sexuality).

The Role of the Nurse

Nursing care for patients with bladder cancer depends on the type of treatment. Immediate care focuses on the postoperative care of the surgical site (wound healing, infection). Subsequently, care shifts to monitoring for complications from surgery (fistulas, bowel or ureteral obstruction). Teaching self-care skills (perineal care, lower-extremity care on side of the node dissection, voiding techniques) are important in preparation for discharge. Management of side effects of cytotoxic therapy (oral hygiene, skin care, safety precautions for neurotoxicities, infection precautions, pulmonary hygiene, and perineal care), and management of responses to Bacillus Calmette-Guerin therapy (allergic reactions, fever, arthralgia, and prostatitis in males) are important for continued care.

Conclusions

Although more than 90% of individuals with bladder cancer have localized disease at the time of diagnosis, up to 80% experience recurrences. Both treatment modalities and the potential consequences of the treatments have implications for individuals diagnosed with the disease in terms of survival and quality of survival. The availability of a multidisciplinary team of care providers is crucial to treatment planning, care during therapy, rehabilitation, and long-term surveillance.

■ Renal Cancer

Incidence

Each year, about 35,710 new cases of renal cancer are diagnosed (22,080 in men and 13,630 in women) in the United States, and about 12,480 people (7,780 men and 4,610 women) die of this disease. Renal cell carcinoma, which occurs in the parenchyma of the kidney, is the most common type of renal cancer. The median age at diagnosis for individuals with renal cancer is 57 years, and the disease is rare in people under the age of 35. The incidence of renal cancer is two times greater in males than in females.

Risk Factors

Multiple risk factors exist for renal cancer. Lifestyle factors, including cigarette smoking, obesity, use of analgesics containing phenacetin, and urban residence, are associated with a higher incidence of renal cancer. Occupational and environmental risk factors for renal cancer include exposure to asbestos, cadmium, gasoline, and lead acetate. The role of genetics in the development of renal cancer has been studied over the past two decades. Inherited forms of renal cancer have been associated with a translocation of the short arm of chromosome 3. The familial form is consistent with an autosomal dominant pattern of inheritance. Individuals with von Hippel-Lindau disease, a cancer syndrome, are also at greater risk for renal cancer.

Detection

Hematuria is the primary presenting symptom of individuals with renal cancer. Additional symptoms may include the presence of a dull, aching flank pain; a palpable abdominal mass; and fever. Most patients with renal cancer are diagnosed when the disease is relatively localized. Symptoms consistent with advanced disease include weight loss, anemia, and hypercalcemia.

Diagnosis

A thorough evaluation is required to determine whether the symptoms are due to benign renal cysts or a malignancy. Diagnostic tests include a battery of radiographic studies: renal ultrasound, computed tomography, and angiography; excretory urography; and a kidney-ureters-bladder study. Magnetic resonance imaging also has a role in the diagnosis of renal cancer. Finally, a fine-needle biopsy of the lesion may be obtained. Most renal cancers are renal cell adenocarcinomas (85%).

Staging

Staging of renal cancer is based on clinical examination and degree of spread of the disease beyond the kidney. The American Joint Committee on Cancer recommends the use of the TNM classification for renal cancer.

Treatment

Treatment of individuals with renal cancer is based on the stage of disease. For early-stage disease, nephrectomy, simple or radical, is the accepted and often curative therapy. For selected patients with bilateral tumors or only one functioning kidney, partial nephrectomy, thus avoiding dialysis or transplantation, may be curative. For individuals who are not surgical candidates, external radiation therapy or arterial embolization provide palliative therapy.

For patients with more advanced disease, radical nephrectomy with resection of the renal vein and vena cava is recommended with or without lymphadenectomy. Although preoperative or postoperative external radiation therapy has been used in the treatment of individuals with advanced disease, no survival benefit has been demonstrated other than palliation of symptoms. Patients who are not surgical candidates may undergo arterial embolization for palliation.

The use of cytotoxic drug therapy in patients with renal cancer is of limited benefit. Responses do not exceed 10%. However, approximately 15% of selected patients have demonstrated responses, some of which are durable, to immunotherapy with interleukin-2 or interferon alfa. Given the poor response rate to systemic cytotoxic and immunologic therapy, potential entry to clinical trials should be discussed with each patient with advanced disease.

The Role of the Nurse

Nursing care for patients with renal cancer depends on the type of treatment being administered. Immediate care focuses on postoperative care (pain management, wound healing, monitoring remaining renal function, atelectasis, infection, and bleeding) (see Unit V for specific symptoms). For patients who will be anephretic after surgery, care focuses on counseling regarding diet, importance of fluid intake, dialysis demands, or transplantation options. Patients receiving radiation therapy require monitoring for acute side effects of therapy (myelosuppression, skin changes, and inflammation of tissues within radiation field) and teaching of self-care skills to reduce the severity of predictable side effects. Monitoring for side effects of immunotherapy (fever, fatigue, liver dysfunction, myelosuppression, flulike symptoms, depression, and respiratory distress) and teaching patients self-care skills to decrease the impact of treatment side effects on quality of life are key roles for nurses.

Conclusions

Renal cancer is an uncommon cancer. The disease is treatable, even in advanced stages. Surgery remains the primary therapy for curative intent, although in rare cases of renal cancer, spontaneous regressions have been observed. The use of immunotherapy in the treatment of renal cancer offers new hope to patients with the disease.

■ Resources

- American Cancer Society: 800-ACS-2345 or *www.cancer.org*
    - Bladder cancer: *http://www.cancer.org/docroot/CRI/CRI_2x.asp?sitearea=&dt=44*
    - Penile cancer: *http://www.cancer.org/docroot/CRI/CRI_2x.asp?sitearea=&dt=35*
    - Testicular cancer: *http://www.cancer.org/docroot/CRI/CRI_2x.asp?sitearea=&dt=41*

Bibliography

Abeloff, M.D., Armitage, J.O., Lichter, A.S. & Niederbuber, J.E. (Eds.) (2000). *Clinical oncology,* 2nd Edition. New York, NY: Churchill-Livingston.

American Joint Committee on Cancer (2002). *AJCC cancer staging manual,* 6th Edition. New York, NY: Springer.

Bast, R.C. Jr., Kufe, D.W., Pollock, R.E., Welch-Selbaum, R.R., Holland, J.F. & Frei, E. (Eds.) (2000). *Cancer medicine,* 5th Edition. Hamilton, Ontario: B.C. Decker, Inc.

DeVita, V.T., Hellman, S. & Rosenberg, S.A. (Eds.) (2001). *Cancer: Principles and practice of oncology,* 6th Edition. Philadelphia, PA: Lippincott Williams & Wilkins.

National Cancer Institute. (06/03/2003). Bladder cancer (PDQ): Treatment. Retrieved June, 2003 from *http://www.cancer.gov/cancerinfo/pdq/treatment/bladder/healthprofessional/*

National Cancer Institute. (06/20/2003). Penile cancer (PDQ): Treatment. Retrieved June, 2003 from *http://www.cancer.gov/cancerinfo/pdq/treatment/penile/healthprofessional/*

National Cancer Institute. (06/06/2003). Renal cell cancer (PDQ): Treatment. Retrieved June, 2003 from *http://www.cancer.gov/cancerinfo/pdq/treatment/renalcell/healthprofessional/*

National Cancer Institute. (6/18/2003). Testicular cancer (PDQ): Treatment. Retrieved June, 2003 from *http://www.cancer.gov/cancerinfo/pdq/treatment/testicular/healthprofessional/*

National Cancer Institute. (06/06/2003). Urethral cancer (PDQ): Treatment. Retrieved June, 2003 from *http://www.cancer.gov/cancerinfo/pdq/treatment/urethral/healthprofessional/*

Walsh, P.C., Retik, A.B., Vaughan, E.D., et al. (Eds.) (2002). *Campbell's urology,* 8th Edition. Philadelphia, PA: W.B. Saunders.

Yarbo, C.H., Frogge, M., Goodman, M., & Groenwald, S. (Eds.) (2000). *Cancer nursing: Principles and practice,* 5th Edition. Boston, MA: Jones and Bartlett.

CHAPTER

20

Gynecologic Malignancies

Virginia R. Martin

Gynecologic cancers account for 13% of all cancers in women. Screening is particularly effective for many of these cancers because it is possible to identify preinvasive and in situ cancers that are curable. However, there are still several gynecologic cancers for which we do not have valid and reliable screening, and therefore, these continue to be diagnosed at an advanced stage. The multifaceted care of women with gynecologic cancer at either end of this spectrum is both rewarding and challenging to nurses.

■ Endometrial Cancer

Incidence, Etiology, and Risk Factors

Endometrial cancer is the most common cancer of the female genital tract. In the United States, it is estimated that 40,320 new cases will be diagnosed in 2004, and 7,090 women will die from this disease. Endometrial cancer is predominantly a disease of postmenopausal women. The endometrial lining of the uterus changes as a result of the influence of estrogen and progesterone. Endometrial hyperplasia develops when the endometrium is hyperstimulated by estrogens; it is classified as either hyperplasia without atypia or hyperplasia with atypia, the latter being a precursor to endometrial cancer.

The primary risk factors for endometrial cancer are those that create an environment of prolonged or unopposed estrogen stimulation of the endometrium, such as obesity, exogenous estrogen, early menarche, late menopause (after age 52), nulliparity, diabetes, hypertension, older age, polycystic ovary syndrome, estrogen-secreting ovarian tumors, and positive family history. Rates for endometrial cancer are highest in North America and are low in Southern and Eastern Asia and most of Africa.

Prevention and Detection

In 2001, the American Cancer Society concluded that there was insufficient evidence to recommend screening women at average risk for endometrial cancer. Endometrial sampling is not a practical or cost-effective screening method for all women. Instead, the American Cancer Society recommended that because endometrial cancer is triggered by the presence of symptoms (usually bleeding), at the onset of menopause, women at average and increased risk should be informed about risks and symptoms of endometrial cancer. Women at high risk (those with or at risk for hereditary nonpolyposis colon cancer, a genetic condition associated with colorectal and endometrial cancer) should begin annual screening at age 35, and endometrial sampling is often recommended

Diagnosis, Evaluation, and Staging

The most common sign of endometrial cancer is vaginal bleeding. It is never normal for any postmenopausal woman to have vaginal bleeding. Sampling of the endometrium and the cervical canal is the essential diagnostic step. Endocervical curettage and endometrial biopsy can be performed in the physician's office. A surgical fractionated dilatation and curettage requires anesthesia and is indicated if an endometrial biopsy is nondiagnostic. The next step after diagnosis is to determine the extent of the disease by imaging studies. A transvaginal ultrasound, computed tomography, or magnetic resonance imaging may be used to image the uterus. Before 1988, endometrial cancer staging was performed clinically, but the International Federation of Gynecology and Obstetrics (FIGO) subsequently adopted a pathological staging classification system (Table 20–1). The surgical classification of endometrial cancers is based on uterine size, cervical involvement, and tumor grade. Prognostic factors include tumor grade, high-risk pathology (papillary serous or clear cell), extrauterine involvement, and depth of myometrial invasion. Progesterone receptor positivity is a highly significant prognostic factor, and aneuploidy and HER2/*neu* positivity are poor prognostic factors. Endometrial cancers are graded as follows: grade 1, well differentiated; grade 2, moderately differentiated; and grade 3, poorly differentiated. Seventy-five percent of patients are diagnosed in the early stages.

TABLE 20–1 ■ FIGO Staging of Endometrial Carcinoma

Stage	Substage	Description
Stage I:		Cancer is limited to the *corpus* (body) of the uterus, and has not spread to lymph nodes or distant sites.
	Stage IA:	Cancer is limited to the inner lining of the uterus (endometrium).
	Stage IB:	Cancer has spread less than halfway through the muscular wall of the uterus (myometrium).
	Stage IC:	Cancer has spread more than halfway through the myometrium but has not spread beyond the body of the uterus.
Stage II:		Cancer has spread from the body of the uterus to the lower part of the uterus next to the vagina (cervix) but has not spread to lymph nodes or distant sites.
	Stage IIA:	Cancer is in the body of the uterus and involves the endocervical mucosa.
	Stage IIB:	Cancer is in the body of the uterus and has spread to the supporting connective tissue of the cervix (cervical stroma).
Stage III:		Cancer has spread outside the uterus but remains confined to the pelvis.
	Stage IIIA:	Cancer has spread to the serosa (outer surface) of the uterus or to the fallopian tubes or ovaries (adnexa), or there are cancer cells in the peritoneal fluid.
	Stage IIIB:	Cancer has spread to the vagina.
	Stage IIIC:	Cancer has spread to pelvic and/or para-aortic lymph nodes.
Stage IV:		The cancer has spread to the mucosa of the urinary bladder or the rectum, and/or has spread to lymph nodes in the groin, and/or has spread to organs away from the uterus, e.g., the bones or lungs.
	Stage IVA:	Cancer has spread to the mucosa of the rectum or bladder. It may or may not have spread to lymph nodes but has not spread to distant sites.
	Stage IVB:	Cancer has spread to distant sites, e.g., the bones or lungs.

Key: FIGO = International Federation of Gynecology and Obstetrics.

Treatment

The treatment plan must be individualized and must take into account prognostic factors determined by surgical staging. The mainstay of treatment is surgery (see Chapter 6, Surgical Oncology). Surgical intervention consists of a total abdominal hysterectomy and bilateral salpingo-oophorectomy, sampling of the peritoneal fluid, biopsy of any extrauterine lesions, and sampling or excision of suspicious lymph nodes (pelvic and para-aortic). Laparoscopic surgical approaches are still under investigation. Women are classified after surgical staging as being at low risk, intermediate risk, or high risk for recurrence. Low-risk patients (stage IA) undergo surgery only. Those at intermediate risk (stages IB, IC, IIA, and IIB) may be offered external-beam radiation therapy, possibly with brachytherapy at the vaginal cuff. Women with high-risk endometrial cancer receive an individualized plan that may or may not include surgery, radiation therapy, and/or chemotherapy or hormonal therapy with progestins. The chemotherapeutic agents used most frequently are doxorubicin, cisplatin, carboplatin, and paclitaxel (see Chapter 7, Chemotherapy). These agents may be used alone or in combination. If endometrial cancer recurs, treatment is palliative and may be a combination of radiation therapy, chemotherapy, and progestins.

Side Effects, Complications, and the Role of the Nurse

After surgery, women with endometrial cancer are at a high risk for complications because they may be older, obese, and/or diabetic. These complications include thrombophlebitis, pulmonary embolus, wound separation, and pneumonia immediately after surgery. Return of bowel function may be slower, and lower-extremity edema can be a potential complication from lymph node dissection. Complications from radiation therapy may include diarrhea, dysuria, nausea, and urinary frequency. Antidiarrheal agents, urinary analgesics, and antiemetics may be offered for symptom management. Side effects for specific chemotherapy agents must be reviewed and a plan developed to manage the acute toxicities. Psychosocial assessment of needs must be included because these women need support when they are confronted with a new cancer diagnosis, including alleviation of fears related to treatment and concern about their sexuality (see Unit V for specific symptoms).

■ Cervical Cancer

Incidence, Etiology, and Risk Factors

Cervical cancer incidence is estimated at 10,520 new cases and is projected to cause 3,900 deaths in 2004. The incidence of cervical cancer has dropped dramatically in countries worldwide where an organized screening and treatment program is available. Cervical cancer is preceded by a preinvasive condition known as squamous intraepithelial lesion or cervical intraepithelial neoplasia. Over time, the preinvasive condition may progress to carcinoma in situ and then invasive cervical cancer. The prolonged natural history of the disease makes it an ideal disease for screening interventions. The average age of a woman with preinvasive disease is 10 to 15 years younger than that of a woman with cervical cancer.

There is a strong causal relationship between human papillomavirus (HPV) and cervical cancer. In fact, high-risk types of HPV DNA are present in 93–100% of squamous cell carcinomas of the cervix. HPV is transmitted during sexual activity. Most HPV infections are transient and result in no cellular changes or low-grade intraepithelial lesions. Studies have shown that infection with high-risk HPV types may lead to low-grade or high-grade intraepithelial lesions. High-grade lesions progress to cervical carcinoma if there is no intervention. Even though HPV is the most important risk factor, epidemiologic studies have identified several other factors, a finding that helps explain why HPV infections resolve spontaneously in some women and progress to invasive cancer in others. These factors are early age at first coitus, multiple sex partners, cigarette smoking, vitamin deficiencies, hormonal status, presence of other sexually transmitted diseases, and immunosuppression. Some of these factors (e.g., multiple sexual partners) are likely to reflect risk of acquiring HPV and other sexually transmitted diseases, whereas others (e.g., cigarette smoking, vitamin deficiencies, and immunosuppression) appear to increase risk independently or synergistically with HPV infection. Carcinoma in situ and preinvasive forms of the disease are highly curable. At the onset of the disease, cellular growth is slow. Once it is invasive, it grows rapidly.

Prevention and Early Detection

About half of the cervical cancer cases found in the United States are diagnosed in women who have never been screened. This highlights the need for reaching women and teaching them about the importance of screening.

The most-used screening method is the Papanicolaou smear. As an alternative form of cervical screening cytology, the liquid-based Papanicolaou test has been introduced in the past several years. Colposcopy is direct visualization of the cervix after acetic acid is applied. Any abnormal cells appear white after the acetic acid is applied. Table 20–2 lists American Cancer Society screening guidelines for cervical cancer.

Evaluation and Staging

The signs of early disease include a thin, watery discharge that usually is blood tinged. As the disease progresses, the patient has frequent episodes of bleeding especially after sexual intercourse. A foul smelling discharge, pain, and edema are late signs of disease.

TABLE 20–2 ■ American Cancer Society Guidelines for Early Detection of Cervical Cancer

- All women should begin cervical cancer screening about 3 years after they being having vaginal intercourse, but no later than when they are 21 year old. Testing should be done every year with the regular Papanicolaou (Pap) test or every 2 years using the newer liquid-based Pap test.
- Beginning at age 30, women who have had 3 normal Pap test results in a row may get tested every 2 to 3 years. Women who have certain risk factors should continue to be tested.
- Another reasonable option for over 30 is to get tested every 3 years (but not more frequently) with either the regular or the liquid-based Pap test, plus the DNA test for human papillomavirus.
- Women 70 years of ago or older who have had 3 or more normal Pap test results in a row and no abnormal Pap test results in the previous 10 years may choose to stop having Pap tests. Some women need to continue testing.
- Women who have had a total hysterectomy may also choose to stop having Pap tests, unless the surgery was performed for cervical cancer.

Initial evaluation of the patient takes place in the office with a clinical appraisal and may include colposcopy and/or biopsy as well as endocervical curettage. The diagnosis is confirmed with an examination under anesthesia that often includes a cystoscopy and/or proctosigmoidoscopy. The clinical staging is based on the FIGO classification system (Table 20–3), taking into account the clinical extent of the disease, which includes the cervical biopsy findings, the class of cytologic interpretation, and the histologic grade.

Treatment

The choice of therapy is dictated by the FIGO stage of the disease. Patients with intraepithelial neoplasia can be treated and cured with an ablative or excisional approach. The choice often depends on several factors, including the site of the lesion, the grade of the lesion, the desire for childbearing, and the cost. Methods include cryotherapy surgery, loop electrosurgical excision procedure, cold knife conization, and hysterectomy. Table 20–4 outlines treatment approaches based on stage of disease.

Side Effects and Complications

In the immediate postoperative period, complications include infection, pain, fluid and electrolyte imbalance, bleeding, infection, pneumonia,

TABLE 20-3 ■ FIGO Staging of Cervical Carcinoma

Stage 0:	Carcinoma in situ.	
Stage I:	Cancer has invaded the cervix but has not spread anywhere else.	
	Stage IA1:	The area of invasion is less than 3 mm deep and less than 7 mm wide.
	Stage IA2:	The area of invasion is between 3 mm and 5 mm deep and less than 7 mm wide.
	Stage IB1:	The cancer is no larger than 4 cm.
	Stage IB2:	The cancer is larger than 4 cm.
Stage II:	Cancer has spread beyond the cervix, but it is still within the pelvic area.	
	Stage IIA:	Cancer has spread beyond the cervix to the upper part (but not the lower third) of the vagina.
	Stage IIB:	Cancer has spread to the parametrial tissue next to the cervix.
Stage III:	Cancer has spread to the lower part of the vagina or the pelvic wall. The cancer may be blocking the ureters (tubes that carry urine from the kidneys to the bladder).	
	Stage IIIA:	Cancer has spread to the lower third of the vagina but not to the pelvic wall.
	Stage IIIB:	Cancer extends to the pelvic wall and/or blocks urine flow to the bladder.
Stage IV:	Cancer has spread to nearby organs or other parts of the body.	
	Stage IVA:	Cancer has spread to the bladder or rectum.
	Stage IVB:	Cancer has spread to distant organs beyond the pelvic area.

Key: FIGO = International Federation of Gynecology and Obstetrics.

TABLE 20-4 ■ Treatment Approaches for Cervical Cancer

- Stage 1A1: radical abdominal hysterectomy or vaginal hysterectomy
- Stage 1B—IIA: radical abdominal hysterectomy with bilateral pelvic lymphadenectomy and para-aortic lymphadenectomy, or radiation therapy and chemotherapy
- Stage IB2 and IIA: Cisplatin alone or in combination with 5-fluorouracil and radiation therapy
- Stage IIA and greater: radiation therapy and chemotherapy
- Recurrent disease: single-agent or combination chemotherapy, possible pelvic exenteration

deep vein thrombosis, and pulmonary embolism. Long-term complications include bladder dysfunction, lymphedema, lymphocysts, and sexual dysfunction. Radiation side effects include skin reactions, diarrhea, vaginal injury, and more rarely, fistula formation. Chemotherapy side effects depend on the drug regimen used but in general cause anorexia, fatigue, nausea and vomiting, and bone marrow suppression (see Unit V for specific symptoms).

The Role of the Nurse

Nurses have a role in educating young people about the risks associated with being sexually active at an early age. This includes the importance of seeing a health care professional if they are sexually active. Information about the correlation of smoking with cervical cancer should be presented. Educating women about screening and providing screening services are critical to early detection.

Nurses are key in developing the plan of care to manage the side effects of treatment. The patient is less likely to be distressed and more able to maintain control during treatment if she has received education and preparation from the nursing professional. It is especially important for the nurse to assess sexual functioning baseline and to provide thorough information about preventing vaginal injury. Vaginal dilators and lubricants are helpful in maintaining vaginal function for intercourse or for posttreatment follow-up pelvic examinations (see Chapter 33, Sexuality).

■ Ovarian Cancer

Incidence, Etiology, and Risk Factors

Ovarian cancer is the most lethal of the gynecologic cancers. It is estimated that 25,580 women will be diagnosed in 2004, and 16,090 women will die. It is the fifth leading cause of death in women of all ages. The disease occurs more frequently in the later decades of life. The etiology of ovarian cancer continues to be investigated, but theories of causation are emerging. These include the ovulation hypothesis, which relates ovarian risk to incessant ovulation, and the pituitary gonadotropin hypothesis, which implicates elevations in gonadotropin/estrogen levels. Some evidence indicates that chronic inflammatory processes may be related to ovarian cancer. Other causative processes include talc/asbestos exposure, endometriosis, and pelvic inflammatory disease. Protective measures, such as tubal ligation, oral contraceptives, and hysterectomy, may reduce the risk of the disease. There are three major pathological categories of ovarian tumors (epithelial, stromal, and germ cell) and more than 30 subtypes. Epithelial tumors constitute 85%–90% of tumors.

The risk factors are classified as genetic, environmental, and endocrine. About 10% of cases occur in women with a family history of cancer.

Prevention and Early Detection

Screening is currently not recommended for the asymptomatic population. It is recommended that all women have a complete family history taken and an annual rectovaginal pelvic exam as part of their routine care. High-risk individuals should have a rectovaginal pelvic exam, CA, ca 125 blood test, and transvaginal ultrasound on at least an annual basis.

Evaluation and Staging

The most frequently reported symptoms of ovarian cancer are increased abdominal size, abdominal bloating, abdominal pain, indigestion, and changes in bowel or bladder habits. It is hoped that educating women about the signs and symptoms of ovarian cancer will improve survival. About 75% of women are diagnosed at an advanced stage of the disease. An ovarian mass should be investigated by ultrasound, a computed tomographic scan, and CACA 125. Staging is based on the FIGO system and is outlined in Table 20–5. Stage of disease, amount of tumor left behind after surgery, grade of tumor, histology, absence or presence of ascites, performance status, and age are all prognostic factors of importance.

TABLE 20–5 ■ FIGO Staging of Ovarian Carcinoma

Stage I:	Cancer is limited to the ovary (or ovaries).
Stage II:	Cancer involves one or both ovaries and has involved pelvic organs, e.g., the uterus, fallopian tubes, bladder, the sigmoid colon, or the rectum, and/or pelvic fluid cytology is positive.
Stage III:	Cancer involves one or both ovaries with peritoneal implants (small bowel, omentum, surface of the liver) outside the pelvis and/or retroperitoneal or inguinal nodes are positive.
Stage IV:	The cancer involves one or both ovaries. Distant metastasis to the inside of the liver, the lungs, or other organs located outside of the peritoneal cavity has occurred. Positive pleural fluid cytology is also evidence of stage IV disease.

Key: FIGO = International Federation of Gynecology and Obstetrics.

TABLE 20–6 ■ Ovarian Cancer Treatment Options

- Stage IA and IB: surgery alone
- Stage IC and higher: surgery followed by combination chemotherapy

Treatment

Ovarian cancer treatment has two major challenges: most cases are in the late stage at diagnosis, and the relapse rate is 80%. Table 20–6 lists treatment options by stage of disease. Surgery is the mainstay of treatment for ovarian cancer. The surgical goal is to leave no tumor larger than 1 cm behind. The procedure includes an abdominal hysterectomy, bilateral salpingo-oophorectomy, scraping of the inner surface of the diaphragm, peritoneal cytology, omentectomy, multiple peritoneal biopsies, pelvic and para-aortic lymph node sampling, and multiple random biopsies. Minimal residual disease is associated with improved survival.

The current standard chemotherapy after surgery is paclitaxel and platinum for six cycles. Newer agents, such as gemcitabine, topotecan, and liposomal doxorubicin, are being evaluated.

Ovarian cancer that recurs is a chronic disease in which symptoms can be managed for a prolonged period of time but cure is not a realistic possibility. Treatment for recurrent disease often starts with one or more of the agents used in primary therapy if the disease-free interval is greater then 6 months. Other chemotherapy agents used include ifosfamide, hexamethylmelamine, 5-fluorouracil, oral etoposide, gemcitabine, vinorelbine, topotecan, liposomal doxorubicin, and hormonal therapy.

Side Effects and Complications

Most patients recover quickly from surgery without complications and begin chemotherapy soon after surgery. Side effects depend on the drugs used but may include hair loss, nausea and/or vomiting, diarrhea, myelosuppression, arthralgias and myalgias, and neurotoxicities. As the disease progresses, the main problems are ascites, bowel obstruction, malnutrition or cachexia, and/or lymphedema. Most problems relate to the abdominal area where the disease tends to stay (see Unit V for specific symptoms).

The Role of the Nurse

Nurses must teach healthy women to continue yearly screening visits to their physicians beyond the reproductive years. A yearly pelvic examination is important—it may lead to an early diagnosis of ovarian cancer. Once a diagnosis is made and treatment is begun, nurses are partners with patients in their care and must teach them about the potential side effects of treatment and complications that should be reported immediately. The focus of nursing care is to promote optimal quality of life for patients with advanced disease (see Chapter 37, End of Life). Significant time should be allowed for assessment of coping skills and emotional needs as part of the care plan for each patient (see Chapters 27 [Anxiety and Depression in the Oncology Setting] and 35 [Psychosocial-Spiritual Responses to Cancer and Treatment: Living with Cancer]).

■ Gestational Trophoblastic Neoplasia

Etiology and Risk Factors

Gestational trophoblastic neoplasia (GTN) refers to all neoplastic disorders arising from the chorionic portion of the placenta and can occur after any gestational event, including a partial or complete hydatiform mole, placental site trophoblastic tumor, invasive mole, and gestational choriocarcinoma. Advanced maternal age and previous molar pregnancy are the most significant risk factors. Bleeding in the first trimester of pregnancy is a common sign, along with a discrepancy in the size and the date of the pregnancy.

Evaluation and Staging

Ultrasound is a reliable and sensitive technique for diagnosis. An enhanced computed tomographic scan of the pelvis, abdomen, lungs, and brain is performed to complete the work-up. Human chorionic gonadotropin (hCG) level is elevated in all patients with GTN. The hCG level is directly related to the number of viable tumor cells. Suction curretage is the preferred method for evacuation while hysterectomy may be considered in a woman no longer interested in fertility. GTN is both staged and scored based on prognotic factors.

There are three classification systems for metastatic gestational tumors (Door, 2002).

Treatment

The treatment after evacuation for nonmetastatic disease and what is called low-risk metastatic disease is single-agent chemotherapy consisting of methotrexate or dactinomycin (see Chapter 7, Chemotherapy). Both agents have comparable remission rates, 90%–100%. The hCG titers are monitored until three consecutive negative titers have been obtained. For patients with high-risk metastatic disease, a combined-modality approach may be needed, including multiagent chemotherapy and possible surgery. Often, the agents combined are methotrexate, actinomycin, etoposide, cyclophosphamide, and/or vincristine. Treatment is continued for several cycles after the hCG level normalizes. With aggressive therapy, high-risk patients have a 75% cure rate.

The Role of the Nurse

Nursing intervention includes education about the unusual disease process and treatment. Often, psychosocial support is an important component of nursing care because grief over the loss of a pregnancy and fear of disease and treatment are concurrent issues for these young patients (see Chapter 35, Psychosocial-Spiritual Responses to Cancer and Treatment: Living with Cancer). Women who have had a complete or partial molar pregnancy can anticipate a normal outcome of a subsequent pregnancy, although avoiding pregnancy during the first year after treatment is recommended.

■ Conclusion

Caring for women with gynecologic cancer poses many challenges for nurses. Nurses assume primary roles in helping women to assess their cancer risk and to understand all personal, environmental, and genetic factors relating to their individual risk profile. Nurses help women obtain information about the disease and the treatment plan and also provide information about the potential complications and side effects of treatment. The patient with gynecologic cancer is less likely to be distressed and more able to maintain control during treatment if she receives education and preparation from the nurse.

■ Resources

- American Cancer Society: 800-ACS-2345 or *www.cancer.org*
  - Cervical cancer: *www.cancer.org/docroot/CRI/CRI_2x.asp?sitearea=&dt=8*
  - Endometrial cancer: *www.cancer.org/docroot/CRI/CRI_2x.asp?sitearea=&dt=11*
  - Ovarian Cancer: *www.cancer.org/docroot/CRI/CRI_2x.asp?sitearea=&dt=33*

- Gynecologic Cancer Foundation: information hotline 800-444-4441 or *www.wcn.org/gcf*
- National Cancer Institute 800-4-CANCER or *www.cancer.gov*
  - Cervical cancer: *www.nci.nih.gov/cancerinfo/types/cervical/*
  - Endometrial cancer: *www.nci.nih.gov/cancer_information/cancer_type/endometrial/*
  - Ovarian cancer: *www.nci.nih.gov/cancerinfo/types/ovarian/*
- National Ovarian Cancer Coalition: 888-OVARIAN or *www.ovarian.org*
- Ovarian Cancer National Alliance: 202-452-5910 or *www.ovariancancer.org*
- SHARE: Self Help for Women with Breast or Ovarian Cancer: 212-719-1204
- Society of Gynecologic Oncologists: 312-644-6610 or *www.sgo.org*

Bibliography

Door, A. (2002). Less common gynecologic malignancies. *Seminars in Oncology Nursing, 18,* 207–222.

Fischer, M. (2002). Cancer of the cervix. *Seminars in Oncology Nursing 18,* 193–199.

Martin, V. R. (2002). Ovarian cancer. *Seminars in Oncology Nursing 18,* 174–183.

Porter, S. (2002). Endometrial cancer. *Seminars in Oncology Nursing 18,* 200–206.

Smith, R.A., Cokkindes, V., & Eyre, H. (2003). American Cancer Society Guidelines for the Early Detection of Cancer, 2003. *CA: A Cancer Journal for Clinicians 53,* 27–43.

Spinelli, A. (2002). Preinvasive disease of the cervix, vulva, and vagina. *Seminars in Oncology Nursing 18,* 184–192.

Other Cancers

Deborah L. Volker

This chapter discusses the less common cancers, including esophageal, gastric, pancreatic, hepatic, thyroid, melanoma, head and neck, and multiple myeloma. Although these cancers occur less frequently than others, they may present even greater challenges to patients and caregivers because many are especially difficult to treat and, in most instances, carry a poor prognosis.

■ Esophageal Cancer

Incidence

Cancer of the esophagus is a disease of middle to older age, with three times as many cases occurring in men than in women. In the United States, there are about 14,000 new cases per year, and the incidence continues to rise each year. There is a disproportionate rate of occurrence in African Americans, with a rate two times higher than that of whites; however, these rates vary according to histologic subtype of disease. The most common histologic types of esophageal cancer are squamous cell carcinoma (more common in African Americans) and adenocarcinoma (more common in white men). The incidence of esophageal cancer fluctuates widely worldwide by geographic area and histologic type, with most cases arising in developing countries. Unfortunately, the 5-year survival rate for esophageal cancer is poor (approximately 13%); 13,000 deaths from this cancer are predicted in the United States each year.

Risk Factors and Prevention

The exact cause of esophageal cancer is unknown, but many cases are associated with chronic irritation of the esophageal tissue. Adenocarcinoma is associated with Barrett's esophagus, in which epithelial changes occur in the lower esophagus secondary to chronic persistent gastroesophageal reflux disease (GERD). Esophageal cancer may have a genetic component because numerous tumor suppressor genes have been associated with the disease. Other risk factors include tobacco, alcohol, esophageal strictures associated with lye ingestion, aclasia, a genetic condition, tylosis (characterized by hyperkeratosis of the palms and soles), and Plummer-Vinson syndrome. Numerous nutritional factors, such as high temperature of foods, and smoked, nitrate-cured, and salt-cured foods, have been linked with esophageal cancers.

Measures to prevent esophageal cancer include avoidance or limited intake of alcohol, cessation of smoking and smokeless tobacco products, and management of GERD with antireflux medications and measures.

Detection and Diagnostic Evaluation

The value of endoscopic screening for individuals with GERD is debatable. Although GERD and Barrett's esophagus are linked with adenocarcinoma, the absolute risk remains low enough to question the cost-benefit ratio of widespread screening. The typical patient with esophageal cancer is a man in his 50s or 60s with a history of cigarette smoking and heavy alcohol use. Obesity may be another factor. Patients usually experience a 3- to 6-month history of progressive weight loss and dysphagia before diagnosis. They often present with locally advanced disease. Other presenting symptoms may include pain on swallowing, anorexia, and supraclavicular adenopathy. Patients with advanced disease may experience hoarseness, melena, shortness of breath, and cough due to tracheoesophageal fistula.

Diagnostic evaluation begins with a barium esophagogram, which reveals a narrowing of the esophagus. Endoscopy and biopsy must then follow to determine the invasiveness of the tumor, the integrity of the esophageal wall, and the tumor tissue type. Once the diagnosis is confirmed, the extent of disease is evaluated via computed tomography (CT) scan of the chest, abdomen and pelvis, bone scan, and bronchoscopy. Additional techniques may include endoscopic ultrasonography and laparoscopy. Such staging is important in order to identify patients who can benefit from surgical resection of the tumor and those with metastatic disease who would not benefit from surgery, and to assess response to treatments. Staging of esophageal cancer follows the American Joint

Committee on Cancer (AJCC) tumor, node, metastasis (TNM) system. Unfortunately, most esophageal cancers are not detected until the tumor is large and invasive because the esophagus is quite distensible and thus compensates for partial blockage by the tumor.

Treatment

Treatment goals (cure versus palliation) are based on the clinical stage of the disease and the feasibility of surgical resection of the tumor. Surgery, radiation therapy, and chemotherapy are all useful treatment modalities, with surgery being the primary approach whenever possible. Usually, local tumor control is best achieved by surgical resection (see Chapter 6, Surgical Oncology). Because the esophagus has no mesenteric support structure, tumor resection with end-to-end anastomosis (as is performed in many colorectal malignancies) is not feasible. Instead, most tumors require a partial esophagogastrectomy (removal of the affected part of the esophagus, the remaining distal end, and the upper portion of the stomach). The remaining esophagus is then reconstructed with the use of the stomach or a segment of intestinal tissue.

Chemotherapy and radiation therapy may be used both for palliation and as a part of the primary treatment program in conjunction with surgery. Cisplatin, 5-fluorouracil, and mitomycin are effective drugs; clinical trials involving other compounds are underway (see Chapter 7, Chemotherapy). Radiation therapy is indicated for relief of the obstructive effects of bulky tumors (see Chapter 8, Radiation Therapy).

Other palliative techniques may be used to maintain esophageal patency and improve dysphagia. These may include esophageal dilatation, insertion of a stent, direct tumor ablation using laser techniques, and photodynamic therapy.

Side Effects/Complications

Complications of surgical resection include anastomotic leaks, fistulae, and respiratory complications. Chemotherapy-related side effects are drug specific. Potential complications of radiation therapy include fistula, stricture, hemorrhage, radiation pneumonitis, and pericarditis. Patients may experience side effects of esophageal radiation, including esophagitis and local skin reactions. Radiation side effects vary according to the anatomic structures in the therapy field.

The Role of the Nurse and Rehabilitation

Nursing care is particularly challenging because most patients present with advanced disease and because treatments cause numerous complications. The goals of care include educating patients about treatment options and their side effects and assisting patients with managing complications of the disease and treatments. Difficulty managing oral secretions is particularly problematic, and it can precipitate respiratory complications caused by aspiration, as well as malnutrition (see Unit V for specific symptoms). Social isolation can be another problem arising from difficulty in managing oral secretions. Some patients may require placement of a feeding tube for nutritional support and need to learn management of feedings and tube care. Throughout the course of the disease, nurses play a key role in helping patients and families cope with the many challenges and fears associated with a debilitating, often terminal, disease.

■ Gastric Cancer

Incidence

Although about 22,000 new cases of gastric cancer arise in the United States each year, the incidence has decreased substantially over the past several decades. Conversely, gastric cancer represents the second leading cause of cancer deaths worldwide and is a major health problem in many South American, Eastern European, and Asian countries. In the United States, stomach cancers are more common in males than females, and a disproportionate number of cases occur in African Americans. Although the incidence of stomach cancer has declined, the death rate is still substantial, at 12,000 per year. Changes in quality of food preservation and an increased intake of vitamin C have been suggested as important factors in the decline in the incidence of stomach cancers. As with many other types of cancers, stomach cancer can be cured when it is diagnosed and treated at an early stage. Currently, the 5-year survival rate for gastric cancer in the United States is approximately 20%.

Risk Factors and Prevention

Although the etiology of stomach cancer is not well understood, several dietary factors are linked with the disease. Smoked or salted foods, foods contaminated with aflatoxin (e.g., some grains or peanuts), and low intake of fruits and vegetables are all associated with stomach cancer. The increased use of refrigeration, resulting in less need to add preservatives (e.g., salt, pickling) to food, may well account for the declining stomach cancer mortality rates over time. The bacterium associated with peptic ulcers, *Helicobacter pylori,* may also be a primary risk factor for gastric cancer. Other potential risk factors include pernicious anemia, peptic ulcers, adenomatous gastric polyps, hypochlorhydria, achlorhydria, atrophic gastritis, and low socioeconomic status. Preventive measures for stomach cancer include following: a diet rich in fruits and vegetables and low in cured foods. Although studies are ongoing, eradication of *H. pylori* infection via antibiotic regimens may become an important and reasonably easy means to diminish risk for gastric cancer. Individuals with the precursors described in the previous paragraph should have regular medical follow-up and receive an endoscopy should symptoms arise.

Detection and Diagnostic Evaluation

Typically, stomach cancer does not produce detectable symptoms until it has advanced to a late stage. The most common symptoms include loss of appetite, stomach pain, bleeding, dyspepsia, dysphagia, early satiety, and vomiting. Because many of these symptoms mimic benign gastric ulcers and other common stomach disorders, patient may self-treat with antacids and other over-the-counter remedies and delay seeking medical intervention for several months. As the disease progresses, weight loss, weakness, anemia, melena, and hematemesis may occur.

Diagnosis is usually confirmed by upper gastrointestinal barium studies and tumor visualization and biopsy via endoscopic gastroscopy. Abdominal CT is also useful for evaluating liver, nodal, and other extragastric involvement. Staging of disease follows the AJCC TNM system; endoscopic ultrasound with biopsy and diagnostic laparoscopy may also assist with staging.

Treatment

Surgical resection of the tumor and any involved nodes may be curative in early stages of the disease. The type of surgery selected depends on the location and the extent of the tumor; most often, options include distal subtotal gastric resection, proximal subtotal resection, or total gastrectomy. Unfortunately, disease often recurs after surgery; therefore, adjuvant therapies may be considered. When used alone, chemotherapy and radiation therapy do not improve survival rates. However, when used in combination with surgery or each other, these treatments may improve survival. Radiation therapy is especially useful for palliating advanced or recurrent disease. Various chemotherapeutic approaches have been used with varying success.

Side Effects/Complications

Potential complications of radical gastric surgery include infection, anastomotic leak, pneumonia, reflux aspiration, and bleeding. The patient may experience problems associated with having a substantially smaller stomach; these may include nutritional problems and dumping syndrome. Side effects of abdominal irradiation may include nausea, vomiting, cramping, diarrhea, and anorexia. Chemotherapy side effects depend on the agents used (see Unit V for specific symptoms).

The Role of the Nurse and Rehabilitation

For patients undergoing surgery, the focus of nursing care is on early detection and management of the previously mentioned complications. Management of nutritional needs is a major component of rehabilitation (see Chapter 24, Gastrointestinal Symptoms); patients may benefit from small, frequent meals that are protein-rich and low carbohydrate. Postgastrectomy patients are also at risk for anemia caused by poor iron and vitamin B12 absorption. For patients who are diagnosed with advanced disease, the focus of nursing care is on management of symptoms and other challenges associated with end-of-life care (see Chapter 37, End of Life).

■ Cancer of the Pancreas

Incidence

Cancer of the pancreas accounts for about 2% of all new cancers, with approximately 31,000 new cases occurring each year. However, pancreatic cancer is the fourth leading cause of cancer deaths in the United States. An estimated 30,000 Americans will have died of pancreatic cancer in 2003. The incidence increases with age and is more prevalent in males and African Americans. Because most patients are diagnosed with locally advanced or metastatic disease, the 1- and 5-year survival rates for pancreatic cancer are 21% and 4%, respectively.

Risk Factors and Prevention

Cigarette and cigar smoking are known risk factors. Although a high-fat diet has been implicated, the linkage to pancreatic cancer remains unclear. Similarly, a diet rich in fruits and vegetables may offer some protective benefit (see Chapter 1, The Biology of Cancer). Other conditions that may be linked with the disease include obesity, lack of physical activity, diabetes mellitus, chronic pancreatitis, and cirrhosis. Occupations associated with pancreatic cancer include chemists; workers in coal, gas, metal, leather-tanning, and textile industries; and those involving long-term exposure to the pesticide DDT. Of note, numerous sporadic and inherited genetic alterations are associated with pancreatic cancer.

Detection and Diagnostic Evaluation

Because presenting symptoms are so vague, most pancreatic cancers are diagnosed in later stages. Symptoms include weight loss, abdominal pain, and jaundice. Other symptoms may include weakness, food intolerance, depression, anorexia, steatorrhea, diarrhea, and new onset of diabetes. Unless the patient is experiencing obstructive jaundice, physical examination may reveal few or no findings. Diagnostic evaluation is accomplished via spiral CT; other imaging studies, including magnetic resonance imaging, endoscopic ultrasound, positron-emission tomography and endoscopic retrograde cholangiopancreatography (ERCP) may also be useful. Fine-needle aspiration biopsy of the tumor may be substituted for surgery, with laparoscopy to identify metastatic sites. Laboratory tests may include liver function tests and serum amylase. CA-19-9 is a useful tumor marker for diagnosis and prognosis. Most pancreatic cancers are located at the head of the pancreas and are ductal adenocarcinomas. Staging is guided by the AJCC TNM system. Metastatic sites include regional lymph nodes, liver, peritoneum, lung, and viscera.

Treatment

Surgical resection is the only option for long-term survival; however, only 15–20% of patients present with localized disease that is resectable. Surgical approaches include total pancreatectomy or the Whipple procedure (pancreaticoduodenectomy). The Whipple procedure involves removal of the head of the pancreas, duodenum, gastric antrum, bile duct, and gall bladder. In order to decrease post-procedural nutritional problems associated with dumping syndrome, some surgeons will modify the Whipple to preserve the pylorus. If the tumor is advanced, other palliative surgical options are available. Biliary obstruction may be relieved via either a biliary bypass cholecystojejunostomy or a choledochojejunostomy. A gastrojejunostomy may be performed to relieve gastric outlet obstruction. Biliary tract decompression can be accomplished via placement of an endoscopic stent.

Combination therapy with radiation and chemotherapy may prolong survival slightly for some patients; radiation alone is especially helpful for palliating symptoms in advanced cases. Gemcitabine is the standard agent for tumor shrinkage for unresectable disease.

Side Effects/Complications

Although potential surgical complications depend upon the specific operative procedure selected, typical problems include anastomotic leakage, fistula formation, abscess, and pneumonia. As with any major abdominal surgery, infection, hemorrhage, and hypovolemia may occur. Pancreatic resection also results in disruptions of both exocrine and endocrine functions. Metabolism of fat, protein, and glucose may all be disrupted. Similarly, insulin secretion and glucagons production will be altered. Thus, oral pancreatic enzyme supplements and insulin replacement therapy are necessary.

The Role of the Nurse and Rehabilitation

Postoperative care includes careful monitoring and prompt intervention for surgical complications. Rigorous nutritional management is critical, given that the patient now has difficulty absorbing fat and protein. Patients experience marked alterations in dietary habits, necessitating intensive teaching regarding insulin therapy, enzyme supplements, and dietary changes. Most patients do best with small, frequent meals of a bland, low-fat diet rich in carbohydrates and protein. Consultation with a clinical dietician is strongly advised (see chapter 30).

Unfortunately, most forms of pancreatic cancer progress rapidly, and most patients die within the first year after diagnosis. Palliative care via aggressive symptom management is critical. Clinical problems typically include pain, nausea, jaundice associated with pruritus (related to liver damage or ductal obstruction), ascites, hemorrhage, and hepatic failure (see chapter 37).

■ Liver Cancer

Most cancers detected in the liver are metastatic deposits, not primary tumors. Liver metastases are associated with many primary cancers, including lung, breast, kidney, and gastrointestinal tumors. However, primary liver cancer can occur.

Incidence

Liver and biliary cancers combined represent about 18,900 new cases each year in the United States. Mortality is high, with 14,400 deaths annually. Primary liver cancer, or hepatocellular carcinoma, is uncommon in the United States, yet it represents one of the most common cancers among men in the world. Approximately 1 million new cases arise worldwide each year, with most cases occurring in Asia and Africa. The 5-year survival rate for patients with primary liver cancer is only 2%.

Risk Factors and Prevention

A number of environmental and host risk factors are associated with liver cancer (see chapter 1). In particular, viral infection with hepatitis B and hepatitis C is strongly implicated. Other risk factors include cirrhosis and other liver diseases, alcohol, aflatoxins, Thorotrast (a biliary contrast medium), and occupational exposure to carcinogens. Prevention can be achieved through avoidance of risk factors, and in particular, immunization against hepatitis B virus may mitigate incidence rates once it becomes widely available. Hepatocellular cancer rates have dropped among young people in Taiwan where immunization has been practiced since 1984.

Detection and Diagnostic Evaluation

Much like other cancers of the gastrointestinal tract, the onset of liver cancer is insidious. Symptoms may include dull upper right quadrant abdominal pain, fatigue, weakness, constipation or diarrhea, epigastric fullness, anorexia, and weight loss. Abdominal mass and increased girth die to ascites may be present. Typically, serum liver function tests are abnormal. Alpha-fetoprotein (AFP) is typically elevated upon diagnosis and is a useful marker for monitoring response to treatment.

Diagnostic imaging studies include abdominal ultrasound, CT, and magnetic resonance imaging. Radionuclide scanning of the liver is also helpful. Ultimately, needle biopsy under ultrasound or CT is usually performed to confirm diagnosis, but it may be avoided if surgical resection is planned. The AJCC TNM system is used for staging the disease.

Treatment

Surgery, chemotherapy, and radiation therapy are all options for control and potential cure. Localized, early disease is best treated via surgical resection. Liver transplantation is a controversial option for curing liver cancer, but it may be useful for those with unresectable disease but no distant metastases and for those with cirrhosis. Because most patients are not candidates for curative or palliative surgery, local tumor ablative therapy may be offered. Approaches include chemoembolization treatment and percutaneous ethanol injection. The success of chemoembolization is based on the fact that liver cancers obtain their blood supply from the hepatic artery. Regional infusion (via catheter into the hepatic artery) of chemotherapeutic agents can deliver concentrated dosages directly to the tumor. Systemic side effects are minimized because the liver extracts the drugs during first-pass metabolism. Drugs used include floxuridine, 5-FU, doxorubicin, and mitoxantrone. Embolization of the tumor's blood supply via Gelfoam injection may also be useful. Percutaneous ethanol injection also offers good response rates and may be used in conjunction with chemotherapy and surgery (see Chapter 7, Chemotherapy).

Side Effects/Complications

Complications of liver resection may include hemorrhage, infection, metabolic aberrations, biliary fistula formation, abscess, pneumonia, portal hypertension, and coagulation abnormalities. Side effects of chemotherapy depend on the specific agents used. Regional drug administration typically involves temporary (or permanent) placement of an arterial catheter directly into the tumor vasculature. Infusion of drugs via this method can precipitate both hepatic and gastric toxicity.

The Role of the Nurse and Rehabilitation

Nursing care is twofold: a focus on management of treatment-induced complications and supportive care over the disease trajectory (see Units V and VI). Postoperative care after liver resection includes assessment and early intervention for the complications listed earlier. Side effects of chemotherapy depend on the agents used. Because most patients with unresectable liver cancer die within 3–4 months of diagnosis, emphasis must be placed on supportive care of the patient and the family. Clinical problems associated with advanced liver cancer include pain, hepatic failure, ascites, bleeding, infection, weakness, anorexia, weight loss, and pneumonia. Aggressive pain management is critical, coupled with other palliative measures to control discomfort associated with nausea, vomiting, ascites, pruritus, and other manifestations of liver failure.

■ Endocrine Cancers

Collectively, the endocrine gland cancers represent about 25,500 new cases per year. Thyroid cancer is the most common type of endocrine cancer; other types include adrenal carcinoma, pheochromocytomas, pituitary tumors, parathyroid tumors, multiple endocrine neoplasia syndrome, carcinoid tumors, and pancreatic islet cell tumors. The endocrine tumors represent a diverse group of both benign and malignant disorders. Often, clinical manifestations of the tumors are first evident from symptoms associated with either excess or deficient hormone production by the target organ. Given its relative prevalence as opposed to the other tumor types, thyroid cancer is reviewed here.

■ Thyroid Cancer

Incidence

Approximately 22,000 new cases of thyroid cancer arise in the United States each year; however, mortality is low, with about 1,400 deaths per year. Prevalence is greater in women than in men and in whites than in African Americans. Thyroid cancers are classified according to tissue type. Most are either papillary or follicular; other types include oncocytic (Hürthle cell carcinomas), medullary, and anaplastic.

Risk Factors and Prevention

Although the precise origin of thyroid cancer is unknown, numerous risk factors have been identified. A primary risk factor is a history of therapeutic irradiation to the head and neck region for benign conditions in childhood. Other radiation exposure, such as radioactive fallout associated with the Chernobyl nuclear disaster, is linked to higher rates of thyroid cancer in people exposed as children. Other risk factors may include both dietary iodine deficiency and excess, as well as certain genetic changes. In particular, a small percentage of thyroid cancers are strongly linked to familial genetic mutations.

Detection and Diagnostic Evaluation

Most typically, thyroid cancer is evidenced by a mass detected on physical examination. The presence of other symptoms is unlikely unless the disease is advanced. Symptoms such as hoarseness, dysphagia, shortness of breath, and hormonal irregularities indicate later-stage disease. The diagnosis is confirmed via tissue examination obtained by fine-needle biopsy. Thyroid cancers are staged via the AJCC TNM system.

Treatment

Surgical resection via total or subtotal thyroidectomy is the treatment of choice. Radiation therapy may also be used as an alternative or in addition to surgery. Typically, radiation is administered by oral ingestion of a radionuclide solution of ^{131}I; this is termed *ablative therapy,* in that it inactivates any remaining thyroid tissue, and it may be used in place of surgery for metastatic disease or as an adjunct to destroy any residual thyroid function. External-beam irradiation may be useful for the treatment of recurrent cancers previously treated with ^{131}I.

Side Effects/Complications

Potential complications of thyroidectomy include hemorrhage, impaired airway, and either temporary or permanent vocal cord paralysis. Because the parathyroid glands may be damaged by surgical manipulation, hypocalcemia can occur. Most patients tolerate ^{131}I treatment fairly well; potential complications include nausea and vomiting, fatigue, headache, inflamed salivary glands, and bone marrow suppression. Side effects of external-beam irradiation include skin erythema, mucositis, dysphagia, and anorexia (see Unit V for specific symptoms).

The Role of the Nurse and Rehabilitation

The focus of nursing care depends on the treatment selected. After surgery, the focus of care is on maintaining airway patency and monitoring for bleeding, symptoms of hypocalcemia, and vocal cord impairment. Patients with little or no residual thyroid function after treatment will require thyroid hormone replacement therapy for the rest of their lives.

Replacement therapy must be discontinued 4–6 weeks before the administration of ^{131}I in order to allow thyroid hormone levels to drop and thyroid-stimulating hormone levels to rise. Thyroid-stimulating hormone allows glandular uptake of ^{131}I. Care considerations for ^{131}I therapy include explaining and maintaining radiation precautions. It is important to remember that all body fluids are radioactive for several days after ^{131}I therapy (see Chapter 8, Radiation Therapy, for a review of radiation precautions.) The amount of time that these precautions should be maintained varies according to the dose of ^{131}I administered. Patients receiving high doses of ^{131}I require hospitalization in isolation. Antiemetics may be needed to prevent nausea and vomiting, and patients need support and encouragement, especially while in isolation. The focus of care for patients receiving external-beam radiation therapy includes oral hygiene to prevent or relieve discomfort from mucositis, appropriate skin care measures for the irradiated field, nutritional support, and management of fatigue.

■ Melanoma and Skin Cancer

Incidence

Skin cancer is the most commonly occurring cancer in the United States. More than 1 million new cases of basal cell or squamous cell skin cancers arise each year, and more than 55,000 cases of melanoma will occur in 2004. Fortunately, nonmelanoma skin cancers are highly curable, whereas melanoma is more difficult to treat and more lethal than nonmelanoma skin cancers. The 5-year survival rate for melanoma is 89%.

Risk Factors and Prevention

All skin cancers are associated with exposure to ultraviolet light; people with red hair or fair skin that does not tan are at particular risk. Other risk factors for nonmelanoma skin cancers include long-term sun exposure or tanning booths and family or personal history of skin cancers. Additional risk factors for melanoma include family or personal history of melanoma, history of severe sunburn occurring early in life, multiple melanocytic (atypical or dysplastic) nevi, advancing age, giant congenital melanocytic nevi, xeroderma pigmentosum, and chronic immunosuppression. Prevention of skin cancers includes limiting sun exposure (e.g., wearing protective clothing and avoiding sun during peak hours), using sunscreen, and avoiding tanning beds and sun lamps. However, the usefulness of sunscreens in preventing melanoma has come into question because sunscreens enhance susceptibility by allowing individuals to increase sun exposure without burning.

Detection and Diagnostic Evaluation

Early detection of skin cancer is critical because most types can be cured if they are treated in the early stages. The American Cancer Society recommends that adults practice skin self-assessment monthly and have suspicious lesions evaluated promptly. The warning signs of melanoma are summarized in the "ABCD" rule: **A** for asymmetry, **B** for irregular borders, **C** for color (pigmentation that is not uniform), and **D** for growing diameter of a lesion. Suspicious lesions should undergo biopsy, with the specific biopsy technique depending on the type of skin cancer suspected. Melanoma is staged using the AJCC TNM criteria; except for very limited disease, lymph node biopsy and possible dissection may be warranted. Although melanoma can metastasize to any body tissue, metastases most often occur in the brain, lung, and liver.

Treatment

All skin cancers must be removed. For nonmelanoma skin cancer, treatment approaches depend on individual lesion and patient characteristics. Options include excision, electrodesiccation and curettage, cryotherapy, Mohs micrographic surgery, or radiation therapy. For melanoma, treatment approaches depend on disease stage and includes wide local excision, sentinel lymph node biopsy, or therapeutic lymph node dissection; other adjuvant treatments, such as chemotherapy and immunotherapy, may be warranted for stage III and IV disease. Radiation therapy is useful for palliating symptomatic metastatic disease. Use of tumor vaccines and gene therapy hold promise for future treatment options.

The Role of the Nurse and Rehabilitation

Given the preventable nature of skin cancers, the nurse's role in teaching the public prevention and early detection measures cannot be overstated. Those individuals who do develop skin cancer are particularly vulnerable to developing more skin cancers and must learn to protect skin from further exposure to ultraviolet light. Care of individuals with melanoma is based on disease stage and treatment used. Although most people who have a wide surgical excision or lymph node biopsy do not experience subsequent problems; however, a regional lymph node dissection could result in lymphedema and risk for infection in the affected extremity (See Chapter 31, Skin and Hair Changes, for lymphedema care considerations.). Individuals with metastatic disease may experience complete remissions with treatment via chemotherapy, immunotherapy, and radiation therapy (see Unit V for nursing care information).

■ Head and Neck Cancer

Incidence

Cancer of the head and neck accounts for about 5% of all cancers and 2% of cancer deaths in the United States; squamous cell carcinoma of the head and neck is the most common type of head and neck malignancy. Major sites include the oral cavity, pharynx, paranasal sinuses, larynx, thyroid gland, and salivary glands. Head and neck cancer is much more common outside the United States, especially in Southeast Asia, China, and India. Cancers of the thyroid gland are discussed previously in this chapter.

Risk Factors and Prevention

Head and neck cancers primarily arise in older men. However, cancers of the tongue and oral cavity are occurring at earlier ages and are believed to be linked to use of smokeless tobacco. Tobacco products and alcohol are primary risk factors for head and neck cancer; others include chewing betel nuts; chronic use of snuff or marijuana; nutritional deficiency; occupations such as nickel refining, woodworking, and steel and textile work; viruses, such as Epstein-Barr and human papillomavirus; and genetic predisposition. Given that most head and neck cancers are associated with tobacco and alcohol use, avoiding tobacco and limiting alcohol consumption are primary prevention strategies.

Detection and Diagnostic Evaluation

Signs and symptoms of head and neck cancers depend on the site affected. Examples include a lump or thickening in the neck, a sore that does not heal, dysphagia, a persistent red or white patch on the oral mucosa, change in voice quality, airway obstruction, unresolved sinusitis, ear pain, and weight loss. Oral lesions in early, very curable stages may be first identified by a dentist or primary care provider. Diagnostic tools include tissue biopsy, CT, ultrasound, and magnetic resonance imaging. Depending on the cancer site, an examination under anesthesia may be necessary. Head and neck cancers are staged using the AJCC TNM system.

Treatment

Surgery and radiation therapy are the primary treatments for head and neck cancers; chemotherapy may also be useful in more advanced cases. A wide variety of surgical approaches may be used; the choice is based on the site and the extensiveness of disease. Because the overall survival rate of squamous cell head and neck cancers remains at 50%, clinical trials with novel approaches to treatment, such as gene therapy, are now underway.

The Role of the Nurse and Rehabilitation

Postoperative nursing care of patients who have undergone surgery for head and neck cancers focuses on airway maintenance, prevention of infection, promotion of nutrition, establishment of alternative communication tools if need be, and psychological support. Given the prevalence of heavy alcohol and tobacco use in this patient population, nurses must be vigilant regarding potential withdrawal symptoms and must intervene appropriately with aggressive symptom management. Given the vital nature of head and neck structures (e.g., eyes, ears, tongue, jaw, throat, and larynx) extensive surgery, radiation therapy, and chemotherapy may leave the patient with substantial rehabilitation needs. A multidisciplinary approach is vital and may require the expertise of speech pathologists and nutritionists. For example, patients may need to learn swallowing techniques that decrease risk of aspiration, techniques for communicating after laryngectomy, dietary alterations to improve safety and efficiency of swallowing, exercises to strengthen muscles that aid in speech and swallowing, use of oral prosthetics, and so on. Alterations in physical appearance, ability to eat, and sense of self-esteem and body image all require intensive support from all members of the team.

■ Multiple Myeloma

Incidence

Multiple myeloma is a cancer of the B lymphocyte cell line and is characterized by proliferation of malignant plasma cells and overproduction of immunoglobulin molecules. More than 14,000 new cases and 11,000 deaths occur annually. Multiple myeloma is a disease of older age (median onset, 71 years) and has a higher incidence in men and African Americans.

Risk Factors and Prevention

Although the etiology of multiple myeloma is not clear, risk factors may include family history and ionizing radiation exposure.

Detection and Diagnostic Evaluation

Most people with multiple myeloma present with bone pain secondary to destruction by plasma cell infiltration of the bone marrow. Lytic lesions may occur throughout the skeleton and result in fractures. Patients may also have hypercalcemia secondary to bone destruction. Anemia is a common presenting symptom, along with increased susceptibility to infection due to cellular and humoral immune dysfunction. Renal insufficiency may be present secondary to renal tubule damage caused by excess production of light-chain monoclonal immunoglobulins. Excess immunoglobulins may also cause a hyperviscosity syndrome characterized by fatigue, changes in mental status and vision, angina, and bleeding disorders. Diagnostic evaluation includes serum and urine electrophoresis studies to detect abnormal immunoglobulins, complete blood count and blood chemistry studies, bone marrow aspiration and biopsy, and skeletal survey.

Treatment

Chemotherapy is used to treat multiple myeloma; useful drugs include alkylating agents and prednisone. Because patients tend to experience relapse after conventional approaches to chemotherapy, use of high-dose chemotherapy and hematopoietic stem cell transplantation may be warranted. Thalidomide is also a useful drug. Patients who experience hyperviscosity syndrome may require plasmapheresis to reduce circulating immunoglobulins. Erythropoietin is a useful adjunct for managing anemia; bisphosphonates are useful for managing lytic bone lesions and persistent hypercalcemia.

Nursing Considerations and Rehabilitation

The focus of nursing care depends on the clinical complications patients experience and the treatment selected. Patient teaching regarding risk of infection, management of treatment-related side effects, safety (fracture precautions), fluid and electrolyte imbalance, fatigue and need to maintain mobility, and risk of hypercalcemia are paramount. Pain management is crucial for those experiencing bony lytic lesions (see Unit V for specific symptoms).

■ Conclusion

With the exception of thyroid cancer, the malignancies presented in this chapter are difficult to treat and create challenging patient care problems. Many patients with these cancers may be eligible for clinical trials and need considerable assistance as they struggle with treatment decisions. Because many people are diagnosed in late stages of the cancers covered in this chapter, nurses must be particularly versed in palliative care and hospice options (see Chapter 37, End of Life). Regardless of treatment outcome, patients and families require strong supportive care skills from all members of the interdisciplinary team.

■ Resources

- American Cancer Society: 800-ACS-2345 or *www.cancer.org*
  This website is designed for both health care professionals and lay people. It contains a wide variety of resources, such as medical information, treatment decision tools, news updates, support services, how to find a treatment center, treatment decision tools, and online publications.

  - Esophageal: *www.cancer.org/docroot/CRI/CRI_2x.asp?sitearea=&dt=12*
  - Pancreatic: *www.cancer.org/docroot/CRI/CRI_2x.asp?sitearea=&dt=34*
  - Hepatobiliary: *www.cancer.org/docroot/CRI/CRI_2x.asp?sitearea=&dt=25*
  - Thyroid: *www.cancer.org/docroot/CRI/CRI_2x.asp?sitearea=&dt=43*
  - Melanoma/skin: *www.cancer.org/docroot/CRI/CRI_2x.asp?sitearea=&dt=39*
  - Multiple myeloma: *www.cancer.org/docroot/CRI/CRI_2x.asp?sitearea=&dt=30*
- National Cancer Institute (NCI): 880-4-CANCER or *www.cancer.gov*
  This website is particularly useful for learning more about specific types of cancers, support resources for patients and families, clinical trials, and NCI publications for both professionals and lay people.
  - Esophageal: *www.nci.nih.gov/cancerinfo/types/esophageal/*
  - Gastric: *www.nci.nih.gov/cancerinfo/types/stomach/*
  - Pancreatic: *www.nci.nih.gov/cancerinfo/types/pancreatic/*
  - Hepatobiliary/Liver: *www.nci.nih.gov/cancerinfo/types/liver/*
  - Thyroid: *www.nci.nih.gov/cancerinfo/types/thyroid/*
  - Melanoma/skin: *www.nci.nih.gov/cancerinfo/types/melanoma/*
  - Head and neck: *www.nci.nih.gov/cancerinfo/types/head-and-neck/*
  - Multiple myeloma: *www.nci.nih.gov/cancerinfo/types/myeloma/*
- Oncolink: *www.oncolink.com*
  Sponsored by the University of Pennsylvania, Oncolink provides information about types of cancers, treatment options, and helpful resources for both patients and professionals.

Bibliography

Lenhard, R., Osteen, R., & Gansler, T. (Eds.). (2001). *Clinical oncology*. Atlanta, GA: American Cancer Society.

Mazzaferri, E., & Kloos, R. T. (2001). Current approaches to primary therapy for papillary and follicular thyroid cancer. *Journal of Clinical Endocrinology and Metabolism, 86*, 1447–1463.

Yarbro, C. H., Frogg, M., Goodman, M., & Groenwald, S, L. (Eds.). (2000). *Cancer nursing principles and practice* (5th ed). Sudbury, MA: Jones & Bartlett.

UNIT V

Introduction to the Experience and Management of Symptoms

Cynthia R. King

From diagnosis to death, patients with cancer are likely to experience many symptoms that may affect their physical and psychological well-being and their quality of life. These symptoms may include myelosuppression, pain, nausea and vomiting, diarrhea, fatigue, changes in sleep, anxiety and mood disorders, dyspnea, cognitive changes, anorexia and weight loss, alopecia and skin changes, infertility, and changes in self-image. These symptoms may affect adults and/or children.

Nurses greatly affect the management of the symptom experience. Appropriate control and management of symptoms by nurses can significantly improve the quality of life (QOL) for patients and families.

■ Definitions

It is important for nurses to understand some of the key definitions related to symptoms and the symptom experience. A *symptom* is different than a *sign*. A symptom involves an individual's subjective experience of disease, or changes in physical, psychological, social, or spiritual well-being. Nurses must ask the patient and family about the symptom to understand the patient's perception of the experience (e.g., pain or fatigue). A sign is objective and observable (e.g., pale skin). A symptom may be continuous or intermittent, and the distress caused by the symptom can affect the individual's QOL and coping abilities.

The *symptom experience* is the individual's perception and response to the symptom occurrence and distress caused by the symptom. The *symptom occurrence* involves three factors: the *frequency, duration,* and *severity* of the symptom. The frequency involves the number of times the event occurs within a given time frame (e.g., 8 hours, 1 week). The duration is how long the symptom continues, and the severity is the amount and degree of discomfort associated with the symptom. *Symptom distress* is the amount of physical or mental upset, anguish, or suffering experienced because of the symptom. Symptom distress is important because it is directly related to the impact of symptoms on the patient and, thus, on the patient's QOL. When symptom distress is relieved, it may help promote recovery in the patient and improve QOL. Both symptom severity and distress may be measured by self-reporting tools.

■ Assessment

Symptoms

One of the most essential aspects of the nurse's role in symptom management is assessment. It is important to use accurate, reliable, and valid methods to assess the symptom experience. It is also vital to evaluate the symptom experience through a report from the individual being assessed. Some important components to assess include location, frequency, duration, and severity of the symptom, as well as distress caused by the symptom. The pieces of information gained from the assessment help determine treatment options, whether a symptom is controlled, and how much relief a patient is getting.

Each of the chapters in Unit V describe reliable and valid assessment methods for specific symptoms experienced by individuals with cancer. One of the most commonly used assessment scales is the numeric scale of 0–10. For example, if a patient is experiencing pain, the nurse may ask "How much pain do you have now?" in order to assess intensity, with 0 meaning no pain and 10 meaning severe pain. Nurses should also ask "How distressing is the pain to you?" (0 = not distressing at all and 10 = the worst distress possible). By asking both questions, nurses may learn that a patient rates his or her pain as mild or moderate but describes the pain as very distressing because it is affecting the entire QOL (physical, psychological, social, and spiritual well-being).

Another way to measure symptoms is with a descriptor scale. For example, a nurse might ask "How much fatigue did you experience in the past 24 hours?" Individuals with cancer then may choose words such as none, mild, moderate, or severe. Nurses may also decide to use instruments designed to measure a single symptom, like the Piper Fatigue Scale or Rhodes Index of Nausea and Vomiting. It is also important to assess symptoms in a specific time frame. If a nurse asks "Do you have nausea and vomiting?" the patient may only answer for the past 15 minutes. Because symptoms may be intermittent or continuous it is helpful to evaluate the patient's usual pattern over several days or weeks.

When nurses perform an assessment of symptoms, it may be helpful to use a symptom checklist. This helps prevent missing any symptoms (e.g., fatigue, anorexia, and dyspnea). Because symptoms may be experienced secondary to the disease process or treatment modalities, nurses must consistently perform evaluations of symptoms throughout the cancer trajectory (e.g., diagnosis to recovery and survivorship or the terminal phase).

Quality of Life

Because symptoms may severely affect the individual's entire life, it is valuable to assess QOL. *Quality of life* refers to an individual's sense of well-being, encompassing physical, psychological, social and spiritual dimensions. The cancer symptom experience (symptom occurrence and symptom distress) may affect all components of QOL. The overall goal of evaluating QOL is to measure the effectiveness of treatment, nursing interventions, and self-care activities, as well as to improve patient care. Self-report measures are preferred because QOL is subjective.

QOL can be assessed by asking one overall question, like "How do you rate your overall quality of life now?" (0 = poor to 10 = excellent) or by using a QOL tool that measures several dimensions, including symptoms (e.g., QOL-BMT Cancer Rehabilitation Evaluation System, Symptom Distress Scale).

There is currently no one specific reliable and valid instrument that measures all aspects of each possible symptom experienced by individuals with cancer. It is up to clinical nurses to assess as accurately as possible the patient's total symptom experience for each symptom.

Symptom Management

Appropriate management of symptoms often requires a variety of approaches for relief. More specific information related to symptom management is provided in the chapters in this section. One approach that may be helpful for certain symptoms is drug therapy (e.g., for pain, nausea and vomiting, depression, anxiety). However, other physical and psychological modalities play a significant role in relieving symptoms. Dietary or nutrition measures may be used to help with nausea/vomiting and weight loss/anorexia. Adequate fluid intake may be recommended for patients with fatigue or mucositis.

Self-Care and Patient/Family Teaching

Unless individuals with cancer are adequately prepared with knowledge regarding ways to manage symptoms, they may experience severe distress, reduced treatment dosages, treatment delays, increased morbidity, and decreased QOL. Patients and families must be provided with information regarding potential symptoms, risks for developing specific symptoms, and ways to participate in care (self-care). Patient education and self-care activities should be individualized based on the symptom experience. Patients and families should be taught to monitor for the development of symptoms. This may be done easily in a daily log.

Preventing and alleviating symptoms for patients with cancer demands a proactive stance by clinical nurses. Decreasing or preventing symptoms and distress requires nurses to use all possible drug and nondrug methods. The prevention and treatment of symptoms such as pain, nausea/vomiting, and fatigue can help improve the overall QOL of individuals with cancer.

Web sites:

- *www.ons.org*
- *www.cancersymptoms.org*
- *www.cancerfatigue.org*
- *www.cancer.org*
- *www.oncolink.org*
- *www.cancer.gov*

Resources:

- Amercian Cancer Society: 800-ACS-2345 or *www.cancer.org*
- National Cancer Institute (NCI) 880-4-CANCER or *www.cancer.gov*

Bibliography

Ferrell, B.R., Grant, M.M. (2003). Quality of life and symptoms. In C.R. King and P.S. Hinds (Eds.). Quality of Life: From Nursing and Patient Perspectives: Theory, Research and Practice (2nd ed.). Sudbury, MA: Jones and Bartlett.

Rhodes, V.A. & Watson, P.M. (Eds.). (1987). Symptom distress. Seminars in Oncology Nursing, 3(4), 242–247.

CHAPTER

22

Myelosuppression

Genevieve Hollis

Margaret H. Crighton

Myelosuppression, a common problem for patients with cancer, refers to a state in which one or more blood cell lines are decreased. It is the most common cause of treatment delays and dose reductions for patients undergoing cancer treatment. These treatment delays and dose reductions may interfere with the effectiveness of cancer therapies. Myelosuppression can also result in life-threatening oncologic emergencies. Because of its physical and psychosocial manifestations, myelosuppression can negatively affect the patient's quality of life.

In this chapter, the pathophysiology of this complex and potentially life-threatening phenomenon is reviewed. Subsequent sections in this chapter outline the complications of myelosuppression, as well as the physical and psychosocial symptoms experienced by the myelosuppressed patient. Evidenced-based management strategies are also presented.

■ Overview of Hematopoiesis

Hematopoiesis is the process by which white blood cells (WBCs), red blood cells (RBCs), and platelets are produced from pluripotent stem cells (Figure 22–1). Pluripotent stem cells are found primarily in the bone marrow. These cells differentiate and become committed to producing a single blood cell lineage, creating a series of actively proliferating "progenitor" cells. Each type of blood cell has a different life

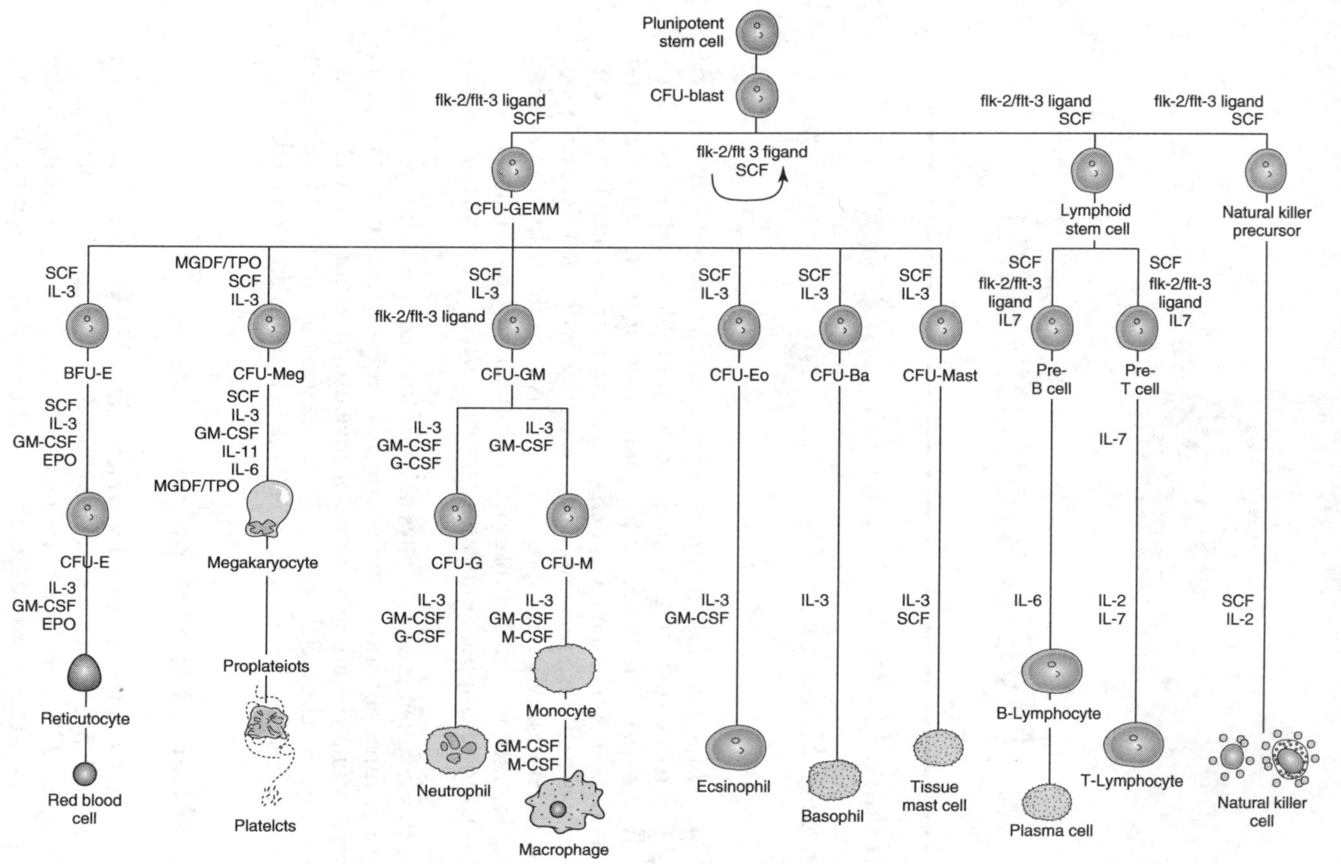

FIGURE 22–1 ■ Hematopoietic tree

Source: Published with permission of Amgen, Inc.

TABLE 22–1 ■ Normal Blood Values[a]

Blood Cell	Normal Range	Life Span (Half Life)
White blood cells	4–10.5 K/mm^3	6–8 hours
Neutrophils	55%–70% of WBC	
Segs	40%–60% of WBC	
Bands	0%–3% of WBC	
Lymphocytes	20%–40% of WBC	
Monocytes	4%–8% of WBC	
Eosinophils	1%–3% of WBC	
Basophils	0%–1% of WBC	
Red blood cells	4.6–6.2 MIL/mm^3 (males)	120 days
	4.2–5.4 MIL/mm^3 (females)	
Hemoglobin	14–18 g/dl (males)	
	12–16 g/dl (females)	
Hematocrit	42%–52% (males)	
	37%–47% (females)	
Platelets	150–400K/mm^3	5–10 days

[a]Values may vary slightly by laboratory

Source: Data from Baquiran, 2001; Pagana & Pagana, 2003; Walch, 1996.

span, ranging from hours to days (Table 22–1). Given the relatively short life span of mature blood cells, "committed progenitor" cells are constantly stimulated to produce large numbers of new cells daily. Hematopoietic growth factors (also known as colony-stimulating factors) are a family of cytokines that regulate the proliferation, differentiation, and viability of these cells. Synthetic versions of some hematopoietic growth factors have been developed and are used in the clinical management of myelosuppression.

■ Causes of Myelosuppression

Hematopoiesis can be impaired as a side effect of cancer therapies, such as chemotherapy and radiation therapy. Chemotherapy works by interfering with the division of rapidly dividing cells, such as cancer cells. Progenitor cells also undergo constant rapid cell division and consequently are inadvertently damaged by chemotherapy. This damage renders progenitor cells temporally unable to produce new blood cells. Because mature circulating blood cells are not destroyed, blood counts do not begin to decrease until 10–14 days after therapy, depending on the natural life span of the blood cell (Table 22–1). This time period of predicable count suppression is referred to as the *nadir.* Blood counts generally recover within 2–3 weeks after therapy, when stem cells have been able to replace the previously damaged progenitor cells. Radiation therapy can cause myelosuppression when the irradiated field involves a large portion of the skeleton, especially major bone marrow production sites, such as the pelvis and sternum.

Myelosuppression can also occur as a manifestation of the disease itself. In leukemia, the malignant cell is derived from the hematopoietic system. As the leukemic cells expand within the bone marrow, normal blood cell production is suppressed. Lymphomas and solid tumors, such as breast cancer and lung cancer, frequently involve the bone marrow and impair blood cell production.

■ Clinical Implications of Myelosuppression

In order to predict the level of myelosuppression a patient may experience, clinicians conduct a detailed risk assessment before the initiation of cancer therapy. This includes a review of the myelosuppressive potential of the proposed therapy because some chemotherapy agents are more myelosuppressive than others (Table 22–2). Higher chemotherapy and radiation doses and combination chemotherapy or chemotherapy/radiation therapy regimens are associated with an increased risk of myelosuppression. The risk of myelosuppression is also increased in patients with a history of prior cancer treatments or with direct bone marrow involvement with disease because of the decreased bone marrow reserve that exists under these circumstances. Elderly patients and those with poor nutritional status have an increased risk because of their decreased ability to repair cellular damage. Some patients experience prolonged exposure to the chemotherapy agent if they are unable to metabolize the drug because of renal or hepatic dysfunction or if the drug is initially sequestered in physiologic effusions (ascites, pleural effusions) and then slowly released into the systemic circulation. Health care providers should use these risk factors to identify patients who have a greater potential for developing myelosuppression and its complications in order to initiate heightened surveillance and preventive strategies.

Laboratory studies are obtained to serve as a baseline for comparison over the course of therapy. This includes a complete blood count (CBC) as well as electrolytes and renal and liver functions. Throughout the course of treatment, CBCs are routinely obtained to assess for the

TABLE 22–2 ■ Myelosuppressive Potential of Chemotherapeutic Agents[a]

Mild	Moderate	Severe
Altretamine	Amsacrine	Busulfan
Bleomycin	Chlorambucil	Carboplatin
Cladribine	Cisplatin	Carmustine
Dacarbazine	Cyclophosphamide	Cytarabine
5-Fluorouracil	Etoposide	Dactinomycin
Mitomycin C	Fludarabine	Daunorubicin
Pentostatin	Gemcitabine	Doxorubicin
Plicamycin	Idarubicin	Hydroxyurea
Streptozocin	Ifosfamide	Lomustine
Vincristine	Mechlorethamine	Paclitaxel
Vinorelbine	Melphalan	Docetaxel
	6-Mercaptopurine	Vinblastine
	Methotrexate	
	Mitoxantrone	
	Procarbazine	
	6-Thioguanine	

[a]Degree of myelosuppression may vary, depending on other risk factors, including dose and schedule.

Source: Baquiran, 2001.

development of myelosuppression. If myelosuppression occurs, it should be graded according to the Common Toxicity Criteria for Adverse Events (Table 22–3).

Myelosuppression is classified according to which blood cell line is affected. Specifically, leukopenia is a decrease in the total number of WBCs, neutropenia is a decrease in the number of neutrophils, anemia is a decrease in the number of RBCs and thrombocytopenia is a decrease in the number of platelets (see Table 22–1 for a review of normal blood values). An understanding of the distinct and important functions of each blood cell provides a foundation for identifying the specific complications that can result from a decreased number of these cells, focused assessment parameters, and management strategies targeted toward decreasing the incidence and the severity of these complications.

Leukopenia and Neutropenia

WBCs are an important part of the immune system and serve as part of the host defense against invading organisms. Neutrophils are a specific

TABLE 22–3 ■ Common Toxicity Criteria for Adverse Events v3.0: Blood and Bone Marrow

Blood Cell	Grade			
	1	**2**	**3**	**4**
Leukocytes (WBCs)	LLN—3000/mm³	<3000–2000/ mm³	<2000–1000/mm³	< 1000/mm³
Neutropenia (ANC)	LLL—1500/ mm³	<1500–1000/ mm³	<1000–500/mm³	< 500/mm³
Hemoglobin	LLN—10 g/dl	< 10–8 g/dl	< 8–6.5 g/dl	< 6.5 g/dl
Platelets	LLN—75,000/mm³	<75,000–50,000/mm³	< 50,000–25,000/mm³	25,000/mm³

Key: ANC = absolute neutrophil count; LLN = lower limits of normal; WBC = white blood cell.

Source: NIH, NCI, 2003.

type of WBC that move to the site of infection and phagocytize ("eat") organisms. When WBCs, especially neutrophils, are decreased, patients are at risk for developing infection. Patients are considered to be neutropenic when their absolute neutrophil count (ANC) falls below 2000/mm^3, but their risk of developing an infection is significantly greater when the ANC is less than 1000/mm^3.

The most common cause of morbidity and mortality in cancer patients is infection. In the patient with neutropenia, infection can occur from sources outside the body (exogenous) or inside the body (endogenous). In most cases, it is the patient's own natural body flora that cause infections. The most common infective organisms are gram-positive organisms, such *Staphylococcus aureus* and *Streptococcus pneumoniae,* but gram-negative-related infections (e.g., *Escherichia coli* (*E. coli*), *Pseudomonas aeruginosa,* and *Klebsiella pneumoniae*) are on the rise in some medical centers. Patients who are neutropenic for extended periods of time or receive broad-spectrum antibiotics are at risk of developing invasive fungal infections from *Candida* or *Aspergillus* species. Causative agents in viral infection include the herpes simplex viruses, respiratory syncytial virus, parainfluenza, and influenza types A and B.

Several factors are important in predicting the potential for a patient to experience an infectious episode while neutropenic. The lower the ANC and the longer the patient has a low ANC, the more likely he or she is to become infected. (Figure 22–2 demonstrates how to calcu-

FIGURE 22-2 ■ Calculating Absolute Neutrophil Count (ANC)

1. Locate the neutrophils on the CBC
   - "segs" (segmented neutrophils)
   - "bands" (young neutrophils)
2. Add percentages of the segs and the bands
3. Multiply the answer (the percent)with the total WBC

$$\frac{\%\text{segs} + \%\text{ bands}}{100} \times \text{Total WBC} = \text{ANC}$$

Example:

WBC = 2.6 (total number of WBCs is 2600)

Segs = 15 (15% neutrophils)

Bands = 5 (5% young neutrophils)

$$\frac{15 + 5 \times 2600}{100} = 520$$

Key: CBC = complete blood count; WBC = white blood cell

Source: From the National Comprehensive Cancer Network & American Cancer Society Fever and Neutropenia Treatment Guidelines for Patients with Cancer.

late the ANC.) A rapidly declining ANC increases the infection risk. Other factors important in determining a patient's risk for infection include impaired cell-mediated or humoral immunity resulting from corticosteroid immunosuppressive therapy or hematologic malignancies, or loss of protective barriers such as altered skin and mucous membranes. These elements of the patient's condition should be considered in the patient assessment.

Assessment Patients at risk for neutropenia, or who are currently neutropenic, require vigilant monitoring for early signs and symptoms of infection. Without neutrophils, the usual signs and symptoms of infection, such as erythema, pustulation, and swelling, may be considerably diminished or absent. Fever, generally greater than 38.5° C (100.5° F), is the hallmark and is often the only sign of infection. Patients may not seem very sick clinically. Within this context, subtle changes in a patient's condition become very significant. This is especially true for older adults, who even when not neutropenic, have less ability to mount an immune response in the face of infection. In addition to asking patients about painful oral lesions, burning with urination or flank pain, cough or sore throat, nausea, vomiting, diarrhea, or perirectal discomfort, the nurse should pay attention to subtle changes in mental status and functional status. The nurse should be sure to ask patients if they have been around anyone who is sick, and if they have done any recent travel or been exposed to any infections that they know of.

The patient's physical examination should consist of vital signs and careful examination of all body systems because common sites of infection include almost every part of the body. Particular attention should be paid to the oral cavity, sinuses, lungs, skin folds, venous access insertion sites, bone marrow aspiration sites, and rectum. Pain may be the only indicator of infection.

Clinical Management Measures to prevent infection should be implemented for all patients at risk for developing neutropenia. The single most important intervention is frequent and thorough hand washing by all those who come in contact with the patient. Other neutropenic precautions include avoiding crowds and people with a cold or the flu, as well as children who have been recently vaccinated. Patients are frequently instructed to practice meticulous oral hygiene, bathe at least once a day, and avoid sharing dishes, cutlery, towels, and anything else that might harbor germs. They are told not to eat certain foods, such as raw milk products, raw or uncooked meat, eggs, uncooked fruits and vegetables, and unpasteurized juice and beer. Hospitalized patients are generally not permitted to have fresh flowers or plants in their rooms. In many cases, the patient is admitted to a private room with signs alerting staff and visitors to the importance of vigilant hand washing. Staff and visitors may also be required to wear a mask, gown, and gloves.

Most of these restrictions and precautions are theoretically rather than evidence based. Recently, dietary restrictions in particular have come under debate. Cancer patients need diets that are high in calories, protein, and vitamins in order to promote immune function and tissue repair. Dietary restrictions theoretically decrease bacteria in the food and gut, but they are a burden for patients because they decrease food choice and increase a sense of restriction. For older adults, who experience chemosensory changes with age, this could be especially problematic. The effect can be decreased oral intake at a time when patients need optimal nutrition.

Because the only sign of infection is often just a fever, a temperature greater than 38.0° C (100.5° F) is an oncologic emergency in the neutropenic patient and must be addressed immediately. Mortality rates from febrile neutropenia can be as high as 70% if antibiotics are not administered within the first 48 hours of a febrile episode. When a neutropenic patient becomes febrile, a diagnostic evaluation follows and includes a CBC with differential and serum electrolytes. Renal

TABLE 22–4 ■ Risk for Complications from Febrile Neutropenia

Higher-Risk Patients	Lower-Risk Patients
• Are already in the hospital when they become febrile • Have comorbid disease • Have impaired renal or liver function • Have uncontrolled cancer • Neutropenic for > 1 week • Have pneumonia • > 65 years old • Status post stem cell transplantation	• Do not have "high risk" criteria • Are outpatients • Do not have an infection related to their IV or central line • Can perform most ADLs and IADLs independently • Do not have leukemia • Have a normal chest x-ray study

Key: IV = intravenous; ADL = activity of daily living; IADL = instrumental activity of daily living.

Source: From the National Comprehensive Cancer Network & American Cancer Society Fever and Neutropenia Treatment Guidelines for Patients with Cancer.

function tests (blood urea nitrogen and creatinine) and liver function tests are performed and frequently influence future antimicrobial selection and dose. Bacterial and fungal blood cultures are taken from a peripheral vein and a central venous catheter, if present. Cultures are also taken from any other suspected site of infection. Urinalysis and imaging studies, such as a chest x-ray study, are obtained as indicated by the history and physical. Treatment of infection usually begins with broad-spectrum antibiotic therapy and shifts to drugs with specific activity once an organism has been identified.

In the past several years, great efforts have gone into the development of models in order to determine which febrile neutropenic patients are at risk for complications (Table 22–4). These models help with decision making in terms of where and how to treat patients with febrile neutropenia. High-risk patients or those with overt signs of infection are more likely to be treated as inpatients and given intravenous antibiotics. Low-risk patients without focal signs of infection may be treated as outpatients with oral antibiotics. Those who are treated as outpatients must have 24-hour access to medical care. The shift to treatment of low-risk patients in the outpatient setting can preserve their quality of life and help keep down the high costs associated with hospitalization.

It is possible to treat the neutropenia itself with granulocyte colony-stimulating factors, such as filgrastim (Neupogen) and pegfilgrastim (Neulasta), which stimulate the body to make neutrophils. They have been shown to decrease the duration and the severity of neutropenia but have not decreased mortality rates. In accordance with current recommendations, clinicians often do not administer filgrastim during the first cycle of chemotherapy unless the patient is at particular risk (e.g., if the patient is expected to have delayed count recovery) or does indeed become febrile. If this is the case, filgrastim is then administered prophylactically—before the patient becomes febrile—during subsequent cycles of chemotherapy. There has been a growing debate around the value of these growth factors to prevent febrile neutropenia. Recent research suggests that it may be clinically and economically beneficial to routinely administer filgrastim as primary prophylaxis for febrile neutropenia in some cases. The next revision of these guidelines will likely reflect the mounting evidence that supports the broader application of filgrastim as a mode of prophylaxis against febrile neutropenia.

For patients receiving myelosuppressive chemotherapy, the starting dose of filgrastim is 5 mcg/kg/day. It is given once daily by subcutaneous injection but can also be given as a slow intravenous infusion. Filgrastim therapy should commence no sooner than 24 hours after chemotherapy and should continue for 10–14 days until the postnadir ANC is greater than 10,000/mm^3. A CBC with differential should be obtained before filgrastim therapy is initiated, and it should be checked twice a week while the patient is receiving the drug.

Pegfilgrastim is a long-acting granulocyte colony-stimulating factor that needs to be administered as a subcutaneous injection only once during each chemotherapy cycle. It should be given at least 24 hours after chemotherapy and should not be given if there are less than 2 weeks before the next cycle of chemotherapy. For adults who weigh more than 45 kg, the typical pegfilgrastim dose is 6 mg.

Anemia

RBCs (erythrocytes) carry oxygen to body tissues. Because the average life span of an RBC is 120 days (versus hours for a neutrophil), anemia tends to develop slowly in patients receiving cancer therapies. Anemic patients experience a wide range of symptoms because of decreased body tissue oxygenation and from physiologic compensatory mechanisms, such as increased heart rate and shunting of blood to vital organs. Specific signs and symptoms of anemia include fatigue, dyspnea, chest pain, weakness, palpitations, syncope, headache, decreased cognition, pallor, and in severe cases, a systolic murmur. The definition of clinically significant anemia is being reexamined. Often, clinicians have viewed lower grades of anemia as an expected sequela of cancer and its treatment and have treated only severe (hemoglobin [Hb] less than 8.0g/dl) cancer-related anemia. Recent research has demonstrated a significant association between even mild-to-moderate (Hb from the low level of normal to 8.0g/d) anemia with fatigue, reduced functional status, and diminished overall quality of life. Other research raises the possibility that anemia may also affect treatment outcomes in some settings, such as radiation therapy for cervical, head and neck, ovarian, and vulvar cancers.

Assessment Patients at high risk for developing anemia and its associated symptoms need to be screened throughout their treatments. This includes frequent determination of Hb with a CBC as well as an assessment of the signs and symptoms anemia described previously. When anemia is detected, a peripheral smear should be reviewed. Consideration needs to be given to noncancer or non-treatment induced causes of anemia, such as bleeding, hemolysis, nutritional deficiencies, medications, and anemia of chronic disease. If clinically indicated, additional tests may be performed, including stool for guaiac testing; reticulocyte count; iron studies; and lactate dehydrogenase, bilirubin, serum creatinine, serum B12, and folate determinations.

Clinical Management After the detection and assessment of anemia, clinical decisions about when and how to treat it depend on a detailed risk assessment to determine whether immediate correction is required. This risk assessment includes the severity of the anemia and its acuity, with a rapidly developing anemia often being associated with more significant symptoms. Patients with a history of cardiac or pulmonary disease or those currently experiencing chest pain or dyspnea on exertion are of particular concern and may require immediate correction with an RBC transfusion.

Erythropoietin is an erythrocyte colony-stimulating factor that is produced primarily by the kidney in response to tissue hypoxia. It stimulates RBC production by progenitor cells in the bone marrow. It has been shown to significantly improve Hb levels in most treated patients, improve the clinical symptoms associated with anemia, and decrease the number of RBC transfusions. Erythrocyte colony-stimulating factors include epoetin alfa (Procrit) and darbepoetin alfa (Aranesp). Treatment guidelines recommend that these agents be used when the Hb is less than 10–11g/dl for symptomatic patients who do not require immediate correction. These agents may also be used in anemic patients who are currently asymptomatic but are at high risk for developing symptoms. This group includes patients who have undergone transfusion within the previous 6 months, have a history of receiving myelosuppressive therapy or radiation therapy to greater than 20% of skeleton, and the elderly.

The starting dose of epoetin alfa is 10,000 units three times a week or 40,000 units weekly by subcutaneous injection. If there is no increase in Hb by 1g/dl within 4 weeks, the dose should be increased to 20,000 units three times a week or 60,000 units weekly. If there is still no increase in Hb, epoetin alfa treatment should be discontinued. Darbepoetin alfa is a long-acting erythropoietic-stimulating agent. Its starting dose is 2.25 mcg/kg weekly by subcutaneous injection. If there is no increase in Hb by 1g/dl within 6 weeks, the dose should be increased up to 4.5 mcg/kg weekly. If there is still no response, darbepoetin alfa treatment should be discontinued. It is also possible to administer darbepoetin alfa at 3.0 mcg/kg every 2 weeks. For patients who are responding to either epoetin alfa or darbepoetin alfa, treatment should be continued until a target Hb of 11–12 g/dl is reached. The nurse should follow the package inserts for dose titration guidelines.

Cancer patients often experience a "functional iron deficiency" where there are sufficient iron stores in the bone marrow but low serum iron levels. Consequently, iron is not provided rapidly enough to meet the demands of epoetin alfa- or darbepoetin alfa-induced erythropoiesis. Serum ferritin level less than 100 ng/ml or a transferrin saturation level less than 20% indicates a functional iron deficiency, and oral iron supplementation should be considered when patients are receiving these products.

Thrombocytopenia

Platelets perform a vital role in hemostasis by sticking to blood vessel walls at the site of injury and forming a plug. They also assist with the conversion of fibrinogen to fibrin, which is important in the formation of blood clots. At any given time, up to one third of platelets are found in the spleen. Because platelets have an average life span of 5 to 10 days, thrombocytopenia typically occurs after the WBC nadir. As the platelet count drops, the risk of bleeding and hemorrhage increases. Thrombocytopenia is defined as a circulating platelet count of less than $100{,}000/mm^3$.

Assessment Patients at high risk for thrombocytopenia are monitored closely throughout their treatments. This includes frequent determination of platelet counts with a CBC as well as assessment for signs and symptoms of bleeding and hemorrhage, including bruises, petechiae (tiny purplish-red spots visible under the skin), epistaxis, oozing from the gums, prolonged and/or heavy menses, melena, "coffee ground" emesis, and hematuria. Other important assessment parameters include frank bleeding from venipuncture sites or cuts. Signs of intracranial bleed include headaches, blurred vision, disorientation, changes in mental status, and changes in pupil size and reactivity to light. As clinically indicated, additional testing may include bleeding times and testing of stools, urine, and emesis for occult blood.

Management Thrombocytopenic patients are often placed on bleeding precautions in an attempt to prevent bleeding or injury. These precautions include avoiding falls and contact sports, using stool softeners to avoid straining, avoiding rectal suppositories and enemas, using a soft tooth brush and avoiding dental floss, and not using scissors, razors, or blades for grooming. Any medications that may alter platelet function, such as anticoagulants, aspirin-containing drugs, and nonsteroidal anti-inflammatory drugs, should be avoided. Patients are also encouraged to use water-based lubricants during sexual intercourse and to avoid sexual intercourse if the platelet count is less than 50,000/mm^3. Premenopausal women are often given oral contraceptives to suppress ovarian function and prevent menstrual bleeding. Additionally, patients are instructed to report any of the signs and symptoms of bleeding and hemorrhage listed earlier.

Platelet transfusions are administered to the thrombocytopenic patient who is actively bleeding. Prophylactic platelet transfusions are also administered to thrombocytopenic patients to reduce the risk of bleeding of hemorrhage when the platelet count falls below a predefined threshold level. Current guidelines recommend a threshold of 10,000/mm^3 for most cancer patients receiving treatment. A threshold of 20,000/mm^3 is recommended for patients experiencing high fevers, hyperleukocytosis, rapid fall of platelets, or coagulation abnormalities. Patients receiving aggressive therapy for bladder tumors as well as those with demonstrated necrotic tumors should also have a threshold of 20,000/mm^3. Bone marrow aspirations and biopsies can be performed safely in patients with counts less than 20,000/mm^3. A platelet count of 40,000–50,000/mm^3 is sufficient to perform major invasive procedures safely, in the absence of associated coagulation abnormalities. A common problem for patients who have received multiple platelet transfusions, especially from random donors, is the development of antiplatelet antibodies, which diminishes the effectiveness of transfused platelets and can lead to transfusion reactions. Using leukoreduced blood products for patients who are expected to require multiple platelet transfusions during their treatment courses could reduce the development of these antibodies.

Oprelvekin (Neumega) is a thrombopoietic growth factor that stimulates the production of platelets. In a limited number of studies, it has been shown to decrease the need for platelet transfusions in patients receiving myelosuppressive chemotherapy for nonmyeloid malignancies, especially if they had required a platelet transfusion after the previous chemotherapy cycle. It is not indicated after myeloablative chemotherapy. The recommended dose of oprelvekin is 50 mcg/kg given once daily subcutaneously. The first dose should be given 6–24 hours after the completion of chemotherapy, and treatment should continue until the postnadir count is greater than 50,000/mm^3.

■ Psychosocial Management

Although myelosuppression is typically regarded as a physiologic event, it is a multidimensional one, also affecting the psychosocial realms of patients' lives. Those who become myelosuppressed face fear and uncertainty as they wait to see if they develop a fever and infection or bleeding complications. The physical and social isolation myelosuppressed patients encounter may be a significant burden and requires interdisciplinary intervention.

Patient Education

Nurses play a primary role in teaching patients and families the knowledge and skills needed to safely receive cancer treatments. Assessment of the patient's learning needs, barriers to learning (e.g., visual or hearing problems, cultural issues, and illiteracy), and preferred method of instruction (e.g., lecture, reading, videos, or computers) aid in the development of an effective teaching plan. Patients should be aware of how and why myelosuppression occurs as a result of their disease and/or treatment and when it is expected to occur. Awareness of signs and symptoms that should be reported to the health care team any time of day or night is of crucial importance so that complications such as infection or bleeding can be treated promptly. The nurse should be sure to ask patients if they have a thermometer. Do they know how to use it? Can they read it? Patients and families should be aware of neutropenia and thrombocytopenia precautions that they can take to minimize complications associated with myelosuppression. Teaching patients and family member's skills such as subcutaneous injection of colony-stimulating factors can significantly reduce the morbidity and mortality associated with the disease and treatment. Energy-conservation techniques as well as a prescription for regular exercise can be very helpful to the patient experiencing fatigue secondary to anemia. Patients and family members can greatly benefit from a frank discussion of the psychological toll that myelosuppression can have on the patient and his or her loved ones.

Conclusion

Myelosuppression is a complex phenomenon experienced at some level by virtually all cancer patients during of the course of their illness. With the publication of practice guidelines, management strategies are increasingly evidenced based. Recent research has contributed to the emerging appreciation among oncology health care providers of the direct impact that myelosuppression has on a patient's quality of life. The nurse, as a member of the multidisciplinary team, has a crucial role in the assessment and management of myelosuppression. Awareness of the potential for myelosuppression, thorough assessment of the patient with special attention to signs and symptoms of complications, assistance in the prevention and treatment of complications, and education of the patient and caregiver about myelosuppression form the cornerstone of high-quality care.

Resources

Treatment Guidelines:

- National Comprehensive Cancer Network (NCCN) and American Cancer Society (ACS) Cancer-related fatigue and anemia treatment guidelines for patients: 800-ACS-2345 or *www.nccn.org* or *www.cancer.org*
- National Comprehensive Cancer Network (NCCN) and American Cancer Society (ACS) NCCN Fever and neutropenia treatment guidelines for patients with cancer: 800-ACS-2345 or *www.nccn.org* or *www.cancer.org*

Professional Organizations and web sites:

- American Cancer Society Side Effects of Chemotherapy: *www.cancer.org/docroot/ETO/content/ETO_1_4X_What_Are_The_Side_Effects_of_Chemotherapy.asp?sitearea=ETO*
- Oncology Nursing Society's Hematologic Toxicities Resource Area: *www.ons.org/xp6/ONS/Login/Splash.xml*

Bibliography

Baltic, T., Schlosser, E., & Bedell, M. K. (2002). Neutropenic fever: one institution's quality improvement project to decrease time from patient arrival to initiation of antibiotic therapy. *Clinical Journal of Oncology Nursing, 6,* 337–340.

Baquiran, D.C. (2001). *Cancer Chemotherapy Handbook,* 2nd ed. Philadelphia: Lippincott.

Barber, F. D. (2001). Management of fever in neutropenic patients with cancer. *Nursing Clinics of North America, 36,* 631–644.

Byars, L. (2002). Neutropenia risk assessment and management in the ambulatory care setting. *Oncology Supportive Care Quarterly, 1,* 27–39.

Gillespie, T. W. (2002). Effects of cancer-related anemia on clinical and quality of life outcomes. *Clinical Journal of Oncology Nursing, 6,* 206–211.

National Comprehensive Cancer Network & American Cancer Society Fever and Neutropenia Treatment Guidelines for Patients with Cancer (2002). Retrieved July 27, 2003 from *http://www.nccn.org*

National Comprehensive Cancer Network (2003). Clinical practice guidelines in oncology: Cancer and treatment-related anemia, version 1. 2003. Retrieved July 27, 2003 from *http://www.nccn.org*

National Comprehensive Cancer Network (2003). Clinical practice guidelines in oncology: Fever and neutropenia, version 1. 2002. Retrieved July 27, 2003 from *http://www.nccn.org*

Pagano, K.D, Pagana, T.J. (2003). *Diagnositic and Laboratory Test Reference,* 6th edition. St. Louis: Mosby.

Schiffer, C., et al. (2001). Platelet transfusion for patients with cancer: clinical practice guidelines of the American Society of Clinical Oncology. *Journal of Clinical Oncology, 19*(5), 1519-1538.

Wallach, J. (1996). *Interpretation of Diagnostic Tests,* 6th ed. Boston: Little, Brown and Company.

CHAPTER

23

Cancer Pain

Ellen Lavoie Smith

Pain is a common problem among cancer patients, occurring as a result of malignancy and anticancer treatment. Approximately 30%–50% of patients undergoing active treatment for solid tumors and 70%–90% of those with advanced cancers experience chronic pain. The most widely accepted definitions of pain acknowledge the subjective nature of the experience, as well as its influence on physiologic and emotional health. The American Pain Society has adopted the following definition, "Pain is an unpleasant sensory and emotional experience associated with actual or potential tissue damage, or described in terms of such damage" (Mersky, 1994). Pain does not predictably correlate with tissue injury. Thus, the patient's self-report is the single most reliable indicator of pain.

Although 90% of cancer pain can be managed with simple methods, this success rate has not been actualized. There is no doubt that uncontrolled pain can result in many physiologic changes, as well as anxiety, anger, and depression. Social relationships, spiritual and sexual health, and the ability to perform daily activities are threatened when pain is pervasive. Adequate pain assessment and treatment can potentially minimize or alleviate these problems.

■ Cancer Pain Types

Knowledge of the source and mechanism of pain is crucial in determining the most effective treatment strategy. Two pain classifications have been defined based upon the underlying pathophysiology; nociceptive and neuropathic pain. Nociceptive pain originates from bone, joint, muscle, skin, connective tissue, or viscera/organs, such as the liver, pancreas, or intestine. Nociceptive pain usually has an aching or throbbing quality. Neuropathic pain originates from either the central or the peripheral nervous system, and it is typically described as a burning, tingling, or electric shock-like pain. Common cancer-specific causes of neuropathic pain include phantom limb pain, in which patients sense discomfort in a nonexistent limb after amputation or painful peripheral neuropathy caused from neurotoxic chemotherapy.

Cancer patients frequently experience both chronic and acute pain, each warranting unique assessment and treatment strategies. Pain that persists or recurs frequently is termed *chronic. Acute* pain occurs intermittently and has an anticipated end. Acute pain occurring despite the use of ongoing analgesics is termed *breakthrough* pain.

■ Cancer Pain Syndromes

Approximately 75% of chronic pain syndromes are caused by the tumor itself, and the remaining syndromes are associated with cancer treatment toxicities or other comorbid conditions. Acute pain can be associated with cancer-specific diagnostic or therapeutic procedures, such as lumbar puncture, bone marrow biopsy, and thoracentesis. Table 23–1 outlines acute pain syndromes associated with cancer treatment. Table 23–2 lists both acute and chronic pain syndromes specifically caused by tumors.

Assessment

Pain assessment should be routinely performed on every patient and should be thought of as the "5th vital sign." The nurse should ask the patient, "Where is your pain?" When a precise pain etiology cannot be defined, the nurse should not assume that pain is absent or less severe. Pain is subjective; the nurse's responsibility is to acknowledge and respect the patient's word.

Next, the nurse uses a rating scale to describe pain severity. Using a severity scale before and after analgesic administration can provide valuable information regarding the efficacy of a particular drug, dose, and/or dosing schedule. Figure 23–1 is an example of a numeric visual analogue scale that is very suitable for clinical practice. This rating scale is easily and quickly understood by patients, is available in many languages, and is simple for the nurse to administer. The patient is asked to rate his or her pain on a 0–10 numeric scale, with 0 representing no pain and 10 indicating the worse pain the patient has ever experienced.

TABLE 23–1 ■ Acute Pain Syndromes Associated with Cancer Treatment

Acute Pain Associated with Chemotherapy, Hormonal Therapy, or Immunotherapy	**Acute Pain Associated with Radiation**
Oropharyngeal mucositis or esophagitis	Oropharyngeal mucositis or esophagitis
Intravenous line placement	Radiation enteritis or proctitis
Painful peripheral neuropathy	Brachial plexopathy after breast irradiation
Bone pain	Skin reaction/irritation
Myalgias and arthralgias	Bone pain after radiopharmaceuticals
Headache	
Painful gynecomastia	
Fluorouracil-induced angina	
Pain from infection	
Pain from bleeding or bruising	

Source: Portenoy, R., & Lesage, P. (1999). Management of cancer pain. *Lancet, 353,* 1695–1700.

TABLE 23–2 ■ Tumor-Related Acute and Chronic Pain Syndromes

Acute Pain Syndromes	**Chronic Pain Syndromes**
Pathological fractures	Rostral retroperitoneal syndrome
Bleeding into tumor	Malignant pelvic and perineal pain
Superficial wounds or abscesses	Peripheral mononeuropathies
Headache	Polyneuropathies
	Plexopathy
	Radiculopathy
	Epidural spinal cord compression
	Phantom pain after limb amputation
	Tumor invasion into joints and soft tissue
	Hypertrophic osteoarthropathy
	Bowel, ureter, or bladder obstruction
	Hepatic distention

Source: Portenoy, R., & Lesage, P. (1999). Management of cancer pain. *Lancet, 353,* 1695–1700.

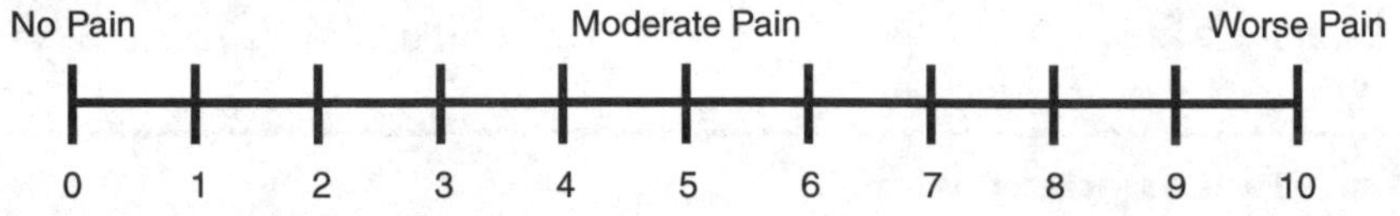

FIGURE 23–1 ■ Numeric rating scale.
Source: McCaffery, M. & Pasero, C. (1999). *Assessment: Underlying complexities, misconceptions, and practical tools*, in *Pain: Clinical manual*, M. McCaffery and C. Pasero, Editors. Mosby: St. Louis. 62–63.

TABLE 23–3 ■ Common Pain Assessment Questions

On a diagram of the body, shade the areas where you feel pain. Put an X on the area that hurts the most.
When does the pain start?
Is it worse or better at certain times of the day?
What makes the pain better or worse? (e.g., body position, certain activities, eating, bowel movements)
Have you tried anything in particular to relieve the pain, e.g., medicines, heat, cold, position changes, rest?
How do others know when you have pain? Do you talk about it, or do you sometimes try to hide it?
How does pain affect your ability to do your normal activities? (e.g., work, sleep, eat, bathe, cook, have sexual relations)
Does the pain make you feel nervous, sad, angry, irritable, or worried?
What concerns/worries do you have about taking pain medicine? Are you worried about becoming "hooked," or addicted to pain medicine?

For children younger than 7 years or for cognitively impaired patients, a similar scale depicting faces can be used.

Assessment Tools In addition to pain severity scales, the Initial Pain Assessment Tool and the Brief Pain Inventory are examples of pain assessment tools that can be used to comprehensively guide the nurse through the assessment process. Table 23–3 summarizes key questions from these tools.

When assessing neuropathic pain, make certain to use neuropathic pain descriptors, such as in the following example, "Does your pain have a burning, picky, or electric shock-like quality?" Using the correct words to convey neuropathic pain is especially important because patients may not otherwise recognize or describe this unique, uncomfortable sensation as "pain," even when it is very severe and distressing. Assessment tools have been developed to assess neuropathic pain.

Challenges to Assessment Nurses and other health care professionals often inappropriately believe that they know more about the patient's pain than the patient does. When a patient's pain cannot be linked with a specific cause, or when the patient exhibits behaviors interpreted as "drug seeking," biases or misconceptions regarding addiction can make pain assessment more complex. Knowledge of the following opioid-associated phenomena can assist the nurse who is assessing the need for modifications in the pain treatment plan.

Opioid addiction: A psychological dependence on opioid analgesics characterized by a pattern of compulsive drug use for purposes other than pain relief. Patients who take opioid medications for pain, regardless of how much is taken, are not addicted.

Physical dependence: Physiologic adaptation of the body to opioids. Withdrawal symptoms occurs if opioids are discontinued abruptly but can be minimized or avoided with gradual dose de-escalation.

Tolerance: A decrease in one or more of the opioid effects (analgesia, sedation, respiratory depression). Over time, increased opioid doses may be needed in order to maintain the same level of pain relief.

Most importantly, less than 1% of patients who take opioid medications for pain become addicted. It is critical that patients who are fearful of addiction understand that the risks of poorly managed pain far outweigh the risks of becoming addicted.

Cognitively impaired or unconscious patients can be more difficult to assess. The nurse must not assume that these patients do not have pain just because they cannot communicate verbally. The nurse should watch for nonverbal indicators of pain, such as facial expressions, restlessness, moaning, and crying.

The nurse must be aware that various ethnic groups express pain differently; thus, assessment strategies may require modification. In addition to using assessment tools and educational materials written in the appropriate language, nurses must work closely with patients and families to define treatment goals that take into consideration culturally specific patient values.

Treatment

Treatment of pain with one or several drugs is often an effective approach. Combined regimens take advantage of more than one drug mechanism of action when pain has several causes. For example, severe pain from bone metastasis is most effectively treated with a nonsteroidal anti-inflammatory drug (NSAID) *and* an opioid because each

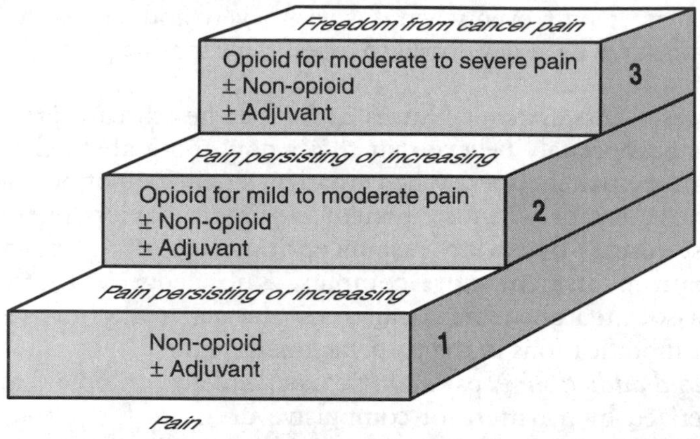

FIGURE 23–2 ■ World Health Organization Analgesic Ladder.
Source: Jacox, A., Car, D., Payne, R., Berde, C., Brietbart, W., Cain, J., Chapman, C., Cleeland, C., & Ferrell, B. (1994). Management of cancer pain: Clinical practice guideline No. 9. (AHCPR publication no. 94-0592). Rockville, MD: Agency for Health Care Policy and Research, US Department of Health and Human Services, Public Health Service.

drug is more powerful when it is combined with the other than when the drugs are used alone. Ultimately, lower drug doses are required and analgesic side effects are minimized. The World Health Organization analgesic ladder (Figure 23–2) provides a model by which analgesics should be considered in a step-wise approach based on pain severity and the individual's response to drug therapy. Patients with mild pain should initially receive drugs from the first level: an NSAID, acetaminophen, and/or an adjuvant drug. Opioids may be used alone or added to level 1 drugs when pain is more severe or not well controlled.

Pharmacologic Therapy Drugs may be chosen from three main classes: (a) NSAIDs or acetaminophen, (b) opioid analgesics, and (c) adjuvant analgesics. Tables 23–4 and 23–5 list drug examples, mechanisms of action, and common side effects from each main class.

NSAIDs, acetaminophen, and opioids Pain relief is optimized and analgesic doses minimized when pain is anticipated and prevented. Therefore, around-the-clock dosing works best for patients with persistent, daily pain. The nurse must choose the simplest, least invasive, yet feasible administration route. The nurse converting the regimen from one opioid to another calculates the equianalgesic dose on the basis of drug potency and route. (See AHCPR or APS guidelines for equianalgesic dosing recommendations.) In patients with chronic pain, continuous-release oral

TABLE 23-4 ■ Common Nonsteroidal Anti-Inflammatory Drugs and Opioids

Drug Class	Generic Name	Action	Side Effects
NSAIDs	Aspirin, ibuprofen, Ketoprofen, Naproxen, celecoxib, choline magnesium, indomethacin, trisalicylate, rofecoxib	Used to treat mild pain caused by inflammation. Inhibits cyclooxygenase, an enzyme that catalyzes conversion of arachidonic acid to prostaglandin. Prostaglandins sensitize nerve receptors, resulting in pain.	Heartburn, nausea, diarrhea, constipation, flatulence, epigastric, and/or abdominal pain. Long-term use can lead to renal and hepatic toxicity, bleeding, and gastric ulceration. Concurrent use with alcohol or steroids should be avoided.
	Acetaminophen	Has minimal anti-inflammatory effects but can decrease pain from inflammation.	Use cautiously in patients with liver disease or when combined with alcohol. Doses exceeding 4000 mg/day can result in liver and kidney damage.
Opioids (mu agonists)	Codeine, hydromorphone, levorphanol, methadone, morphine, oxycodone, meperidine, fentanyl Combination opioid/NSAID preparations: codeine (with aspirin or acetaminophen), oxycodone (with aspirin or acetaminophen), hydrocodone (with aspirin or acetaminophen)	Used to treat moderate to severe pain, or when NSAIDs or acetaminophen are contraindicated. Relieve pain by binding to opioid/mu receptors, blocking substance P. Substance P, when released by damaged cells, sensitizes nerve receptors. No ceiling dose except when using meperidine.* (High doses or long-term use causes toxic metabolite accumulation, leading to dysphoria, agitation, and seizures.	Constipation, sedation, nausea, pruritus, urinary retention, myoclonus, biliary spasm, respiratory depression.

Key: NSAID = nonsteroidal anti-inflammatory drug.

Source: Modified from American Cancer Society web site. *http://www.cancer.org/docroot/MIT/content/MIT_7_2x_Pain_Control_A_Guide_for_People_with_Cancer_and_Their_Families.asp)*

or transdermal drug formulations or intravenous, subcutaneous, or intraspinal drug administration techniques result in stable drug levels and a constant baseline of analgesia. Breakthrough or as-needed dosing of an immediate-release analgesic is frequently necessary to treat episodic pain that occurs despite the use of a long-acting administration method. Patient-controlled analgesia allows self-administration of intravenous, subcutaneous, or intraspinal analgesics via a preprogrammed computerized pump.

Adjuvant Drugs These drugs (see Table 23–5) are used to enhance the analgesic effect of opioids; to treat specific pain types, such as neuropathic pain; or to treat other symptoms that can make pain worse. Chemotherapeutic drugs used to treat the tumor can have the secondary effect of decreasing pain.

Under no circumstances should a placebo be used to treat cancer pain.

Nonpharmacologic Management Nonpharmacologic approaches can be used concurrently with analgesics to optimize pain relief. Cutaneous stimulation via application of superficial heat or cold, massage, pressure, and vibration can help alleviate pain. Increased nutrients and oxygen are concentrated in an area through heat's vasodilating effects. Heat can also be effective in decreasing joint and muscle stiffness. Cold can be effective in causing local vasoconstriction, reducing inflammation and edema. Massage can ease general aches and pains, as well as have a relaxing effect. Although immobilization may be necessary to prevent or allow healing of pathological fractures, in general, prolonged immobility should be avoided. Patients should be encouraged to remain as active as possible to avoid joint stiffness, contractures, overall muscles weakness, and other complications of immobility. Patient repositioning, passive range-of-motion exercises, and attention to proper body alignment are important strategies for the nurse caring for a bed-bound patient. Counterstimulation via transcutaneous electrical nerve stimulation or acupuncture is believed to activate endogenous pain-modulating pathways by direct stimulation of peripheral nerves. Biofeedback, guided imagery, hypnosis, music, art, aromatherapies, or other distraction techniques can be helpful. Finally, emotional support gained through counseling or involvement in a support group may also benefit the patient whose life is significantly disrupted by pain.

Invasive Therapies Although noninvasive techniques should always be considered before invasive approaches, in some circumstances, an invasive approach is the best option. Radiation therapy to a painful primary or metastatic tumor can result in dramatic relief in radiosensitive cancers. In addition to external-beam and brachytherapy techniques,

TABLE 23-5 ■ Common Adjuvant Drugs

Drug Class	Generic Name	Action	Side Effects
Anti-depressants	Amitriptyline, nortriptyline, desipramine	Help to control tingling or burning from nerve injury caused by the cancer or cancer therapy. Also used to treat depression.	Dry mouth, sleepiness, constipation, orthostatic hypotension, blurred vision, and, urinary retention. Patients with heart disease experience arrhythmias.
Anti-histamines	Hydroxyzine, diphenhydramine	Helps to control nausea, insomnia, and pruritus.	Drowsiness.
Antianxiety drugs	Diazepam, Lorazepam	Used to treat muscle spasms that accompany severe pain. Also lessen anxiety.	Drowsiness. May cause urinary incontinence.
Amphetamines	Caffeine, dextroamphetamine, methylphenidate	Enhance opioid effectiveness and reduce the drowsiness they cause.	Irritability, tachycardia, decreased appetite.
Anti-convulsants	Carbamazepine, clonazepam, gabapentin, phenytoin	Help control tingling or burning from nerve injury caused by the cancer or cancer therapy.	Liver toxicity, bone marrow suppression. Gabapentin may cause sedation and dizziness.
Steroids	Dexamethasone, prednisone	Relieve pain caused from bone metastasis, spinal cord and brain tumors, and inflammation.	Edema; hyperglycemia, stomach irritation; rarely, confusion; altered behavior; and sleeplessness.
Bisphosphonates	Pamidronate, etidronate, zoledronic acid	Decrease pain from bone metastasis.	Flulike symptoms, renal toxicity, injection site erythema, electrolyte abnormalities.

Source: Modified from American Cancer Society web site. *http://www.cancer.org/docroot/MIT/content/MIT_7_2x_Pain_Control_A_Guide_for_People_with_Cancer_and_Their_Families.asp*)

strontium 89 and samarium 153 are systemically administered radiopharmaceuticals, which are absorbed in areas of high bone regeneration. Through the use of these agents, radiation can be delivered to many painful bone metastases all at once. Bone marrow suppression is the major toxicity.

Other invasive procedures include nerve blocks, in which the peripheral nerve is destroyed through injection of a neurolytic agent. Peripheral nerves, nerve roots, or pain-conducting nerve tracts located in the spinal cord can also be surgically severed. However, because of the permanent nature of these approaches, these procedures should be reserved for circumstances in which other therapies are ineffective, poorly tolerated, or clinically inappropriate.

■ Nursing Care

Side Effect Management

In addition to the nurse's role in pain assessment and treatment, management of analgesic side effects is a key component of any successful pain management plan. Constipation, a common side effect of opioid medication, can be managed through the use of laxatives, stool softeners, adequate fluids, dietary management, and ambulation. Administration of adjuvant medications to treat nausea and pruritus can improve patient compliance to analgesic regimens. Sedation and respiratory depression are typically transitory. However, opioid dosage and schedule modifications may be required. Central nervous system stimulants may counteract problematic sedation.

Patient and Health Professional Education

The patient and family must understand the importance of reporting pain and adhering to the treatment plan. The nurse should make certain that the patient knows the medication name, how to take it, and when and how to manage side effects. Also, it is important to address patient concerns regarding addiction, as well as the social, cultural, or religious implications of their pain and its treatment. Finally, the nurse should make certain the patient understands not to stop opioids abruptly and to plan ahead so as not to run out of medication. Several excellent patient and family teaching tools are available.

Just as an informed patient is central to effective pain management, so must health care professionals be knowledgeable about pain. Although this may be difficult to believe, previous research has revealed that physicians and nurses lack knowledge about the most effective pain relieving strategies. Therefore, clinicians must not assume that others know more than they do. Nurses must keep abreast of pain-specific evidence-based literature and advocate for patients by teaching themselves and their colleagues about pain.

Communication and Collaboration

Whether nurses are employed in an inpatient or an outpatient setting, they should document the details of the pain assessment and treatment plan. Pain severity scores should be recorded alongside other vital signs. The patient's self-defined goal for pain relief, response to the prescribed regimen, side effects, and any special considerations should be documented so that others may provide excellent continuity of care. Outpatients should be taught to document pain scores both before and after analgesic use, as well as the drug taken, the dose, and the dosing interval, and to bring this information to their next appointment. Lastly, nurses must collaborate with colleagues when designing, implementing, and evaluating the nursing care plan. Multidisciplinary input is particularly important for complex pain problems.

■ Resources

Treatment guidelines:

- National Comprehensive Cancer Network (NCCN) and American Cancer Society (ACS) NCCN Cancer Pain Treatment Guidelines for Patients: 800-ACS-2345 or *www.nccn.org* or *www.cancer.org*

Books:

- American Cancer Society (2001). *American Cancer Society's guide to pain control: Powerful methods to overcome cancer pain.* Atlanta, GA: American Cancer Society.

Professional organizations and web sites:

- Agency for Health Care Research and Quality: *www.ahrq.gov*
- American Academy of Pain Management: *www.aapainmanage.org/*
- American Pain Society: *www.ampainsoc.org/*
- Hospice Net-Pain: *www.hospicenet.org/html/what_is_pain.html*

- National Center for Complementary and Alternative Medicine: *www. altmed.od.nih.gov*
- Oncology Nursing Society: *www.cancersymptoms.org/symptoms/pain/*

Bibliography

American Pain Society. (1999). *Principles of analgesic use in the treatment of acute pain and cancer pain* (4th ed.). Glenview, IL.

Jacox, A., Car, D., Payne, R., Berde, C., Brietbart, W., Cain, J., Chapman, C., Cleeland, C., & Ferrell, B. (1994). *Management of cancer pain: Clinical practice guideline No. 9*. (AHCPR publication no. 94-0592). Rockville, MD: Agency for Health Care Policy and Research, US Department of Health and Human Services, Public Health Service.

McCaffery, M. & Pasero, C. (1999). *Assessment: Underlying complexities, misconceptions, and practical tools,* in *Pain: Clinical manual,* M. McCaffery and C. Pasero, Editors. Mosby: St. Louis. 62–63.

Mersky, H. & Bogduk, N., eds. (1994). *Classification of chronic pain: Description of chronic pain syndromes and definitions of pain terms,* in *Pain,* 2nd ed. IASP Press: Seattle. 222.

Portenoy, R., & Lesage, P. (1999). Management of cancer pain. *Lancet, 353,* 1695–1700.

CHAPTER

24

Gastrointestinal (GI) Symptoms

Deborah Fleming

The gastrointestinal (GI) system is frequently affected by cancer and/or its treatment. Several of the more common complications are discussed in this chapter, with an emphasis on assessment, treatment, and nursing care guidelines.

■ Assessment

Using a head-to-toe approach, assessment of the GI system begins with the oral cavity and mucosa and ends with the large intestine and rectum. The nurse should obtain a history of comorbidities, previous infections, and disease symptoms. Information pertaining to each symptom help in the assessment of risk for developing complications during treatment. Table 24–1 summarizes key data the nurse should obtain during a history. Table 24–2 lists assessment data to obtain during treatment through patient interview and physical assessment.

■ Complications

Disruption of the GI System Lining

The lining of the GI system begins in the oral cavity and follows the tract in its entirety through to the anus. The cells of the GI tract are

TABLE 24–1 ■ Assessment History Data

Assessment Area	Symptoms/Issues to Assess
Oral cavity	HSV, thrush, tooth decay, dental hygiene, gum disease, halitosis
Esophagus	Painful swallowing, dysphagia, heartburn, bleeding
Upper abdominal area	Nausea, vomiting, appetite changes, ascites, bleeding, distension
Lower abdominal area	Bowel movements, diarrhea, constipation, bowel obstruction, colostomy, ileostomy, discharge, bleeding, fistula

Key: HSV = herpes simplex virus.

TABLE 24–2 ■ Assessment during Treatment

Assessment Area	Interview Questions	Physical Assessment
Oral cavity	Sores in mouth? Difficulty swallowing? Oral dryness? Blood in saliva or gums?	Examine oral cavity: buccal membranes, surface and underneath tongue, gums
Esophagus	Heartburn? Indigestion? Pain in chest area? Dysphagia? Painful swallowing?	Examine back of throat; severe symptoms may warrant invasive exam by physician
Upper abdominal area	Hiccups? Abdominal distension? Nausea/vomiting?	Listen for bowel sounds, palpate for ascites/distension
Lower abdominal area	Last bowel movement? Constipation? Diarrhea? Blood in stool?	Listen for bowel sounds, assess skin in perianal area

rapidly reproducing cells, or very frequently entering and exiting the life cycle. Because of this, they are particularly vulnerable to the effects of chemotherapy and radiation therapy. Other treatments, used frequently for supportive care in the cancer setting, can also lead to breakdown of the mucosal lining. Table 24–3 summarizes the factors that can lead to mucosal breakdown.

Mucosal breakdown is defined using three terms that delineate the area affected. *Mucositis* and *stomatitis* describe oral cavity disruption. *Esophagitis* describes breakdown or infection of the esophageal lining. *Enteritis* delineates erosion of the lining of the intestines.

TABLE 24–3 ■ Factors that Lead to Mucosal Breakdown

Chemotherapy	Antibiotics
Radiation therapy given directly over the area of mucosal lining	Compromised host immunity
Direct tumor invasion of the tissue	Decreased platelet count

TABLE 24–4 ■ Risk factors for Mucositis/Stomatitis

Smoking	Poor dental health
Drinking alcohol	Poorly fitted dentures
High-dose chemotherapy	History of HSV, yeast, candida or any infection of the oral cavity
Chemotherapy antimetabolites: 5-FU, MTX, ARA-C	Steroids
Radiation therapy to the area	AIDS

Key: AIDS = acquired immunodeficiency syndrome; ARA-C = cytosine arabinoside; HSV = herpes simplex virus; 5-FU = 5-fluorouracil; MTX = methotrexate.

Signs and symptoms of mucositis/stomatitis vary and can be progressive. At onset, the oral cavity usually develops erythema. The patient may experience a process in which the imprint of the teeth is visible on the tongue and buccal membranes. This is described as geographic mucosa, and it may be painful. Lesions may follow within hours or days and be infectious; infections include bacterial, yeast, and viral. A mucositis grading scale for assessment is found in the introduction to this section. Risk factors for developing mucositis/stomatitis are summarized in Table 24–4.

Treatment and the Role of the Nurse Treatment of mucositis begins with prevention, with the initial step being assessment of risk factors. Patients with risk factors are begun on prophylactic measures. Medical measures may include the administration of antivirals, such as acyclovir, and antifungals, such as fluconazole. When the patient is receiving radiation therapy directly to the oral cavity, the medical team may require the removal of teeth in the radiation field. This is done primarily to prevent infection; however, teeth exposed to direct radiation also decay easily. If teeth are not extracted, fluoride gel treatments should be considered. If the patient wears dentures, they should be removed for treatment and not worn for up to 9 months.

TABLE 24–5 ■ Nursing Interventions for the Prevention of Mucositis/Stomatitis

Avoid alcohol and tobacco.
Use normal saline mouth rinses or baking soda in water rinse several times a day.
Avoid over-the-counter mouthwash that may contain alcohol or peroxide.

Nursing measures are extremely important. They focus on infection prevention, comfort, and nutrition maintenance.

Infection prevention begins with proper oral hygiene on a routine basis. For example, the patient at high risk for mucositis, perhaps one who is receiving 5-fluorouracil and radiation therapy to the head and neck area, requires normal saline rinses four times a day using a soft-bristled tooth brush twice daily and flossing until the platelet count becomes low. Preventive measures are summarized Table 24–5.

Assessment frequency of the oral cavity should be increased once treatment has begun. Comfort measures become necessary if mucositis/stomatitis develops. Patients with severe mucositis report high levels of pain, necessitating pain management. Topical and oral analgesic can be used if tolerated. Intravenous therapy should be considered if the patient is hospitalized and unable to swallow. It remains important to keep the oral cavity clean, even after onset of mucositis/stomatitis. Switching from a toothbrush to a sponge-tipped swab may be necessary to prevent pain or bleeding. All lesions must be reported to the physician for possible cultures and administration of antibiotics.

The nutritional status of the patient may become compromised if the patient cannot eat because of pain or swelling from the mucosal breakdown. Consulting with a clinical dietician is recommended for a discussion of alternate routes of nutritional supplement. Patients who are receiving radiation therapy to the oral cavity or esophagus begin taking nutritional supplements at the onset of treatment to help delay the necessity of enteral feedings.

Esophagitis is most often associated with radiation therapy that involves the esophagus in the field. Patients who are receiving aggressive chemotherapy treatments and who experience mucositis/stomatitis should be monitored for esophagitis. Often, all mucosal membranes are involved. Infection in the oral cavity may also travel down the esophagus.

Assessment should include monitoring for signs and symptoms, such as painful swallowing, complaints of heartburn sensation, and pain over the sternal area. The most severe symptom is dysphagia.

Similar to mucositis/stomatitis treatment, nursing care focuses on infection, comfort, and nutrition management. Antibiotics are often used empirically or for the treatment of documented infections. Topical, oral, or intravenous analgesics may be used for comfort, but alternate routes of delivering nutrition must be considered. In some cases, a pause in treatment may be required for healing to occur. Dose adjustments may be necessary to decrease recurrence.

As with esophagitis, enteritis is frequently associated with radiation therapy. Enteritis is characterized by nausea, vomiting, and watery diarrhea. The severity of the diarrhea is usually the measure of the extent of the enteritis.

Treatment includes antiemetics and antidiarrheal agents. Dietary changes include avoiding alcoholic beverages, roughage, and dairy products. Patients who are unable to eat must be started on intravenous nutrition, and the possibility of infectious diarrhea should be ruled out (see Diarrhea).

Nursing care focuses on meticulous intake and output records, fluid replacement, and comfort. Skin care for the prevention of breakdown in the perianal area should be started with gentle cleansers and moisture barrier creams. The area must be frequently assessed for breakdown or sign of infection. Cultures should be obtained of any lesions that develop. In the immunocompromised patient, the only signs of infection may be fever and pain in the anal area.

Xerostomia

Xerostomia refers to a dry mouth. The most common cause in cancer patients is salivary gland failure due to radiation therapy damage. The causes of xerostomia are summarized in Table 24–6.

Xerostomia is not only uncomfortable but also leads to difficulty eating and swallowing. Treatment centers on stimulation of any remaining salivary glands and artificial replacement of saliva. Clinical trials are currently looking at preventive measures.

Treatment and the Role of the Nurse Nursing care focuses on teaching the patient how to increase comfort and ease chewing and swallowing. Table 24–7 summarizes tips for patients with xerostomia.

Halitosis

Halitosis, or bad breath, can occur when disease is present in the oral cavity. Xerostomia, oral infections, and poor oral hygiene can cause halitosis.

TABLE 24-6 ■ Causes of Xerostomia

Radiation therapy to the oral cavity	Antihistamines
Radical head and neck therapy	Opioids

TABLE 24-7 ■ Tips for Patients with Xerostomia

Use hard candies to moisten mouth and stimulate remaining salivary glands.
Carry a water bottle for frequent sipping.
Use nonalcoholic mouthwash frequently to rinse and clean mouth.
Use artificial saliva before meals.
Use moisturizer on lips.
Use gravies and sauces on foods to aid in chewing and swallowing.

Treatment and Nursing Care Treatment and nursing care should focus on hydration and hygiene. Frequent assessment for infection and mucositis is also a priority. Patients should be instructed to brush the back of the tongue frequently and to freshen with mouthwash, breath mints, and charcoal tablets. If infections are present, antibiotics may be necessary.

Dysphagia

Dysphagia, or difficulty swallowing, can occur in the patient who has cancer. It can be caused by a mechanical obstruction from tumor or from severe reflux disease, stricture formation, or esophageal obstruction related to radiation therapy.

Treatment and the Role of the Nurse Treatment of dysphagia should involve a referral to a gastroenterologist for evaluation. For benign causes, dilation can be used. Antireflux medications may be used, and if dysphagia is treatment related, treatment may be postponed. When tumor is the cause, chemotherapy or radiation therapy may be necessary.

Nursing care would include providing comfort and nutrition. A Yankauer suction set-up for patients who are unable to swallow saliva should be at the bedside. Gastrostomy tube feedings may be required for patients who are unable to swallow safely.

Esophageal Achalasia

Esophageal achalasia occurs when the esophageal muscle cannot move food into the stomach. This disorder can present as a paraneoplastic

TABLE 24–8 ■ Conditions Associated with Hiccups

Irritation of the diaphragm: tumor, hepatomegaly, ascites	Uremia
Mediastinal cancers	Esophagitis
Gastric distention	Brain tumors

TABLE 24–9 ■ Remedies for Hiccups

Home Remedies	Medication Categories
Breathing into a paper bag	Antiflatulents
Drinking a glass of water mixed with 2 teaspoons of sugar	Antiemetics
Drinking a glass of cool water through a straw	Anticonvulsants/antiarrhythmics
Holding one's breath	Anesthetics
	Anticonvulsants
	Stimulants
	Sedatives
	Muscle relaxants

syndrome in patients who have gastric cancer. Patients usually experience dysphagia with all foods and liquids.

Treatment and the Role of the Nurse Treatment and nursing care is focused on palliative care. Gastrostomy tubes are necessary if the tumor is unresectable. In some cases, dilation is possible.

Hiccups

Hiccups can cause much distress in the patient with cancer. Although the exact cause of any hiccup is not known, Table 24–8 summarizes conditions associated with hiccups in the patient with cancer.

Treatment and the Role of the Nurse Treatment and nursing care of hiccups are centered on finding a remedy. Many "home" remedies may be tried; however, several medications can also be effective. It has been the author's observation that home remedies seldom work for the patient with cancer who has chronic hiccups. Table 24–9 summarizes remedies for hiccups.

Ascites

Malignant ascites is most commonly caused by the presence of ovarian, colon, gastric, or biliary tract carcinomas. Metastatic disease from other tumors that invade the liver may also cause ascites.

Before treatment can begin, a paracentesis must be performed to help determine the cause of the ascites and evaluate for the possibility of infection. If the ascites is caused by cancer, the treatment is strictly palliation, with the exception of ovarian cancer. Patients with ovarian cancer often have ascites at diagnosis. It is standard treatment for ovarian cancer patients to undergo surgery for the diagnosis and debulking of the disease, regardless of the suspected disease stage.

Palliation of malignant ascites includes administering furosemide and spironolactone and performing large-volume paracentesis. Chemotherapy may be given to help reduce the reproduction of malignant cells, thus slowing the recollection of ascites.

In the case of cancers other than ovarian, nursing care should focus on emotional support and comfort. Fluid and sodium restriction can help decrease fluid retention. Measuring abdominal girth for significant increases may help diagnosis when paracentesis is indicated. Placing the patient in the reverse Trendelenburg position may reduce pressure on the diaphragm. Cancer that has invaded the liver usually indicates a poor prognosis. The nurse must make the appropriate resources available to the patient for support. Clergy, social workers, psychologists, and hospice should be considered (see Chapter 37, End of Life).

Nursing care for the patient with ovarian cancer must focus on education of treatment options and symptom management (see Chapter 20, Gynecologic Malignancies).

Nausea and Vomiting

Historically, nausea and vomiting has been the first thing that enters one's mind when the topic of chemotherapy is mentioned. It can be a serious side effect of chemotherapy and radiation therapy; it can also be caused by several other processes that may be occurring in the patient with cancer. Table 24–10 summarizes risk factors for nausea and vomiting in the patient with cancer.

Distress related to nausea and vomiting can be profound. Patients who experience severe cases of this symptom often delay or withdraw from treatment. Furthermore, vomiting can lead to serious complications. Dehydration, electrolyte imbalances, and esophageal bleeding or tears can all result from prolonged vomiting. These complications can also delay or alter further treatment.

TABLE 24–10 ■ Risk Factors for Nausea and Vomiting

Chemotherapy (see Figure 24-11 for emetogenic potential of specific agents)
Radiation therapy to the abdominal area
Delayed gastric emptying (obstruction)
Opioid-related side effects
Increased intracranial pressure
Metabolic disturbances

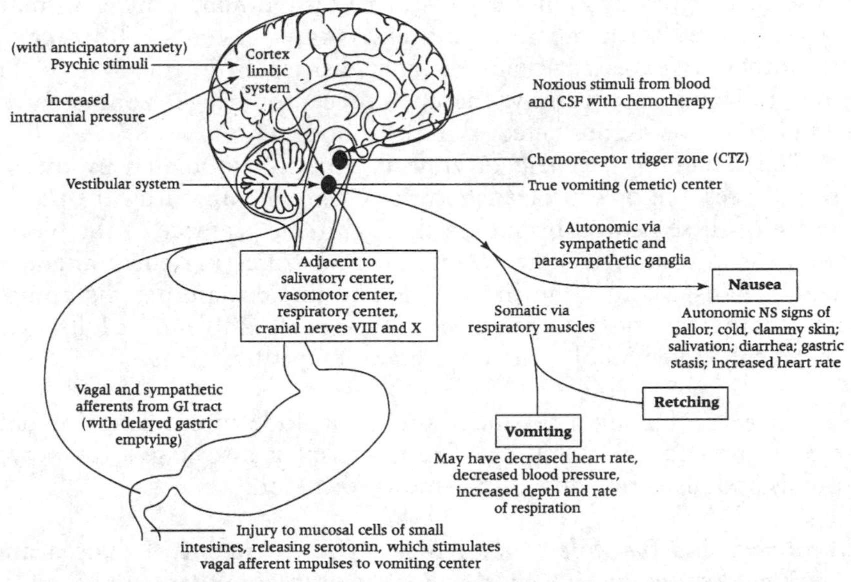

FIGURE 24–1 ■ The Physiology of Nausea and Vomiting.
Source: Burke, M. M., Wilkes, G. M., & Ingwersen, K., et al. (1996). *Chemotherapy and the nursing process*. Sudbury: Jones & Bartlett Publishers. Drawing adapted from original by Gail Wilkes.

Although many patients believe that the nausea and vomiting are caused by an upset stomach, the physiologic controls that lead to vomiting are much more complex. The diagram in Figure 24–1 illustrates the complex and many pathways that can cause nausea and vomiting.

The vomiting center is located in the brain near the brain stem. Its location is close to the centers that regulate salivation and the vasomotor response. This is thought to explain why salivation, respirations, and heart rate all increase with the sensation of nausea. The center receives stimulation through several different pathways. The vagal and sympathetic afferents that originate in the GI tract trigger the vomiting center when delayed stomach emptying occurs. Afferents in the midbrain respond to increased intracranial pressure but can also be triggered by a learned response. The learned response is called anticipatory nausea and vomiting. This occurs when a patient has an experience with treatment that leads to nausea. It is not uncommon for a patient to become nauseated before the chemotherapy is begun because of a learned response from previous treatment. The vestibular system can trigger the nausea center through inner ear disturbances. Although this is primarily associated with motion sickness, some patients who receive chemotherapy experience nausea from disruption in this system. Finally and most importantly, the chemoreceptor trigger zone receives stimulation from toxins detected in the blood.

The chemoreceptor trigger zone is actually stimulated by the increased presence of neurotransmitters. Chemotherapy drugs cause the release of these neurotransmitters through their presence in the blood. The neurotransmitters that are involved in triggering chemotherapy-related nausea and vomiting are serotonin, dopamine, histamine, prostaglandins, and gamma-aminobutyric acid. Table 24–11 lists the emetogenic potential of common chemotherapeutic agents.

Assessment Nursing assessment should include monitoring for patterns in nausea and vomiting. The nurse must also assess for bowel sounds and distention and check emesis for blood.

Treatment and the Role of the Nurse The treatment of nausea and vomiting focuses on prevention. Because the vomiting center can be stimulated in numerous ways, the use of multiple medications with different actions is the best approach. Table 24–12 summarizes how common antiemetics prevent or treat nausea and vomiting.

To effectively block the neurotransmitters from stimulating the chemoreceptor trigger zone, the medications must be given before the administration of the chemotherapeutic agents. In order to sustain the antiemetic effect, the medications must also be given around the clock and not as needed. Waiting until the patient is nauseated can allow too many neurotransmitters to enter the trigger zone, thus making the treatment more difficult.

Nursing care must focus on patient education about properly using antiemetics, maintaining patient nutritional status, and promoting comfort. Patients should be encouraged to take the scheduled medica-

TABLE 24-11 ■ Emetogenic Potential of Common Chemotherapeutic Agents

Incidence	Agent	Onset (hours)	Duration (hours)
Very High (> 90%)	Cisplatin	1–6	24–48+
	Dacarbazine	1–3	1–12
	Mechlorethamine	0.5–2	8–24
	Melphalan—high dose	0.3–6	6–12
	Streptozocin	1–6	12–24
	Cytarabine—high dose	2–4	12–24
High (60–90%)	Carmustine	2–4	4–24
	Cyclophosphamide	4–12	12–24
	Procarbazinc	24–27	variable
	Etoposide—high dose	4–6	24
	Semustine	1–5	12–24
	Lomustine	4–6	12–24
	Dactinomycin	2–5	24
	Picamycin	1–6	12–24
	Methotrexate—high dose	4–12	3–12da
Moderate (30–60%)	Doxorubicin	4–6	6+
	Mitoxantronc	4–6	6+
	Topotecan	—	—
	5-Fluorouracil	3–6	24+
	Irinotecan	—	—
	Mitomycin C	1–4	48–72
	Ifosfamide	4–12	—
	Curboplatin	4–6	12–24
	Paclitaxel	1–6	2–12
	Daunorubicin	2–6	24
	L-Asparaginase	1–4	2–12
	Hexamethylmelamine	1–4	—

Source: Burke, M. M., Wilkes, G. M., & Ingwersen, K., et al. (1996). *Chemotherapy and the nursing process.* Sudbury: Jones & Bartlett Publishers.

tions and not wait until after nausea begins. Taking as-needed nausea medications a half-hour before meals can help decrease nausea during meals. When the patient is hospitalized, the nursing staff should remove the tray tops before entering the room to avoid an overwhelming smell of food that can stimulate nausea. The patient at home should avoid entering the kitchen during the preparation of food. Many patients tolerate cold food or chilled supplements better than hot food. If

TABLE 24-12 ■ Mechanism of Action in Common Antiemetics

Drug/Class	Action
Ondansetron, granisetron, dolasetron mesylate	Serotonin 5-HT_ receptor blocker
Dexamethasone	Inhibits prostaglandin
Diphenhydramine, promethazine	Inhibits histamine
Dronabino	Depresses CNS
Droperidol, haloperidol, perphenazine, prochlorperazine	Inhibits dopamine
Metoclopramide	Blocks dopamine but also stimulates upper GI tract motility to increase gastric emptying
Scopolamine	Blocks cholinergic impulses (motion sickness)
Lorazepam	Depresses CNS

Key: CNS = central nervous system; GI = gastrointestinal.

vomiting persists and the patient is unable to maintain an adequate fluid balance, the use of intravenous hydration or parenteral nutrition may be necessary.

Diarrhea

Diarrhea can occur for several reasons in the patient with cancer. Table 24–13 summarizes the five causes of diarrhea.

Treatment and the Role of the Nurse Before treating diarrhea, the cause of the diarrhea must be determined. If it is infectious diarrhea, antibiotics must be administered and antidiarrheal agents may not be used until the infection is under control.

Diarrhea related to the disease itself may require surgery, chemotherapy, or radiation therapy. When carcinoid syndrome is present, octreotide acetate is administered.

Diarrhea related to treatment is commonly treated with diphenoxylate and loperamide. Treatment-related diarrhea is commonly caused by the deterioration of the mucosal lining known as enteritis. However, irinotecan can cause a cholinogenic effect, resulting in abdominal cramping and diarrhea. Atropine can prevent this effect. In most cases, loperamide is administered with doses of irinotecan to help lessen the severity of the diarrhea. In the case of severe diarrhea caused by

TABLE 24–13 ■ Causes of Diarrhea in the Patient with Cancer

Category	Description
Disease itself	Partial bowel obstruction Endocrine hypersecretion of serotonin Gastrin Vasoactive intestinal protein Prostaglandins (carcinoid)
Disease sequelae	Fecal impaction Anxiety Melena Infection
Prior history of noncancerous diseases	Diverticulitis Inflammatory bowel disease
Cancer treatment	Chemotherapy with antimetabolites, irinotecan Radiation therapy to abdomen, pelvis, lower spine
Drugs used in other symptom management	Laxatives Antacids NSAIDs Nutritional supplements Opiate withdrawal

Key: NSAID = nonsteroidal anti-inflammatory drug.

TABLE 24–14 ■ Nursing Interventions for Cancer-Related Diarrhea

Monitor intake and output: report imbalances and number of stools.
Monitor electrolytes: report abnormal levels and replace as ordered.
Treat pain.
Practice skin care to prevent skin breakdown in perianal or stoma area.
Monitor nutritional status: parenteral nutrition may be necessary if patient is unable to eat.

irinotecan, antimetabolites, or radiation therapy, dose adjustments may be required.

Nursing care must first focus on obtaining a history. Determining the most likely cause of the diarrhea help determine the appropriate interventions. Table 24–14 summarizes nursing interventions.

Gastrointestinal Bleeding

GI bleeding occurs most commonly in patients with primary gastric tumors and secondary gastric lymphoma, but non-cancer related causes can also result in GI bleeding. These causes include stress ulcers, gastritis, peptic ulcer disease, esophageal varices, candida esophagitis and tears, diverticulosis, vascular ectasias of the colon, and colitis. Corticosteroids, commonly used in conjunction with chemotherapy and radiation therapy regimens, are associated with GI bleeding.

GI bleeds can be slow or massive. They can present with hematemesis, coffee ground emesis, melena, or bright red blood per rectum or stoma. The symptoms include abdominal cramping and pain, vomiting, and symptoms of hypovolemia.

Treatment and the Role of the Nurse The most important treatment is always volume repletion. The hemoglobin and hematocrit should be monitored frequently and red blood cells replaced. Oxygen therapy may help maintain tissue oxygen levels. Upper GI bleeds can be treated with nasogastric tube lavage with tepid water. Coagulopathies are not uncommon in patients with cancer. The administration of fresh frozen plasma, platelets, and cryoprecipitate may be necessary to control the bleeding.

Nursing assessment for hypovolemia must be constant. Meticulous intake and output with description of emesis and stool must be recorded. Monitoring blood counts and vital signs and looking for early signs of shock are all part of nursing care.

Bowel Obstruction

Intestinal obstruction in the patient with cancer can be acute or chronic, partial or complete. It can occur in the small or the large intestine. Obstruction occurs when contents are unable to pass through the GI tract. Blockage can occur from fecal impaction, cancerous lesions on the wall of the bowel, external tumors exerting pressure on the bowel, or neuromuscular and vascular disruptions in bowel functioning. Radiation exposure can cause thickening of the bowel wall and can place a patient at risk for an obstruction up to 20 years after therapy. Approximately half of all ovarian cancer patients experience bowel obstruction of some type during their disease and treatment. Other cancers that can cause obstruction are colorectal, gastric, pancreatic, uterine, bladder, cervical, lymphoma, breast, melanoma, and soft tissue sarcoma. Ninety percent of small-bowel obstructions result from surgical adhesions.

Perforation occurs when the intraluminal pressure of the bowel wall surpasses its resistive capability; the result is a rupture of the bowel membrane. This causes spilling of the bowel contents into the peritoneal cavity. This is a life-threatening emergency with a high mortality rate. It is generally treated with immediate surgical repair and antibiotics.

Assessment The patient who is experiencing an intestinal blockage experiences nausea and vomiting, abdominal pain, abdominal distention, and obstipation or watery diarrhea. The patient may have a fever and may appear dehydrated. Assessment should include gathering a history of bowel movements, listening to bowel sounds, and palpating the abdomen for tender or firm areas.

Treatment and the Role of the Nurse Treatment and nursing care include placement of a nasogastric tube to decompress the colon and resolve the distention. Electrolytes must be monitored closely and corrected, and parenteral nutrition should be considered. In many instances, surgery is the only treatment for permanent relief of the obstruction. Surgical intervention is considered a palliative measure, even when the patient is considered terminal. Nursing care should focus on comfort measures, including keeping the mouth clean and moist, managing pain, and providing psychosocial support. If the patient has experienced a perforation, sign and symptoms of septic shock must be monitored.

Constipation

Constipation can occur for many reasons in the patient with cancer. Causes of constipation in the patient with cancer are presented in Table 24–15.

Constipation can interfere with quality of life, cause pain, and decrease appetite. In severe cases, perforation of the bowel can occur.

Assessment and the Role of the Nurse Nursing care is central in the treatment of constipation. It begins with assessment of the patient's dietary habits and bowel movement patterns. It also includes gathering the historical data that could help identify the most likely cause of the constipation. Immediate treatment consists of medications to relieve the constipation. Magnesium citrate, lactulose, and docusate are frequently used, but enemas and suppositories are used very cautiously in the patient who has received cancer treatment, because intestinal walls

TABLE 24–15 ■ Causes of Constipation in the Patient with Cancer

Category	Description
Disease itself	Primary bowel cancer
	Paraneoplastic autonomic neuropathy
Disease sequelae	Dehydration
	Paralysis
	Immobility
	Alterations in bowel elimination patterns
Prior history	Laxative abuse
	Other disease
Cancer therapy	Vinca alkaloids
	Bowel surgery
Medications used to manage symptoms	Opioids
	Antihistamines
	Tricyclic antidepressants
	Aluminum antacids

that have been exposed to chemotherapy and radiation therapy are easily torn if they are disrupted. Immunosuppression and low platelet counts may also be present. These conditions all contraindicate the use of enemas or suppositories. Once the acute constipation in relieved, the nurse should educate the patient about preventive measures and medications. High-fiber diets, adequate fluid intake, and use of a daily stimulant, such as senna, are recommended. These interventions are especially important for the patient who is taking opioids.

■ Conclusion

Complications of the GI system can inhibit quality of life, delay treatment, and threaten life if left untreated. Nursing plays a key role in assessing, preventing, and treating each of these complications. Patient education for the prevention and treatment of GI side effects is crucial to maintaining quality of life and nutritional status.

■ Resources

- American Cancer Society. This internet site gives access to patient education materials as well as resources for patient support. Patient education materials include "Nutrition for the Person with Cancer" and "NCCN/ACS Patient Treatment Guidelines for Nausea and Vomiting." 800-ACS-2345 or *www.cancer.org*

- Oncology Nursing Society. This internet site offers reference materials on many symptoms. It also offers publications of nursing care guidelines. *www.ONS.org*
- CancerSource RN. This internet site allows anyone to register and offers patient education materials that can be personalized for any patient, disease process, treatment, or side effect. *www.Cancersourcern.com*
- National Cancer Institute. This site gives access to clinical trials for disease and symptom management. 800-4-CANCER or *www.cancer.gov*

Bibliography

Casciato, D., & Lowitz, B. (Ed.). (2000). *Manual of clinical oncology* (4th ed.). Philadelphia: Lippincott, Williams & Wilkins.

King, C. (1997). Nonpharmacologic management of chemotherapy-induced nausea and vomiting. *Oncology Nursing Forum, 24(7)*. 41–46.

McCarthy, D., & Weihofen, D. (1999). The effect of nutritional supplements on food intake in patients undergoing radiotherapy. *Oncology Nursing Forum, 269(5)*. 897-900.

Rhodes, V. (1997). Criteria for assessment of nausea, vomiting, and retching. *Oncology Nursing Forum, 24(7)*. 13-20.

Wilkes, G., Ingwersen, K., & Barton-Burke, M. (2001). *Oncology nursing drug handbook*. Sudbury, MA: Jones & Bartlett Publishers.

Wilkes, G. (2001). Hiccups. *www.emedicine.com* Retrieved on July 9, 2003.

CHAPTER

25

Fatigue

Andrea M. Barsevick

Deena Damsky Dell

Individuals with cancer have consistently described fatigue as their most persistent and distressing symptom, regardless of diagnosis, type of treatment, or stage of disease. Cancer-related fatigue has been defined as "a persistent subjective sense of tiredness related to cancer or cancer treatment that interferes with usual functioning" (Mock, 2001). It can have a negative effect on quality of life by reducing the individual's ability to function during treatment as well as lingering after treatment is over. It can also cause treatment delays and may be related to shorter survival.

Over the past decade, fatigue has become better recognized and understood by health care professionals. However, fatigue does not occur as a single isolated symptom. Instead, it often occurs along with several symptoms that challenge the coping of individuals with cancer. Little is known about how symptom combinations or clusters interact or influence patient outcome, but we do know that fatigue, pain, and sleep disturbances negatively influence one another. Fatigue seems to play a central role in increased symptom burden. Perhaps this is because, unlike other symptoms, fatigue has no definitive pharmacologic treatment.

■ Assessment

Although there is not yet an established method for conducting an assessment of fatigue, individuals and organizations have made recommendations. The National Comprehensive Cancer Network, a consortium of 19 comprehensive cancer centers, has established guidelines for the assessment and management of cancer-related fatigue in a two-stage process. Screening for the presence and intensity of fatigue is suggested for every patient with cancer at the initial contact with a health care professional. A quantitative rating on a 0–10 rating scale is easily documented. A rating of 1–3 indicates mild, 4–6 moderate, and 7–10 severe fatigue. Patients unable to put a numeric value on their fatigue may use terms such as mild, moderate, or severe, or they can point to a pictorial representation to indicate how they feel (Figure 25–1). If it is determined that fatigue is absent or mild, no immediate follow-up is required; however, periodic screening assessments of fatigue are recommended.

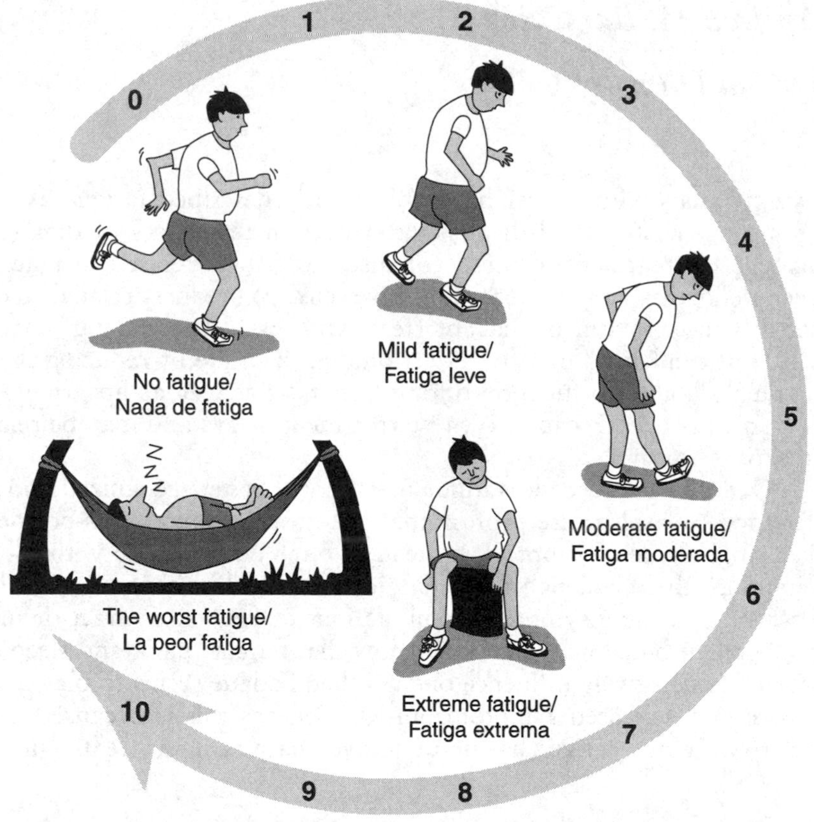

FIGURE 25–1 ■ Fatigue Scale.
Source: From the *National cancer fatigue awareness planning and promotional guide,* 2000. Used with permission by the Oncology Nursing Society.

TABLE 25–1 ■ Assessment of Fatigue

1. Is fatigue related to recurrence or progression of malignancy?
2. What is the treatment regimen and its likelihood of causing fatigue?
3. What medications is the patient taking (including prescribed, over-the-counter, and herbal remedies) that could cause or contribute to fatigue?
4. Does the individual have any noncancer comorbidities (e.g., congestive heart failure, chronic lung disease, renal or hepatic failure, sepsis, or endocrine dysfunction) that could cause or contribute to fatigue?
5. What are the onset, duration, and pattern of fatigue, as well as aggravating or alleviating factors that could provide information about potential cause(s) of the fatigue?
6. To what extent does fatigue interfere with ability to function in usual activities?

If fatigue is present at a moderate or severe level (4 or higher on a 0–10 scale), the National Comprehensive Cancer Network guidelines recommend that a focused history and physical examination be conducted to further evaluate factors that could cause this symptom (Table 25–1).

Addressing these issues provides important information about potential causes and consequences of fatigue. Fatigue can be an important indicator of cancer recurrence or disease progression. An aggressive treatment regimen is often a major source of fatigue. A host of medications, including beta-blockers, opioids, antidepressants, anxiolytics, antihistamines, and antiemetics, can cause fatigue; adjustment of dose or selection of an alternative drug could alleviate the symptom. In addition, the identification and management of comorbidities could alleviate fatigue. Likewise, knowing the pattern of fatigue and its impact on functioning can provide a basis for education and nursing care activities.

In addition to the history and physical examination, it is important to evaluate specific treatable causes of fatigue, including the presence and severity of pain, emotional distress (especially depression), sleep disturbance, anemia, nutritional deficits, and low activity level. The identification and management of one or more of these causes has the potential to reduce or alleviate fatigue.

■ Patient Education

Patient education is an essential component of fatigue management for all cancer patients and their families. Education about the expected intensity, pattern, and duration of fatigue for a given set of circumstances (e.g., type of treatment or disease stage) should be made available to all cancer patients, especially if they are likely to experience fatigue during the course of their disease and/or treatment. Ideally, preparatory information about fatigue is provided before its onset. With this information, patients and their families can plan for the intrusion of this symptom into their lives and modify their usual activities to accommodate it. Without information about fatigue that is expected during treatment, patients and families may inappropriately attribute fatigue to disease progression or treatment failure.

■ Treatment

Several approaches are available for the management of fatigue, including specific pharmacologic and nonpharmacologic interventions. Anemia (see Chapter 22, Myelosuppression) is a treatable cause of fatigue; iron or folic acid replacement can be used to restore iron and red blood cells to the appropriate level if there is a deficiency. Blood transfusions may be used to replace acute blood loss. If the anemia is related to poor nutritional intake, a nutritional consultation should be initiated. Orexigenic (appetite-stimulating) agents may be tried; megestrol acetate and dexamethasone stimulate appetite and weight gain. Dronabinol has been shown to increase appetite as well as mood.

The use of recombinant human erythropoietin is a significant breakthrough in the management of the anemia of chronic disease. Increasing the hemoglobin to a range of 11–13 g/dl has been shown to reduce fatigue and improve quality of life. Two pharmacologic agents have been shown to increase hemoglobin levels and decrease transfusion requirements, especially with early intervention, before the hemoglobin decreases to less than 10 g/dl. Epoetin alfa, a synthetic erythropoietin, may be administered via subcutaneous injection once a week at a dose at 40,000 units. If hemoglobin has not increased by at least 1 g/dl after 4 weeks, the dose should be increased to 60,000 units per week. The recommended pediatric dose (6 months-18 years) is 25-300 units per kilogram via intravenous or subcutaneous injection 3-7 times per week. Darbepoetin alfa, an erythropoiesis-stimulating protein, is administered via subcutaneous injection at a dose of 2.25-4.5 micrograms per kilogram weekly. It should be administered every 2 weeks in patients who were previously receiving Epoetin alpha one time a week. Doses may be adjusted one time a month to maintain a target hemoglobin of 12. Safety and effectiveness in children has not been established. Patients may complain of burning with the injections of erythropoietin alfa or darbepoetin. This is related to the acidity of the solution. Burning can be decreased if the nurse draws a bubble of air into the hub of the syringe. This action prevents the drug from entering the dermal layer.

Other treatable causes of fatigue that are amenable to pharmacotherapy include pain and depression (see Chapters 23 [Cancer Pain] and 27 [Anxiety and Depression in the Oncology Setting]). Research has shown that the presence of unrelieved pain increases fatigue in individuals with cancer and that pain and fatigue together can increase overall symptom burden. Optimal pain management could diminish fatigue. It is also possible that drowsiness induced by pain medications could contribute to fatigue. A careful evaluation and titration of pain medications may be a useful adjunct to fatigue management. According to anecdotal reports, stimulants such as caffeine, methylphenidate, pemoline, dextroamphetamine, and modafinil may be useful in reducing fatigue, but none of these have been tested for efficacy in randomized, controlled trials. As many as 25% of patients with cancer experience clinical depression; fatigue is one of the presenting symptoms of this disorder. Appropriate management of depression with antidepressants and psychotherapy could reduce fatigue and result in increased energy levels.

■ The Role of the Nurse

Not all interventions for fatigue are pharmacologic; many self-care approaches also are effective. Although the idea is counterintuitive, increased physical activity and exercise programs are very effective ways to manage fatigue. Although most studies have focused on females with breast cancer, a few studies that included both men and women have demonstrated similar effectiveness. When individuals receive toxic therapies for cancer, they tend to decrease their activity level, causing a loss of capacity for physical performance. Then they must expend more energy to perform usual activities, resulting in fatigue. Physical exercise programs reduce or eliminate the loss of capacity, thereby preventing fatigue. Based on the body of evidence about the benefits of exercise for patients with cancer, it is reasonable to encourage all individuals to maintain or increase their activity levels during cancer therapy. Walking several times a week has positive results. Patients should be encouraged to set short-term goals (time or distance) and increase activity level as they are able. Caution must be taken in prescribing exercise programs for patients with comorbidities, such as bony metastasis, neutropenia, low platelet count, anemia, or fever. These patients may need to be referred to a physical therapist or physical medicine and rehabilitation practitioner.

If individuals describe themselves as being "mentally fatigued," having a diminished capacity to concentrate or focus attention, they may benefit from restorative therapy. Bird watching, craft activities, or sitting in a natural environment (e.g., a park) are examples of restorative activities. The restorative activity should be something fascinating to the patient and should provide a sense of being removed from his or her current environment. The activity should be performed at least three times a week for 20 to 30 minutes. Studies have shown that patients who engaged in these activities had improved concentration and problem solving and earlier return to work after breast cancer surgery.

Another self-care activity is the use of energy-conservation strategies. Energy conservation is the deliberate planned management of individuals' energy resources to keep them from being depleted. It is used to balance rest and activity so that important activities can be continued. To conserve energy, individuals can set priorities, delegate less important tasks, pace themselves in doing tasks, take extra rest periods, and plan high-energy activities at times of peak energy. Labor-saving devices also help to conserve energy; these may include the use of a bedside commode, walker, energy-saving appliances, and grabbing tools.

Sleep disturbance is a common problem in patients with cancer that can cause or contribute to fatigue. Both insomnia and hypersomnia can compound fatigue. Patients should be taught to avoid stimulants (including caffeine and nicotine) or stimulating activities 3 hours before bedtime, long or late afternoon naps, and alcohol. Alcohol may help induce sleep, but the quality of sleep is poor. Relaxation techniques or a warm bath may help promote sleep.

Issues may arise in the workplace if there is not good communication between employee, employer, and coworkers regarding the nature of cancer-related fatigue. Resources helpful with this issue can be found at the Oncology Nursing Society (*www.cancersymptoms.org*)web site as well as the Job Accommodation Network (*www.JAN.wvu.edu*).

■ Conclusion

The management of cancer-related fatigue begins with an initial screening assessment that can be conducted easily in the context of nursing care. It is important to educate all patients about fatigue if they are likely to experience it during the course of their disease and/or treatment. The presence of moderate or severe fatigue requires a more in-depth history and physical examination. It also requires the assessment of specific treatable causes of fatigue; these could include pain, distress, sleep disturbance, anemia, nutritional deficits, and low activity level. If any of these conditions are present, they should be managed, and a follow-up assessment of fatigue should be conducted. If a specific treatable cause of fatigue is not found or if the fatigue remains unresolved despite treatment, nonpharmacologic therapies should be considered. These include the use of exercise, attention conservation, and energy conservation. Effective fatigue management is the result of regular systematic assessment, education, and targeted therapies.

■ Resources

Treatment guidelines:

- National Comprehensive Cancer Network (NCCN) Fatigue Treatment Guidelines: *www.nccn.org*.
  American Cancer Society (ACS) Fatigue Treatment Guidelines for Patients with Cancer: 800-ACS-2345 or *www.cancer.org*

Professional organizations and web sites:

- American Cancer Society Resources on Fatigue *www.cancer.org/docroot/MIT/MIT_2_2x_Fatigue.asp* or *800-ACS-2345*
- Oncology Nursing Society Cancer Symptoms: *www.cancersymptoms.org/symptoms/fatigue/*
- Job Accommodation Network: *www.JAN.wvu.edu* or 800-ADA-WORK

Bibliography

Cimprich, B. (1993). Development of an intervention to restore attention in cancer patients. *Cancer Nursing, 16,* 83–92.

Curt, G. A., Breitbart, W., Cella, D., Groopman, J. E., Horning, S. J., Itri, L. M., et al. (2000). Impact of cancer-related fatigue on the lives of patients: New findings from the Fatigue Coalition. *Oncologist, 5,* 353–360.

Mills, M., & Graci, G. (2003). Sleep disturbances. In C. H. Yarbro, M. H. Frogge, & M. Goodman (Eds.), *Cancer symptom management* (3rd ed., pp. 111–128). Sudbury, MA: Jones & Bartlett Publishers.

Mock, V. (2001). Fatigue management: evidence and guidelines for practice. *Cancer, 92*(suppl.), 1699–1707.

CHAPTER

26

Sleep Problems

Stacey Young-McCaughan

Various studies have reported that between 45% and 75% of patients with cancer experience difficulty sleeping. Insomnia, or the inability to sleep when desired, is the most frequently reported sleep disturbance. Insomnia can include the inability to initiate sleep, inability to maintain sleep, early awakening, and/or the feeling that sleep is not refreshing. Sleep disturbances can also include hypersomnia, or the inability to stay awake when desired.

Possible causes of insomnia and hypersomnia in patients with cancer include the cancer treatment, symptoms, psychological problems, medications, and environmental distractions (Table 26–1). Because insomnia is the most common sleep disturbance, this chapter focuses on it. Insomnia is often associated with fatigue, pain, depression, and anxiety. Each of these symptoms individually and collectively negatively affect patients' quality of life.

The diagnostic criteria for insomnia are listed in Table 26–2. Symptoms lasting less than 1 month are considered transient or situational, symptoms lasting between 1 and 6 months are considered short-term or sub acute, and symptoms lasting 6 months or longer are considered chronic.

This chapter does not necessarily represent the official position or policy of the Army Medical Department, the Department of Defense, or the U.S. government.

TABLE 26–1 ■ Causes of Sleep Disturbances in Patients with Cancer

	Insomnia	**Hypersomnia**
Cancer treatment	• Steroids	• Bone marrow transplantation • Radiation therapy, in particular, cranial radiation
Symptoms	• Dyspnea • Fever • Hot flashes • Nausea & vomiting • Pain • Pruritus • Urinary frequency	• Delirium
Psychological problems	• Anxiety • Depression • Worry	
Medications	• Alcohol • Benzodiazepines • Opioids • Steroids	• Sleeping medications in patients with impaired hepatic clearance
Environmental distractions	• Light • Noise • Unfamiliar surroundings, e.g., with hospitalization	• Darkness

TABLE 26–2 ■ Diagnostic Criteria for Insomnia

- Sleep latency, or the time to fall asleep, ≥ 30 minutes
- Sleep efficiency, or the time spent in bed asleep as a percentage of the time spent in bed, < 85%
- Sleep disturbance occurring ≥ 3 nights per week
- Sleep disturbance causing impairment of daytime functioning

■ Sleep-Wake Cycle

Sleep is a naturally occurring circadian behavior that is believed to be a restorative process essential for normal metabolic, thermoregulatory,

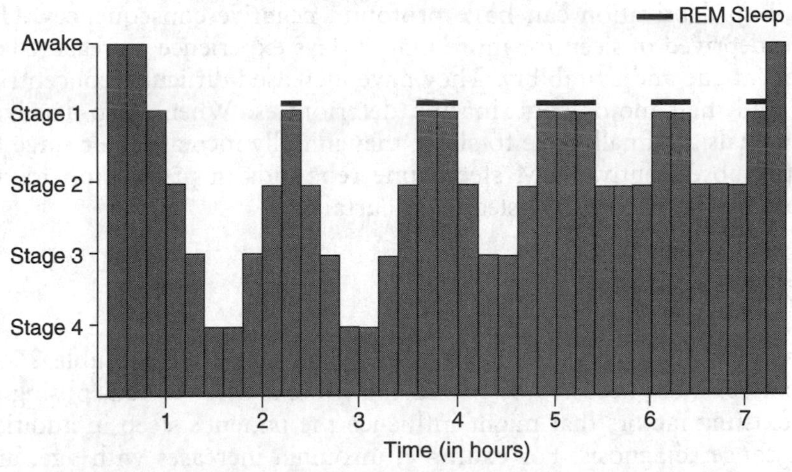

FIGURE 26–1 ▪ Stages of sleep.

and information-processing functions. There are five distinct stages of sleep. Stages I, II, III, and IV are collectively called non-rapid eye movement sleep. The fifth stage is labeled rapid eye movement (REM) sleep.

Each of the sleep stages occurs several times during normal sleep in cycles lasting approximately 90 minutes (Figure 26–1). During non-rapid eye movement sleep, the electroencephalogram (EEG) becomes progressively more synchronized. Temperature drops, as do heart rate, blood pressure, and respiratory rate. REM sleep is characterized by the sudden onset of an asynchronous EEG pattern very similar to the EEG pattern when the person is awake. However, the body is flaccid during REM sleep, except for twitches of the face and the eyes. Sleepers awakened from REM sleep typically report dreaming.

Sleep is regulated by the hypothalamus and brainstem. Triggers for sleep and wake are not clearly understood. Like sleep and wake cycles, body temperature and hormone levels also have 24-hour circadian rhythms and so are postulated to be internal triggers for sleep and wake. Body temperature fluctuates during the day, the highest being about mid-afternoon and the lowest being early morning. As body temperature falls mid-afternoon, many people feel sleepy. Melatonin is one hormone believed to trigger sleep. Melatonin is normally produced by the pineal gland and secretion increases when it becomes dark. This may be one way light and dark are believed to be an external cue for sleep and awake. Many people report sleeping longer during the winter, when it is dark for a longer proportion of the day.

Sleep deprivation can have profound negative consequences. Humans deprived of sleep for more than 2 days experience increasing levels of fatigue and irritability. They have increased difficulty concentrating, and their motor coordination deteriorates. When sleep-deprived individuals are finally able to sleep, they initially increase their stage IV sleep. Subsequently, REM sleep time rebounds in proportion to the amount of time that REM sleep was curtailed.

■ Assessment

Items typically included in a sleep assessment are listed in Table 26–3. This assessment needs to be put in the context of any predisposing or pre-existing factors that might influence the patient's sleep in addition to a cancer diagnosis. For example, insomnia increases with age, and women have twice the prevalence of sleep disturbance than men. A family or personal history of sleep disorders may also put the patient at increased risk for sleep disturbance with a cancer diagnosis.

The best measure of sleep would be one that is unobtrusive and that can assess both sleep and activity over time while the person is performing normal activities of daily living. Three very different, yet valid and reliable, measures of sleep commonly used in both clinical practice and research include a sleep diary, the Pittsburgh Sleep Index, and the wrist actigraph. Each of these measures is described in Table 26–4.

■ Treatment

Treatment of insomnia should first address any known precipitating causes of sleep disturbance. For example, pain should be treated with analgesics, and nausea and vomiting should be treated with antiemetics. After obvious causes of insomnia are addressed, sleeping medications should be considered. Hypnotic medications are the most commonly used treatment for insomnia. Table 26–5 lists commonly prescribed medications.

Nonpharmacologic therapies are as effective as sleeping medications, with between 70% and 80% of patients benefiting from treatment. The most common nonpharmacologic interventions include stimulus control therapy, which aims to establish a regular circadian sleep wake cycle with environmental cues; sleep restriction, which limits the time in bed to sleep; relaxation therapy, which promotes relaxation and sleep; and cognitive therapy, which corrects any misperceptions of sleep and insomnia to establish realistic expectations of sleep. Typical sleep hygiene recommendations are listed in Table 26–6.

TABLE 26-3 ■ Sleep Assessment

- Sleep latency, or the time to fall asleep (normally ≤ 30 minutes)
- Wake after sleep onset
- Total sleep time (normally 6–8 hours per night)
- Sleep efficiency, or the time spent in bed asleep as a percentage of the time spent in bed (normally ≥ 85%)
- Timing and duration of daytime naps
- Feeling that sleep was restorative
- Energy for daily activities
- Use of sleep medications or medications known to affect sleep, e.g., caffeine, alcohol, tobacco, steroids, amphetamines, opioids, and benzodiazepines

TABLE 26-4 ■ Examples of Measures of Sleep

Sleep Measure	Description
Sleep diary	• A qualitative method of sleep assessment. • The patient is cued to comment on time they went to bed, the time they arose in the morning, number and length of awakenings during the night, any medications taken, number and length of daytime naps, energy levels at various times during the day, and so on.
Pittsburgh sleep index	• 19-item instrument scored to produce seven component subscales describing sleep quality, sleep latency, sleep duration, habitual sleep efficiency, sleep disturbance, use of sleeping medications, and daytime dysfunction. • The overall score of the Pittsburgh Sleep Index can range from 0 to 21; the higher the score, the worse the sleep quality.
Actigraph	• A microcomputer that measures movement in three dimensions. The displacement of a sensor beam in the actigraph generates a voltage proportional to the deflection. These changes in voltage are recorded by the actigraph as activity counts per epoch of time. • Data from the wrist actigraph can provide an objective assessment of minutes of awake and sleep time, activity intensity, number and length of nighttime awakenings, number and length of daytime napping, and sleep efficiency.

TABLE 26–5 ■ Commonly Prescribed Medications for Sleep

Medication	Usual Dosage
Benzodiazepines	
Clonazepam (Klonopin)	0.5–1.5 mg at bedtime
Estazolam (ProSom)	1.0–2.0 mg at bedtime
Flurazepam (Dalmane)	15–30 mg at bedtime
Lorazepam (Ativan)	0.5–2.0 mg at bedtime
Oxazepam (Serax)	10–30 mg at bedtime
Quazepam (Doral)	7.5–15 mg at bedtime
Temazepam (Restoril)	7.5–30.0 mg at bedtime
Triazolam (Halcion)	0.125–0.25 mg at bedtime
Sedative-Hypnotic	
Zaleplon (Sonata)	10–20 mg at bedtime
Zolpidem (Ambien)	5–10 mg at bedtime
Antidepressants	
Amitriptyline (Elavil)	25–75 mg at bedtime
Doxepin (Sinequan)	30 –150 mg at bedtime
Trazodone (Desyrel)	50–150 mg at bedtime

TABLE 26–6 ■ Sample Sleep Hygiene Recommendations

- Stay in bed only for the hours intended for sleeping.
- Establish a regular bedtime and wake time.
- Exercise regularly, but not late in the evening.
- Don't worry about getting to sleep.
- Try to deal with worries before bedtime (e.g., writing down worries that need to be addressed at a later time).
- Create your perfect sleep environment (e.g., darkening the room, playing relaxing music, reading before turning off the lights, using progressive muscle relaxation).
- Avoid stimulants (e.g., caffeine, tobacco, heavy or spicy meals).
- Use sleeping medications as prescribed.

■ The Role of the Nurse

Nursing care focuses on (a) assessment to ascertain the cause of the sleep disturbance and (b) patient education, suggesting actions that patients might try to get a restful night's sleep.

■ Resources

Insomnia is just beginning to be recognized as a concern in patients with cancer, and so there is not very much information on sleep disorders specific to this patient population. However, several organizations provide generic information about insomnia and sleep disorders.

- The National Institutes of Health National Heart, Lung, and Blood Institute (NHLBI) hosts a site for both the public and health care professionals with information on sleep and sleep disorders located at *www.nhlbi.nih.gov/about/ncsdr.*
- The American Academy of Sleep Medicine (One Westbrook Corporate Center, Suite 920, Westchester, IL 60154, phone 708-492-0930). Their web site (*www.aasmnet.org/*) has a specific section dedicated to patient information and an extensive listing of other sleep-related web sites.
- The American Sleep Association (614 South 8th Street, Suite 282, Philadelphia, PA 19147, phone 1-443-593-2285) is the national organization of the International Sleep Medicine Association. The aim of the organization is to improve sleep health around the world by educating health care providers and increasing public awareness about sleep health and sleeping disorders. Their web site is located at *www.AmericanSleepAssociation.org.*

Bibliography

Ancoli-Israel, S., Moore, P. J., & Jones, V. (2001). The relationship between fatigue and sleep in cancer patients: A review. *European Journal of Cancer Care,* 10, 245–255.

Mills, M., & Graci, G. M. (2004). Sleep disturbances. In C. H. Yarbro, M. H. Frogge, & M. Goodman (Ed.), *Cancer symptom management* (3rd ed., pp. 111–133). Sudbury, MA: Jones & Bartlett.

Savard, J., & Morin, C. M. (2001). Insomnia in the context of cancer: A review of a neglected problem. *Journal of Clinical Oncology,* 19, 895–908.

CHAPTER

27

Anxiety and Depression in the Oncology Setting

Jeannie V. Pasacreta

Major changes in the understanding and treatment of cancer have led to a wider range of treatment options and longer survival. In addition, new genetic technologies have theoretically moved the crisis that is often associated with diagnosis to the prediagnostic period. Although such advances are quite positive, their impact on the cancer are profound and cannot be overlooked.

The goal of this chapter is to provide information about the assessment and treatment of anxiety and depression in individuals who are faced with cancer, and to delineate psychosocial interventions that are effective in minimizing these troubling symptoms. Practical guidelines for managing patients and identifying those who may require formal psychiatric consultation are offered.

Many health care professionals lack knowledge about the signs and symptoms of depression and anxiety. Often, patients who elicit anxiety and sadness in staff, rather than their objectively depressed or anxious counterparts, are referred for psychiatric evaluation. A lack of attention to systematic assessment and treatment of depression and anxiety may lead to ongoing dysphoria, family conflict, noncompliance with treatment, increased length of hospitalization, persistent worry, and suicidal ideation.

■ Prevalence of Anxiety and Depression along the Cancer Trajectory

Depression and anxiety are the most commonly occurring psychiatric states in patients with cancer. When severe or unremitting, these problems require aggressive assessment and treatment. Psychiatric emergencies require the same rapid intervention as medical crises.

The acute crisis response has been described as a usual response to a cancer diagnosis as well as to other transitions in the disease process (e.g., identification of risk status, beginning of treatment, recurrence, treatment failure, disease progression). The crisis is characterized primarily by symptoms of anxiety and depression. Under favorable circumstances, these psychological symptoms should resolve within a short period . The time period is variable but the general consensus is that once the crisis has passed and individuals know what to expect in terms of a treatment plan, psychological symptoms diminish.

For some patients, psychological distress does not subside with usual interventions. Unfortunately, clinically relevant symptoms and severe psychiatric syndromes are often missed by non-psychiatric care providers. It can be difficult to detect serious psychiatric reactions in patients because several of the diagnostic criteria used to evaluate the presence of severe depression (e.g., lack of appetite, insomnia, decreased sexual interest, diminished energy) may overlap with usual effects of the disease and its treatment. In addition, health care providers may confuse their own fears about cancer with the emotional reactions of their patients and may rationalize a lack of need for treatment (e.g., "I, too, would be extremely depressed if I were in a similar situation."). Because of the high prevalence rates and confusion about the symptoms that warrant aggressive intervention, assessment and treatment guidelines are highlighted in this chapter.

■ Assessment

Anxiety

Anxiety is a vague, subjective feeling of apprehension, tension, insecurity, and uneasiness, usually without a known, specific cause. Normally, anxiety serves as an alerting response that results from a real or perceived threat to a person's biologic, psychological, or social integrity, esteem, identity, or status. A wide variety of signs and symptoms accompany anxiety along the continuum of mild, moderate, severe, and panic levels. Anxiety responses can be adaptive, and anxiety can be a powerful motivating force for productive problem solving. Talking, crying, sleeping, exercise, deep breathing, imagery, and relaxation techniques are all adaptive anxiety relief strategies. Responses to anxiety also can be maladaptive and may indicate a psychiatric disorder, but not all distressing symptoms of anxiety indicate a psychiatric disorder.

Depression

The assessment of depression in any health setting relies on the provider's awareness of risk factors associated with depression and the provider's ability to elicit from the patient key signs, symptoms, and history of illness . In addition to medical comorbidity, risk factors include prior episodes of depression, family history, prior suicide attempts, female gender, age of onset under 40 years, postpartum period, lack of social support, stressful life events, personal history of sexual abuse, and current substance abuse.

The experience of chronic and progressive disease may increase dependency, helplessness, and uncertainty and may generate a negative self-critical view. Cognitive distortions can easily develop, leading to interpretation of benign events as negative or catastrophic. Motivation to participate in care may be diminished, leading to withdrawal. Patients may see themselves as worthless and burdensome to family and friends. Family members may find themselves immobilized, impatient, or angry with the patient`s lack of communication, cooperation, or motivation.

The concept of depression has various meanings. It has been used to describe a broad spectrum of human emotions and behaviors. The spectrum ranges from expected, transient, and nonclinical sadness following upsetting life events to the clinically relevant extremes of suicidality and major depressive disorder. *Depressive syndrome* refers to a specific constellation of symptoms that comprise a discrete psychiatric disorder, such as major depression, dysthymia, organic affective disorder, and adjustment disorder with depressed features. Depressive symptoms describe varying degrees of depressed feelings not necessarily associated with psychiatric illness. In many health care settings, nurses have the most patient contact and are likely to talk with individuals about their physical and emotional problems and detect depression. Recognition of depression begins with knowing that many people who experience depression seek treatment for related somatic symptoms in medical rather than mental health settings.

A diagnosis of major depression in medically ill patients relies heavily on the presence of affective symptoms, such as hopelessness, crying spells, guilt, preoccupation with death and/or suicide, diminished self-worth, and loss of pleasure in most activities, such as being with friends and loved ones. The neurovegetative symptoms that usually characterize depression in physically healthy individuals are not good predictors of depression in the medically ill, because the disease and the treatment can also produce these symptoms.

■ Distinguishing Psychiatric Complications from Expected Reactions

Psychosocial responses to cancer vary widely and are influenced by several factors, including (a) demographic and disease factors, (b) previous coping strategies and emotional stability, and (c) social support. Key predictors of psychosocial adjustment are the coping strategy and the emotional stability of the person before the cancer diagnosis. People with a history of poor psychosocial adjustment before developing cancer are at highest risk for emotional decompensation and should be monitored closely throughout all phases of treatment. This is particularly true of people with a history of a major psychiatric syndrome or psychiatric hospitalization.

The initial response to diagnosis may be influenced profoundly by a person's prior association with a particular disease. Those with memories of close relatives with the same illness often demonstrate heightened distress, particularly if the relative died or had negative treatment experiences. During the diagnostic period, patients may search for explanations or causes for their disease and may struggle to give personal meaning to their experience. Because many clinicians are guarded about disclosing information until a firm diagnosis is established, patients may develop highly personal explanations that can be inaccurate and may provoke intensely negative emotions. Ongoing involvement and accurate information minimize uncertainty and the development of maladaptive coping strategies based on erroneous beliefs.

The availability of significant others for support when dealing with diagnosis and treatment can significantly affect the patient's view of himself or herself. Patients who are able to maintain connections with family and friends report less symptoms of anxiety and depression than those who do not maintain such relationships.

Most patients manifest transient symptoms of anxiety and depression that are responsive to support, reassurance, and information about what to expect from the cancer course and its treatment. Some require more aggressive psychotherapeutic intervention, such as pharmacotherapy and ongoing psychotherapy. Predictive factors for the occurrence of anxiety and depression are listed in Table 27–1. Patients with a previous history of anxiety and depression disorders can have

TABLE 27–1 ■ Predictive Factors of Anxiety and Depression in Patients with Cancer

Past psychiatric history	Advanced disease
Limited social support	Uncontrolled symptoms
Alcohol or drug abuse	Pessimistic outlook on life
Recent losses	Multiple obligations

Adapted from Rowland, with permission

TABLE 27–2 ■ Psychosocial Consequences of Cancer that Can Exacerbate Anxious and Depressive Symptoms

Cancer risk status
Exposure to difficult treatments experiences of family members
Fear of recurrence
Disfigurement
Conditioned nausea and vomiting
Unemployment
Denial of life insurance
Denial of health benefits
Increase in life insurance rates
Difficulty changing health care coverage
Breakdown of marriage/relationship
Decline in participation in leisure activities
Diminution of support from others
Disruption in sexual functioning
Fertility

exacerbation of symptoms due to psychosocial sequelae associated with cancer (Table 27–2).

Guidelines for evaluating the need for a formal psychiatric referral include

- Past history of psychiatric hospitalization or significant psychiatric/personality disorder
- Persistent refusal, indecisiveness, or noncompliance with regard to needed treatment
- Persistent symptoms of anxiety and depression that are unresponsive to usual support from health care providers or family members

- Unremitting fear associated with treatment and procedures or excessive crying and hopelessness that worsen rather than improve with time
- An abrupt, unexplained change in mood or behavior
- Insomnia, anorexia, diminished energy out of proportion to treatment effects
- Persistent suicidal ideation
- Unusual or eccentric behavior or confusion (may be indicative of an organic mental disorder)
- Excessive guilt and self-blame for illness
- Evidence of dysfunctional family coping or complex family issues

Numerous tools have been developed to screen for psychological distress, but they have not been consistently incorporated into clinical care. One tool that is easy to administer, and that patients report as capturing their problems, is the Distress Thermometer. This tool, developed by a team led by Dr. Jimmie Holland at Memorial Sloan-Kettering Cancer Center, is similar to pain measurement scales that ask patients to rate their pain on a scale from 0 to 10 and consists of two cards. The first card is a picture of a thermometer, and the patient is asked to mark the level of distress. A rating of 5 or above indicates that a patient has symptoms in need of further evaluation by a mental health professional and potential referral for services. The patient is handed a second card and asked to identify which items from a six-item problem list relate to the patient's distress, such as illness-related, family, emotional, practical, financial, or spiritual.

■ Management of Anxiety and Depression

Psychosocial interventions can exert an important effect on the overall adjustment of patients and their families to chronic illness and treatment. Several studies have documented the beneficial effect of counseling on anxiety, feelings of personal control, depression, and generalized psychological distress.

Pharmacologic Interventions

Anxiety For patients with excessive anxiety, factors other than a psychological state must first be evaluated. Metabolic abnormalities, pain, hypoxia, and drug withdrawal states can all present as anxiety. Medications such as steroids and antipsychotics, often used to control nausea, can also cause anxiety, characterized by agitation and motor restlessness. After medical or drug-induced causes for anxiety are ruled out, an anxiolytic agent is the treatment of choice. Tricyclic antidepressants are the most effective agents, with the exception of patients who present with panic episodes. Anxiolytic agents are most effective when they are used at adequate dosages and given regularly. These medications may assist the patient to participate in psychotherapy. This therapy can provide more permanent control over psychological symptoms. When anxiety develops in the context of the terminal stages of cancer, it is often secondary to hypoxia or an untreated pain syndrome. Intravenous morphine sulfate is usually an effective palliative treatment in this setting (see Chapter 37, End of Life). Benzodiazepines are the most frequently used for the treatment of anxiety. Buspirone, which is primarily used for generalized anxiety disorder, is attractive for use in oncology settings because it is nonsedating, it does not impair cognition, and its half-life and liver toxicity are unaffected by age. Buspirone has almost no significant interactions with other medications that are commonly used in medical settings.

Cyclic antidepressants are well established as anxiolytic agents that are particularly effective in the treatment of panic disorder and are also effective in the treatment of generalized anxiety disorder. When prescribed for anxiety or for sedation in depressed medically ill patients, their side effects must be carefully monitored. Potentially deleterious side effects include sedation, anticholinergic effects, orthostatic hypotension, and quinidine-like effects. Liver and renal disease may effect metabolism and drug excretion and may require careful dosage titration. Neuroleptics, such as haloperidol in low doses, are used for anxiety with severe agitation or psychotic symptoms.

Anxiolytics are most effective when doses are on a regular schedule. If given on an as-needed basis, anxiety may increase in patients who are already frightened and anxious. Anxiolytic medications help patients gain control over agonizing anxiety. Use of these medications may also help the patient make use of psychotherapy, which can help control symptoms.

All pharmacologic treatments must be monitored for effectiveness and side effects. The effects of benzodiazepines are felt within hours, and a full response can occur within days. Buspirone has no immediate effect, but a full response is expected after 2–4 weeks. The sedating effects of benzodiazepines are associated with impaired motor performance and cognition. Benzodiazepines have dependence and abuse potential, as well as a risk of withdrawal symptoms when they are discontinued. Buspirone has no association with dependence or abuse.

Depression The major categories of antidepressant medications are the tricyclic antidepressants, the heterocyclics/monocyclics, the serotonin reuptake inhibitors, and the monoamine oxidase inhibitors. No one medication is clearly more effective than another. The newer serotonin reuptake inhibitors are associated with fewer long-term side effects than the older tricyclic antidepressants but are more expensive. Monoamine oxidase inhibitors are usually not the first choice because they require dietary restrictions and can have potentially fatal interactions with other medications. Side effects of antidepressant medications are usually dose dependent and short term. Patient education is essential in this area to decrease the possibility of nonadherence to the medication regimen.

The primary medical contraindication to the use of tricyclic antidepressants is the risk of significant cardiac conduction delays, which should be ruled out before the initiation of treatment. The doses of these medications are started low and are increased slowly, over days to weeks, until symptoms improve. Peak dosages are usually substantially lower than those tolerated by physically healthy individuals. Antidepressant medications may take 2–6 weeks to produce their desired effects. Patients may need ongoing support, reassurance, and monitoring before they experience the antidepressant effects of medication. It is essential that patients are monitored closely during the initiation and modification of psychopharmacologic regimens.

A newer class of antidepressants that have achieved rapid and widespread use among the general population are the selective serotonin reuptake inhibitors, such as fluoxetine (Prozac) and sertraline (Zoloft). This class of antidepressants are often desirable because they have fewer anticholinergic, cardiac, or cognitive side effects than tricyclic antidepressants.

In some patients who have a problem that precludes the use of typical antidepressants, a psychostimulant, such as dextroamphetamine or methylphenidate, may be used. Dextroamphetamine is essentially free of side effects. Another advantage of the drug is the rapidity of response, 1–2 hours after the first or second dose. Studies document 48%–80% improvement in depressive symptoms with psychostimulant medication. Psychostimulants can counteract opioid-induced sedation and can improve pain control through a positive action on the patient's mood. Common side effects of psychostimulants include insomnia, anorexia, tachycardia and hypertension, although incremental dosage increases allow adequate monitoring of therapeutic effects versus side effects. In patients with cardiac conduction problems, stimulants may be the treatment of choice.

Antidepressant medications are easily administered and are an effective treatment strategy. Disadvantages include the need for strict adherence to the schedule and the need for repeated health care visits to monitor patient response and adjustment of the dosage, possible adverse side effects and medical reactions, and potential for use in suicide attempts. Patients should be informed that most antidepressant medications must be taken for 3 to 4 weeks before a significant response is achieved. The nurse must be aware that suicidal patients become more energized with medications and appear to look better long before their depressive feelings and suicidal thoughts are relieved. Careful monitoring of suicidal ideation should continue for weeks after the patient appears improved.

Psychotherapeutic Modalities

Depending on the nature of the problem, the treatment modality may take the form of individual psychotherapy, group therapy, family therapy, marital therapy, behaviorally oriented therapy, or some combination A combination of psychotherapy and antidepressant medication is often extremely effective useful in treating depression and anxiety in patients with cancer and can positively affect a range of outcomes, from compliance with medical treatment to quality of life. Table 27–3 outlines the major psychotherapeutic modalities and the advantages, goals, and indications for each.

■ Conclusion

Most patients with cancer experience periods of anxiety and depression at transition points along the clinical course of the disease. For a proportion of patients, severe psychiatric complications may occur, warranting referral to a psychiatric specialist, including psychiatrists, social workers, psychologists, and psychiatric nurses. A variety of psychotherapeutic modalities are useful in helping patients work through the expected emotional responses to cancer, as well as more severe responses. Supportive psychotherapeutic measures should be used routinely because they minimize distress and enhance feelings of control and mastery over self and environment. For these reasons, their value in the care of patients with cancer is paramount. Patients who are not responsive to routine support and information require a referral to a psychiatric specialist.

Throughout the clinical course of cancer, the patient's relationships with health care providers, as well as the presence of a supportive social network, are important factors in ensuring the successful negotiation of the many physical and psychosocial demands imposed by a cancer diagnosis and treatment. As scientific inquiry continues to produce

TABLE 27–3 ■ Psychotherapeutic Modalities in the Oncology Setting

Modality	Selected Indications	Goals and Advantages	Comments
Individual psychotherapy	Prolonged adverse reactions to diagnosis, treatment, and other aspects of chronic illness (e.g., anxiety, depression)	Support patient and enhance ability to cope with distressing feelings. Short-term therapy; focused and goal directed.	Pharmacotherapy and family involvement are useful adjuncts in some cases.
Support groups	Patients desire exposure to others who are experiencing chronic illness	Support patient and enhance coping ability. Usually does not involve a fee. Patients benefit by observing the coping strategies of others.	Expands social network of patients with limited support systems.
Family and marital therapy	Relationship problems secondary to illness (e.g., family tension, role changes, conflict, sexual problems)	Assists couples to clarify problems and solve them together. Addresses role changes in family system.	Problems, issues, and concerns about children can be addressed.
Progressive muscle relaxation, guided imagery, and reiki	Patients desire assistance with control of pain; anxiety; anticipatory and posttreatment nausea and vomiting; fears associated with medical procedures	Increase sense of control and participation in treatment. Individualized to meet patient's preferences and circumstances. Time limited and goal directed. Evaluated in terms of observable changes in symptoms.	Realistic goals should be stated explicitly (some patients view relaxation, guided imagery, and reiki as a cancer cure).

information, sometimes conflicting, regarding the etiology and treatment of cancer, concurrent investigation regarding the psychosocial aspects of the disease is crucial. This line of inquiry will, at the very least, assist in promoting emotional well-being in patients faced with an extreme and unexpected life crisis. At best, expanding the knowledge base relative to the psychosocial aspects of cancer may provide some "missing links" regarding psychosocial adaptation and quality of life and their impact on survival.

■ Resources

- American Cancer Society Resources on Anxiety, Fear, and Depression: 800-ACS-2345 or *http://www.cancer.org/docroot/MBC/MBC_4x_Anxiety.asp?sitearea =MBC*
- National Cancer Institute Anxiety Disorder: *http://www.nci.nih.gov/cancerinfo/pdq/supportivecare/anxiety/ patient/*
- National Institutes of Mental Health Depression and Cancer: *http://www.nimh.nih.gov/publicat/depcancer.cfm*
- Oncology Nursing Society Cancer Symptoms: *www.cancersymptoms.org/symptoms/depression/*

Bibliography

Breitbart, W. (1995). Identifying patients at risk and treatment of major psychiatric complications of cancer. *Supportive Care in Cancer 3,* 45–60.

Cunningham, L. A. (2001). Depression in the medically ill: Choosing an antidepressant. *Journal of Clinical Psychiatry, 55,* 98–100.

Fawzy, F. L., Fawzy, N. W., Arndt, L. A., Pasnau, R. O. (1995). Critical review of psychosocial interventions in cancer care. *Arch Gen Psychiatry, 52,* 100.

Roth, A. J., & Breitbart, W. (1996). Psychiatric emergencies in terminally ill cancer patients. *Hematology-Oncology Clinics of North America, 10,* 235–259.

CHAPTER

28

Respiratory/Dyspnea

Cynthia Chernecky

Dyspnea is defined as shortness of breath, difficulty breathing, breathlessness or tight throat. It is a symptom that is often underdiagnosed and poorly managed. It has no reliable objective measure. The gold standard for assessment is patient self-report. Dyspnea is a common respiratory symptom in lung cancer, in both primary and metastatic disease, and in other pathological processes, such as obesity, chronic obstructive pulmonary diseases, anemia, anxiety, cachexia, and heart failure. Therapy-induced dyspnea can result from surgical thoracotomy, radiation-caused fibrosis of the lungs, and chemotherapy-related pulmonary and cardiac toxicities. Dyspnea in the patient with cancer is usually multifactorial and affects quality of life through decreasing physical and social functioning.

Respiratory symptoms, especially dyspnea, can result from many diseases or conditions, including primary and metastatic lung cancer. An overall assessment includes evaluating the following areas: respiratory, cardiac, neuromuscular, central nervous system, pregnancy, diabetes, obesity, and anemia. There are two subcategories of dyspnea: dyspnea at rest and dyspnea with activity, also known as dyspnea on exertion. Once the type of dyspnea is identified it is quantified in time and/or in relationship to activity and impact on quality of life.

Dyspnea is a predictor of increased likelihood of hospital rather than home death. It is the one symptom that causes the greatest distress for caregivers. Dyspnea causes loss of physical stamina, so that activities such as shopping, getting the mail, bathing, grooming, and dressing can become difficult, if not impossible. This change in activity status can lead to anger, helplessness, frustration, and depression. In particular, there is a fear of dying because "I cannot breathe." This feeling of drowning due to air hunger is real and should be discussed with the patient and caregiver at the appropriate time.

■ Assessment

If dyspnea is not treated, it will progress and continue to have a negative impact on quality of life. Therefore, nurses must recognize the importance of assessing for dyspnea in all patients, along with further assessment for persons who have the potential for lung cancer. Cancer-related dyspnea is usually multifactorial and includes responses from the respiratory center in the brain due to direct or indirect effects of the tumor or treatment as well as other conditions, such as acquired immunodeficiency syndrome, anemia, cachexia, chronic obstructive pulmonary disease, heart failure, hypophosphatemia, lung reduction surgery, obesity, thoracic scoliosis, thyroid toxicosis, and pulmonary emboli. Tumor invasion causes increased resistance during breathing, which leads to increased respiratory work and increased perceived dyspnea. Tumor load can cause decreased lung volume, causing hypercapnia and hypoxia, which increase dyspnea. However, not all patients who are hypoxic are dyspneic and vice versa, so further assessment is imperative.

Persons with lung cancer are the primary group of patients who have respiratory symptoms. There are four major respiratory symptoms and three major associated symptoms in persons with lung cancer. The four respiratory symptoms are dyspnea (shortness of breath), cough, wheezing, and hemoptysis (bloody sputum) (Table 28–1). The three associated symptoms included fatigue, pain, and hypersecretion of mucus.

Of all the respiratory symptoms, dyspnea is the most common, easiest to assess, and most known to have a negative impact on the pa-

TABLE 28–1 ■ 28-1 Respiratory Symptoms

- Dyspnea: the subjective experience described as shortness of breath, breathlessness, unpleasant breathing or tight throat
- Cough: the forceful expiration of air with a partially closed glottis, causing a short sound to be expelled through the mouth
- Wheezing: a musical sound or whistling heard in the chest
- Hemoptysis: the production of bloody sputum from respiratory passages and/or lungs

tient's quality of life. This primary symptom occurs in 21%–90% of all cancer patients, with a predominance of about 80% in patients with lung cancer. Every cancer patient should be assessed for dyspnea because it is a leading symptom of lung cancer as well as a symptom found in lung metastasis from breast, colorectal, and prostate cancers. The assessment of a patient with dyspnea should begin with a thorough history and be followed by a physical examination of the cardiac and pulmonary systems. Dyspnea is perceived as a greater stressor by men than by women, and dyspnea has a greater impact on functional performance in women than in men. For patients at high risk for lung cancer, a specific assessment related to dyspnea should be conducted (Table 28–2). A person should undergo further assessment if he or she has significant occupational exposure to chemicals and second-hand smoke, periods of dyspnea and fatigue, and history of any tobacco use and/or positive family history of lung cancer. An objective assessment should include a history for acute conditions and past comorbid conditions; observation for respiratory symptoms, such as dyspnea, wheezing, mucus production, hemoptysis, and use of accessory muscles to breath; agitation; and tachycardia. Evaluation of laboratory and diagnostic tests help identify the type of disease as restrictive, obstructive, or mixed. Histology from a biopsy determines whether the person has lung cancer. As dyspnea progresses, cognitive changes occur that can endanger safety. The effects of dyspnea are not only change altering for the patient but also increase caregiver burden.

Each patient needs to be asked about dyspnea (Table 28–3), and if the answer is positive, each answer should be quantified by the question, "How often?" and by descriptions of other characteristics.

■ Treatment

There is little research evidence on which dyspnea treatment decisions should be based; most evidence is related to dyspnea at the end of life. Treatment is focused on the comorbid disease or diseases, the type and stage of lung cancer, and the severity of the dyspnea. Examples of treating comorbid diseases include the use of metered-dose inhalers for chronic obstructive pulmonary disease, antibiotics for pneumonia, pleurodesis for pleural effusions, behavioral relaxation for anxiety, and anticoagulants for pulmonary emboli. Lung cancer (see Chapter 14, Lung Cancer) is treated by surgery (see Chapter 6, Surgical Oncology), chemotherapy (see Chapter 7, Chemotherapy), radiation therapy (see Chapter 8, Radiation Therapy) and/or phototherapy, along with efforts to increase respiratory muscle function, such as with exercise, nutrition,

TABLE 28-2 ■ Assessment of Dyspnea

Acute event:	• ARDS, hemoptysis, pneumonia, pneumothorax, pulmonary embolism, COPD, GERD.
Personal lifetime history	• AIDS, anemia, anxiety, ascites, asthma, bronchitis, cachexia, emphysema, heart failure, neuromuscular disease, obesity, pulmonary disease, sarcoidosis, thyroid toxicosis, tobacco use, tuberculosis. • Job history in high risk areas: agriculture, chemical worker, construction, forestry, hairdresser, repair services, entertainment industry.
History last 6 months	• Cancer treatment, cardiac problem, coughing, lung disease/problem, medications (anxiolytics, bronchodilators, corticosteroids, diuretics, MDIs, opioids, oxygen therapy) tobacco use, wheezing. • Use of medications that may alter dyspnea, including MDIs. • Effects of dyspnea on type of activity, length of activity, rest, and body position preferred.
Laboratory test results	• Complete blood count, electrolytes (magnesium, phosphate, potassium), sputum cytology.
Diagnostic test results	• Arterial blood gases, bronchoscopy, Cardiopulmonary exercise test, chest x-ray study, computed tomography, or magnetic resonance imaging of chest, pulmonary function test, pulse oximetry.
Subjective data	• Do you sit up in bed when falling asleep? • Do you stop what you are doing during the day to catch your breath?
Objective data	• Respiratory rate increased, tachycardia, use of accessory muscles to breath, visual analogue scale (VAS) for "Have you had a hard time breathing within the past 2 hours?" VAS can be either a 100-mm line (vertical preferred over horizontal) or 4 forced choices of none, mild, moderate, severe.

Key: ARDS = acute respiratory distress syndrome; COPD = chronic obstructive pulmonary disease; GERD = gastroesophageal reflux disease; MDI = metered-dose inhaler; AIDS = acquired immunodeficiency syndrome.

and acupuncture, thereby decreasing weakness and fatigue. Surgery and radiation therapy can also be used to treat hemoptysis. Surgery for primary lung cancer can lead to dyspnea if enough lung tissue volume is removed. Unilateral lung volume reduction surgery has less of an effect on dyspnea and a lower morbidity than bilateral surgery. Stent placement has been used to successfully manage tracheobronchial ob-

TABLE 28-3 ■ Nursing Symptom Assessment for Dyspnea

1. Do you have shortness of breath or difficulty breathing, breathlessness, or tight throat?
2. How many times does this occur in one day?
3. When does the dyspnea begin?
4. How long does the dyspnea last?
5. Is there anything that makes the dyspnea better?
6. Is there anything that makes the dyspnea worse?
7. What kind of activity produces the dyspnea? (rest, walk, stairs?) Quantify results.
8. Does dyspnea negatively affect your quality of life?
9. Are there other symptoms that occur with your dyspnea, such as pain, cough, wheezing, spitting up blood, or fatigue?

struction, and treatment of malignant pleural effusions has been successfully managed by chest tube drainage, talc, or other irritant poudrage, and a flexible indwelling pleural catheter can be used for periodic drainage in the home setting. Dyspnea may also be treated by use of oxygen therapy, prayer, rest, opioids (usually administered by oral or inhaled [nebulized]), nebulized fentanyl citrate, or nebulized furosemide. Theophyllines have not been shown to be effective in treating dyspnea in patients with lung cancer. The use of ipratropium (Atrovent), in daily doses of > 80 μg (micrograms) in conjunction with exercise, has shown to improve exercise capacity. Associated conditions, such as anemia (see Chapter 22, Myelosuppression) are treated with biologic response modifiers or transfusion, and symptoms such as cough are treated with cough suppressants, radiation therapy, or acupuncture.

Teaching is effective in reducing distress from dyspnea and includes information related to the causes of dyspnea, changes in lifestyle that will not increase stress, effective coping strategies, and the appropriate use of oxygen, especially the common misconception that more oxygen is better. The body normally responds to increased levels of carbon dioxide or low levels of oxygen by increasing the respiratory rate. Therefore, if a patient's oxygen supply is increased, the breathing rate will slow down and the dyspnea will increase. Teaching diaphragmatic breathing and pursed lip breathing can decrease stress, increase relaxation, decrease respiratory rate, and increase tidal volume, all of which help alleviate dyspnea.

Other interventions for dyspnea include relaxing the neck and shoulder muscles, positioning in an upright or slightly inclined backwards position, using diaphragmatic breathing, breathing out for longer than breathing in, and using a fan or open window. Exertional dyspnea, particularly in persons with heart failure, can be relieved by improving muscle function through lower-limb training by use of a standing bicycle or treadmill and leg calisthenics with minute ventilation less than 25 L/minute as measured by a pulmonary function test or spirometer. Ventilatory demand can be reduced by exercise training, chest wall vibration, or chest percussion, or with the use of oxygen, benzodiazepines, and opioids, with a starting dose of morphine of 0.5 mg/hour via subcutaneous or intravenous routes in naive adults.

To help control dyspnea, it is essential that medications are given in a timely manner to maintain adequate blood levels. Appropriate and patient-specific interventions, including periods of rest and use of adjunct medications, are also warranted.

■ The Role of the Nurse

Thorough assessment and documentation are essential to high-quality care in the patient with lung cancer. Management strategies must be implemented for the four components of dyspnea: ventilatory impedance, ventilatory demand, respiratory muscle function, and altered perception (Table 28–4). Assessment should take place at frequent intervals, and the results should be compared with those of the previous

TABLE 28–4 ■ Management of Dyspnea

Outcome	Interventions
Reducing ventilatory impedance	• Smoking cessation. • Use metered dose inhalers (MDI). • Use corticosteroid medications. • Use bronchodilator medications. • Manage pleural effusion. • Initiate brachytherapy radiation therapy.
Reducing ventilatory demand	• Sit in a forward-leaning position. • Sleep using 2 or 3 pillows under your head.
Improving respiratory muscle function	• Do respiratory exercises against resistance by using a hand-held device. • Increase abdominal muscles by doing abdominal breathing exercises.
Altering perception	• Use psychoactive medications.

assessment. The nurse must address factors that contribute to risk for dyspnea or increase the severity of dyspnea, such as continuing to use tobacco, inability to afford medications, and nonadherence with medication regimens or self-management activities. Morphine is effective for treating dyspnea in addition to pain control. The nurse must deal with the issue of the nurse's own fear—as well as the family's—of overdosing patients with opioids.

Nurses also need to remember that as a person comes near to the end of life, he or she retains more carbon dioxide, causing increased periods of sleep, and ultimately coma (see Chapter 37, End of Life). Nursing care includes a focus on psychosocial support for the family and caregivers. The family caregivers may be uninformed about lung cancer, its symptoms, and its treatment. A particular information need is when the family observes the patient being "too sleepy" and wants the morphine "turned down" or "shut off." They must be reassured that this action would not change the underlying problem of carbon dioxide retention, but it would increase symptom distress. Family members may need repeated explanations and reassurance during this time.

A pulmonary rehabilitation program for persons with early-stage disease and/or those with moderate to high activity level should be considered. The benefits of this program can include increased socialization that aids in increasing psychological and social interactions, a decrease in dyspnea, a chance to answer questions and to correct misinformation, and an increase in quality of life. Increasing the body's aerobic capacity, decreasing minute ventilation, lessening fear, and increasing energy through exercise all contribute to the control of dyspnea.

Once dyspnea becomes severe, nursing care includes comfort measures, hospice care, pain control, and support (see Chapter 37, End of Life).

■ Conclusion

Respiratory compromise can affect many areas of a person's life. Symptoms including dyspnea, coughing, wheezing, and hemoptysis have specific interventions that may help relieve the resulting respiratory compromise and reduce distress. Systematic and ongoing evaluation of respiratory symptoms is essential to maintaining an acceptable quality of life.

■ Resources

- Alliance for Lung Cancer Advocacy, Support, and Education (ALCASE), a nonprofit organizations dedicated to helping people with lung cancer: *http://www.alcase.org*
- Winnipeg Health Sciences Centre article on Dyspnea: *http://www.hsc.mb.ca/nursingpractice/July_02.htm*
- Protocol for Incident Dyspnea: *http://www.palliative.info/incidentpain.htm*
- American Thoracic Society Consensus Statement on Dyspnea: *http://www.olivija.com/dyspnea*

Bibliography

Bruera, E., Schmitz, B., Pither, J., Neumann, C. M., & Hanson, J. (2000). The frequency and correlates of dyspnea in patients with advanced cancer. *Journal of Pain and Symptoms Management 19,* 357–362.

Chernecky, C. & Sarna, L. (2000). Pulmonary toxicities. *Critical Care Nursing Clinics of North America, 12,* 281–295.

Sarna, L. (1998). Effectiveness of structured nursing assessment of symptom distress in advanced lung cancer. *Oncology Nursing Forum 25,* 1041–1048.

Wickham, R. (2002). Dyspnea: Recognizing and managing an invisible problem. *Oncology Nursing Forum, 29,* 925–934.

CHAPTER

29

Cognitive Impairment

Catherine M. Bender

Cognitive function is a multidimensional concept that is generally considered to be comprised of eight domains: attention, learning, memory, psychomotor speed, mental flexibility, executive function, visuospatial ability, and language (Table 29–1). These cognitive domains are highly interrelated; a deficit in one may negatively affect other domains. Cognitive function is subjectively perceived. Patients may express cognitive impairments as problems remembering an individual's name or difficulty concentrating when trying to read. Cognitive function is also associated with mood and quality of life. Patients with cognitive impairments may be depressed or anxious and may experience decreased quality of life.

Normal cognitive functioning facilitates intellectual and academic development, occupational achievement, establishment and maintenance of social relationships, and appropriate self-care. Conversely, cognitive impairment affects patients' psychosocial well-being and interferes with understanding and decision making about illness and treatment, including the ability to participate in the consent processes. Cognitive impairment may also interfere with patients' work and with their ability to perform usual daily activities. All of these effects increase the distress experienced by patients' families and caregivers. Cognitive impairment can interfere with patient's abilities to adhere to their recommended treatment regimen and with nurses' ability to accurately assess and manage the patient's cancer-related symptoms.

Cognitive impairment in patients with cancer, referred to informally by patients as "chemo-brain," may result from cancer or its treatment. and may be subtle or dramatic, temporary or permanent,

TABLE 29-1 ■ Domains of Cognitive Function

Attention:	The ability to be receptive to stimuli, to concentrate, and to respond to more than one task at a time
Learning:	The ability to acquire new information
Memory:	The ability to store information for short- and long-term future recall
Psychomotor Speed:	The speed at which mental activities and motor responses are performed
Mental Flexibility:	The ability to shift a course of thought or action according to situational demands
Executive Function:	The ability to plan, problem solve, reason, and strategize
Visuospatial ability:	The ability to recognize visual shapes and forms, to perceive spatial orientation and localization in space
Language:	The ability to speak, verbal expression, verbal fluency, auditory-verbal comprehension, speed and ease of verbal production, reading comprehension, and writing

Source: Bender, C. M., Paraska, K. K., Sereike, S. M., Ryan, C. M., Berga, S.L. (2001). Cognitive function and reproductive hormones in adjuvant therapy for breast cancer: A critical review. *Journal of Pain and Symptom Management, 21,* 407–424. Copyright (2001), with permission from U.S. Cancer Pain Relief Committee.

and stable or progressive. In most patients with cancer, cognitive impairment is reversible. However, in some situations, cognitive impairment is persistent.

Cognitive impairment is also a component of delirium, an acute mental disorder characterized by confusion, disorientation, restlessness, clouding of the consciousness, anxiety, fear, incoherence, illusions, or hallucinations. The symptoms of delirium usually develop over a short period of time and can be short lived and reversible with treatment of the underlying cause.

Cognitive impairment in patients with cancer is typically subtle and most commonly includes deficits in attention, learning, memory, psychomotor speed, mental flexibility, and executive function. Although patients frequently return to their usual family, work, and community roles during or after completing cancer treatment, they may find it more difficult to function effectively, particularly in cognitively challenging environments.

TABLE 29–2 ■ Direct and Indirect Factors Contributing to Cognitive Impairments in Patients with Cancer

Direct factors
Metastases to the CNS
Primary CNS tumors
Indirect factors
Antineoplastic therapies
Infections
Fevers
Nutritional deficiencies
Metabolic/endocrinologic abnormalities
Hematologic abnormalities
Medications (analgesics, antiemetics, antidepressants)
Advancing age
Depression/anxiety
Sleep disorders

Key: CNS = central nervous system.

■ Causes

Cognitive impairment may be the direct result of a primary brain tumor or cancer that has metastasized to the central nervous system, or it may be an indirect consequence of such factors as infection, fever, or metabolic or endocrinologic abnormalities (Table 29–2). In many situations, the cause of cognitive impairment is multifactorial. For example, delirium is most often associated with the use of concomitant medications, such as opioid analgesics in patients with severe pain.

■ Risk Factors

Certain cancer patients are at increased risk for developing cognitive impairment. Factors that increase a patient's risk for cognitive impairment include advancing age, history of neurologic or psychiatric illness or of substance abuse, and prior cancer treatment, particularly radiation therapy to the central nervous system. Patients who receive high doses of chemotherapy or radiation therapy are also at increased risk. Certain forms of cancer treatment, such as biologic therapies, pose a greater risk of cognitive impairment with longer duration of therapy. An example of this is interferon α-2b therapy used to treat patients with melanoma, renal cell carcinoma, and hairy cell leukemia.

■ Assessment

Nurses must be aware of patients who are at increased risk for the development of cognitive impairment. Accurate assessment is challenging because early signs of cognitive impairment are frequently subtle. The causes of the impairment may not be readily apparent, and the impairment may not be detected with the use of standard methods for the assessment of cognitive function. Additionally, subtle changes in cognitive function can be confused with, or confounded by, depression, anxiety, fatigue, or the side effects of certain medications, such as antiemetics and analgesics.

A baseline assessment of cognitive function is needed for all cancer patients. This assessment can be a part of a complete neurologic examination that includes a mental status examination. Additional assessment criteria include the patient's ability to recall recently learned information and to focus on a topic or task at hand. Valid and reliable clinical screening tools are available that aid in the assessment of cognitive function and are relatively simple and quick to administer. Examples of such screening tools include the Folstein Mini-Mental State Exam and the Cognitive Capacity Screening Examination. The Mini-Mental State Exam evaluates attention by asking patients to count backward from 100 by seven. Memory is assessed by identifying three simple objects (e.g., watch, pitcher, and blanket) and asking patients to recall the three objects 15 to 20 minutes later. It is important to alter the methods and sequences used to assess cognitive function over time because patients "learn" the correct answers to questions posed. This can result in inaccurate results.

Although screening measures are useful in detecting global changes in cognitive function, they may not be sensitive to the more subtle cancer-related changes. In these cases, nurses are called on to be observant for changes from a patient's normal or baseline performance. Frequently, patient's family members are the first to notice a change in cognitive function. Patient and family reports of slowed verbal or motor responses or reduced ability to maintain attention or to recall information should prompt a more comprehensive evaluation of cognitive function. Early identification of cognitive impairment can lead to early interventions that may reverse or arrest the problem before more persistent and resistant cognitive impairment develops.

As part of the assessment, nurses inquire about any effect of cognitive impairment on the patient's functional abilities and quality of life, including the ability to maintain responsibilities at work, at home, and in the community. Nurses should evaluate patients for symptoms of depression or anxiety that commonly accompany cognitive impairment. Nurses must also explore the meaning that cognitive impairment has for patients and family members. Some patients and family members may inaccurately fear that cognitive impairment is a sign that their cancer treatment has failed or that their disease has progressed. These fears must be identified so that the actual cause of the impairment can be explored.

■ Treatment

Approaches to the management of cognitive impairment include the treatment of the underlying cause, as well as pharmacologic and behavioral interventions. Pharmacologic management includes use of psychostimulants, antidepressants, and opioid antagonists. The psychostimulant methylphenidate (Ritalin) has been used to manage depression, opiate-induced somnolence, and cognitive impairment. Antidepressants are used in situations in which cognitive impairment is suspected to be related to depression.

Behavioral interventions to manage cognitive impairment include restorative and compensatory strategies. Restorative interventions involve the use of personalized relaxation techniques, such as walking in a natural environment, tending gardens, or observing wildlife, to restore patients' abilities to focus and maintain attention. Compensatory strategies permit patients to circumvent the problems they experience as a result of cognitive impairment and help patients organize information, maintain attention, and encode information for future recall. Compensatory strategies include use of personal digital assistants, use of hand-held recording devices, and integration of procedures to reduce distractions. Vocational rehabilitation may be needed in situations in which cognitive impairment is severe, persists for an extended period of time, or interferes with a patient's ability to maintain employment. The goal of vocational rehabilitation is to improve the productivity level of patients so that they can maintain competitive employment or work at a modified job. Vocational rehabilitation can also be used to help patients with school and volunteer work or with household activities.

■ The Role of the Nurse

The primary nursing goals for the patient with cancer who is experiencing cognitive impairment are to minimize the degree of impairment experienced, maintain or improve the psychological well-being of the patient and the patient's family, maintain patient safety until cognitive function returns to normal, and minimize the effect of cognitive impairment on the patient's quality of life. Efforts to minimize the degree of impairment experienced include ensuring that patients avoid substances such as alcohol and unnecessary medications that may aggravate the loss of cognitive function. Sleep alterations may also exacerbate cognitive impairment. Thus, nurses should help the patient to get sufficient periods of uninterrupted, restful sleep and to plan for rest periods. Patients who experience more severe cognitive impairment can benefit from interventions that help orient the patient to time, such as placing a clock and calendar with the date clearly marked within their range of vision. Continual presence of a family member or significant other may also serve as a means of orienting the patient.

The presence of family members may reassure patients and help minimize the anxiety or depression they may experience as a consequence of cognitive impairment. A psychiatric referral may be necessary to institute appropriate pharmacologic and behavioral management of anxiety or depression (see Chapter 27, Anxiety and Depression in the Oncology Setting). Patients' family members and significant others may need emotional support as they cope with the patient's changes in cognitive function.

Certain precautions are advised when cognitive impairment is serious enough to become a safety concern. For example, patients may need to avoid driving or operating heavy machinery, or they may need to not be responsible for self-administered medications. Patients may be embarrassed and may isolate themselves socially as they contend with the cognitive changes. They and their families need to be reassured that in most cases, cognitive function returns to normal after treatment of the underlying problem. Nurses should pay particular attention to family members' reports of changes in the patient's cognitive impairment.

Patient Education

Nursing care of patients who experience cognitive impairment includes teaching patients and their family members to monitor for indicators (e.g., slowed responses, decreased ability to focus attention or to recall information) of cognitive impairment. Patients experiencing cognitive impairment who have not been taught about the potential for this problem may mistakenly believe that the impairment is a sign of the treatment failure, disease progression, or psychiatric illness. Patients could be reluctant to report the problem because they fear that it will result in premature cessation of their cancer treatment.

Conclusion

Appropriate management of cognitive impairment begins with identification of the cause of the problem. For example, cognitive impairment associated with an infection may be managed by antibiotic therapy. Cognitive impairment related to cancer treatment may be managed by dose reduction, treatment delay, or treatment cessation. Determining the exact cause of cognitive impairment in patients with cancer may be complicated by the fact that the cause is frequently multifactorial. In some situations, patients and their families benefit from psychological counseling as they learn to adjust to the changes they are experiencing in their lives.

Resources

- The American Cancer Society (800-ACS-2345 or *www.cancer.org*) provides information for patients and their families to learn about coping with the physical and emotional changes associated with cancer and cancer treatment. It also provides a means for communicating with other cancer survivors via the Cancer Survivors' Network.
- The National Cancer Institute website (*www.nci.nih.gov*) presents information for health care professionals, patients, and their families about coping with cancer. There is specific information about delirium at *http://www.nci.nih.gov/cancerinfo/pdq/supportivecare/delirium/healthprofessional/*
- The American Society of Clinical Oncology website, *www.plwc.org,* is specifically for persons living with cancer. This website provides an overview of mental confusion (delirium) at *www.plwc.org/plwc/MainConstructor/1,1744,_12-001011-00_17-001029-00_18-0025851-00_19-0027286-00_20-001-00_21-008,00.html*
- The web site *www.pinkribbon.com* is specifically for patients with cancer and their families and includes information about

"chemo-brain." The information is detailed and includes a discussion of strategies for coping with cognitive impairment and a description of related research in this area.
- The Oncology Nursing Society's CancerSymptoms.org website is designed for patients and caregivers to provide information on learning about and managing common cancer treatment symptoms, including cognitive dysfunction at *http://cancersymptoms.org/symptoms/cognitive_dysfunction/*

Bibliography

Folstein, M. F., Folstein, S. E., & McHugh, P. R. (1975). "Mini Mental State," A practical method for grading the cognitive state of patients for clinicians. *Journal of Psychiatric Research, 12,* 189–198.

Jacobs, J. J., Bernhard, M. R., Delgado, A., & Strain, J. J. (1977). Screening for organic mental syndromes in the medically ill. *Annals of Internal Medicine, 86,* 40–46. (Cognitive Capacity Screening Examination).

Rogerio, T., & DeAngelis, L. M. (2000). Altered mental status in patients with cancer. *Archive of Neurology, 57,* 1727–1731.

Walch, S. E., Ahles, T. A., & Saykin, A. J. (1998). Neuropsychological impact of cancer and cancer treatments. In J. C. Holland (Ed.), *Psycho-Oncology* (pp. 500–505). New York: Oxford University Press.

CHAPTER

30

Anorexia and Weight Loss

Jean K. Brown

Weight loss is often the first symptom experienced by individuals with cancer, and additional weight loss along with anorexia (i.e., loss of appetite combined with decreased food intake) may occur during treatment or advanced disease. Some patients experience progressive weight loss with muscle wasting; this is called *cachexia.* Clinical characteristics of cachexia are weight loss of greater than 10% within a 6-month period, intake less than 1.5 times basal energy needs for longer than 1 month, or triceps skin fold and mid-arm circumference measurements that are more than 10% below the reference standard or a change in baseline skin fold and mid-arm circumference of more than 10%. Clinical manifestations of cachexia include anorexia, weight loss, muscle wasting, weakness, fatigue, impaired immunocompetence, decreased physical and motor functioning, and apathy. Poor nutritional status has been strongly associated with increased morbidity and mortality as well as decreased quality of life, especially physical, social, and psychological functioning. Thus, effective management of nutrition-related symptoms, such as anorexia and weight loss, is extremely important for the individual with cancer.

Cancer-related anorexia and weight loss may be the result of direct tumor effects, cancer treatment side effects, or complex indirect systemic effects. Direct tumor effects include anatomic or physiologic consequences of the tumor that alter nutritional intake, digestion, absorption, and metabolism. All cancer treatments destroy and damage tissues. The related breakdown and clearance of damaged cellular byproducts and healing increase metabolic demands. Treatment effects, such as decreased saliva, difficulty chewing or swallowing, impaired digestion, and diarrhea, may have a negative effect on nutritional status. Effective cancer-related symptom management may also cause potential nutritional problems (e.g., pain management with opioids leads to constipation that results in anorexia). Complex indirect effects result from cancer-related metabolic abnormalities that activate the patient's defense system to release cytokines (e.g., tumor necrosis factor and interleukin-6) that cause anorexia and weight loss. Understanding how these mechanisms affect anorexia and weight loss provides the nurse with a framework for the assessment and treatment of both current and potential nutrition-related problems experienced by individuals with cancer.

■ Assessment

Nutritional assessment is a two-step process that includes nutritional screening and, if necessary, comprehensive nutritional assessment. All patients with cancer should be screened at diagnosis and at regular intervals thereafter for current and potential nutrition-related problems. Patients who are found to be at risk or malnourished should undergo a comprehensive nutritional assessment conducted by a qualified health care provider (e.g., dietitian or nutrition support team).

Nutrition screening determines the presence of risk factors for cancer-related nutritional problems. The goal of screening is to identify individuals at nutritional risk in order to prevent or treat malnutrition as early as possible. Even if individuals are not identified as at risk initially, ongoing assessment is needed to identify nutritional problems that may develop later. Factors to be assessed in nutritional screening include current weight, weight change, food intake, symptoms affecting nutrition, functional status, physical examination findings, and projected nutritional problems associated with treatment or disease progression (Table 30–1).

Current weight and weight change must be evaluated with respect to overall body size. Thus, both weight and height must be measured carefully. In measuring weight, it is important to weigh patients with the same amount of clothing (preferably one light layer) each time and to have them remove shoes and heavy objects from pockets. Height should be measured with the head in the Frankfort plane (notch in ear [tragus] and top of cheekbone aligned to be parallel to the floor) and when the patient has taken a deep breath to achieve maximum height. If height cannot be measured, self-reported height and arm span have been shown to be accurate alternatives in adults.

TABLE 30–1 ■ Assessment Indicators, Measures, and Evaluation Criteria for Nutritional Screening

Assessment Indicator	Measure	Evaluation Criteria
Current weight to height	Body mass index (kg/m)	Obese ≥ 30 Overweight 25–29.9 Healthy weight 18.5–24.9 Protein-calorie malnutrition Mild 17.0–18.4 Moderate 16.0–16.9 Severe < 16
Weight change	Percent weight change	> 10% in 6 months is severe
Food intake	24-hour diet history	Food intake usual, more than usual, or less than usual Food intake less than usual accompanied by weight loss
Symptoms and side effects	Symptom checklist	Presence of anorexia, pain, fatigue, taste changes, depression, infection, stomatitis, difficulty swallowing, vomiting, diarrhea, constipation, and difficulty breathing
Functional status	Karnofsky, ECOG, or WHO performance scales	Decreased functional status that interferes with self-care
Physical examination	Subcutaneous fat loss, muscle wasting, edema	Normal/absent, mild, moderate, severe
Projected nutritional problems	Cancer treatment plan, expected disease trajectory, symptom management plan	Future nutritional risks

Key: ECOG = Eastern Cooperative Oncology Group; WHO = World Health Organization.

Although several methods are used to evaluate weight-to-height index, the best approach is the body mass index (BMI). BMI is equal to weight in kilograms divided by height in meters squared (or pounds divided by inches squared and then divided by 0.0014192). Many tables and nomograms are available to quickly determine BMI in the clinical setting (Figure 30–1). BMI is then evaluated to determine whether the

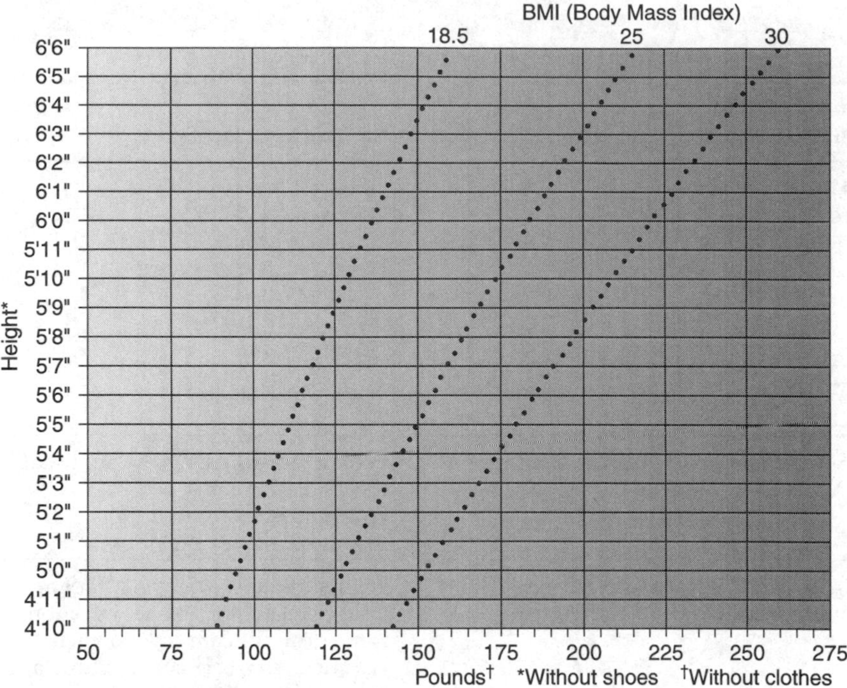

BMI measures weight in relation to height. The BMI ranges shown above are for adults. They are not exact ranges of healthy and unhealthy weights. However they show that health risk increase at higher levels of overweight and obesity. Even within the healthy BMI range weight gains can carry health risks for adults.

Directions: Find your weight on the bottom of the graph. Go straight up from that point until you come to the line that matches your height. Then look to find your weight group.

- **Healthy Weight** BMI from 18.5 up to 25 refers to healthy weight.
- **Overweight** BMI from 25 up to 30 refers to overweight.
- **Obese** BMI or higher refers to obesity. Obese persons are also overweight.

FIGURE 30–1 ■ Determining Body Mass Index (BMI).

patient has a healthy weight, is malnourished, or is overweight or obese. Percent weight change is also a useful assessment. This is calculated by dividing current weight by usual weight, and then multiplying by 100. Weight loss of 10% or more in 6 months is considered severe.

The most efficient method of assessing food intake is to ask patients to recall what they have eaten in the previous 24 hours. It is also useful to ask them if this is typical of what they usually eat, less than usual, or more than usual. If food intake has been less than usual and weight loss is evident, the patient is at nutritional risk. If food intake has been less than 1.5 times the basal energy needs for more than a month, cachexia may be present.

Cancer and treatment-related symptoms and side effects also affect nutritional status and should be assessed. Anorexia is commonly experienced by patients with cancer and is often associated with malnutrition. Other symptoms associated with weight loss in patients with cancer include pain, fatigue, taste changes, depression, infection, stomatitis, difficulty swallowing, vomiting, diarrhea, constipation, and difficulty breathing (see Unit V for specific symptoms). The severity of symptoms and the cumulative effect of symptoms are also associated with malnutrition. A symptom checklist is a useful method of determining the presence and severity of symptoms.

Poor functional status has also been strongly related to weight loss in patients with cancer. This may interfere with the patient's ability to purchase food and prepare meals, thereby further contributing to weight loss. Three commonly used clinical measures to assess physical functioning are the Karnofsky Performance Scale, the Eastern Cooperative Oncology Group Performance Scale, and the World Health Organization Performance Scale. The nutritional screening physical examination should focus on three areas: subcutaneous fat loss, muscle wasting, and presence of edema. Subcutaneous fat loss is indicated by loss of fullness or skin looseness in the shoulders, triceps, chest, and hands. Muscle wasting is best assessed in the deltoid muscles and quadriceps. Edema is indicated by either pitting edema or ascites. Results should be assessed as normal/absent, mild, moderate, or severe.

Projected nutritional problems associated with treatment, symptom management, or disease progression give information regarding potential nutritional risk. As the patient's treatment plan, symptom management, and disease trajectory are reviewed, it is important to consider potential nutritional risks. For example, patients with head and neck cancer may undergo surgery reconstruction and radiation therapy. All of these modalities alter ability to ingest food. Pain symptom management may cause constipation and anorexia (see Chapter 23, Cancer Pain).

The information obtained from nutritional screening is used to determine malnutrition or nutritional risk and the need for a more comprehensive assessment. A BMI below 18.5, a 10% weight loss over 6 months, low food intake, the presence of symptoms affecting nutrition, poor functional status, a loss of subcutaneous fat and muscle, and projected nutritional problems associated with treatment or disease progression are all indicators for a more comprehensive nutritional assessment by a dietitian or nutrition support team.

■ Treatment and the Role of the Nurse

Patients living with cancer have different nutritional needs and issues during treatment, recovery from treatment, and life with advanced cancer. The type of cancer diagnosis and treatment modality has a large impact on the nutritional care needed.

During Cancer Treatment

Nutrient needs are increased during cancer treatment because of cell destruction and healing. In addition, the ingestion, digestion, absorption, or utilization of food can be altered (see Chapter 24, Gastrointestinal Symptoms). Unintentional weight loss and eating difficulties are common but are usually temporary; however, in some patients, these problems can persist. Nutritional interventions are best planned based on projected common problems and should be carefully monitored to accommodate severity and additional problems that may be encountered. Usual eating patterns and food choices may need to be adjusted to accommodate temporary problems, such as dry mouth and difficulty swallowing. If unintentional weight loss is expected or experienced, maintaining energy balance is a high priority. If patients are unable to meet their energy needs with regular food intake, high-energy, nutrient-dense drinks (home made or commercial) and snacks may be helpful supplements to meals. If these interventions are not enough to meet calorie and protein needs, other methods of nutritional support (e.g., enteral nutrition) may be needed temporarily. Table 30–2 lists common nutritional problems and suggested interventions.

Taking dietary vitamin and mineral supplements during cancer treatment is controversial. Some oncologists hypothesize that the antioxidants in these supplements interfere with treatment by repairing some of the cellular damage resulting from chemotherapy or radiation therapy. Other oncologists hypothesize that antioxidants are not powerful enough to repair tumor cell damage, but they may repair and protect normal cells, thereby having a net effect of a more rapid recovery from treatment side effects, such as oral mucositis. Moreover, supplements or fortified foods (e.g., cereals) high in folic acid may interfere with some chemotherapy agents, such as methotrexate. Until more evidence is available, it is best for patients receiving cancer treatment to discuss the use of vitamin and mineral supplements with their oncologist, so that an individualized decision can be made.

Another nutritional issue during cancer treatment is food safety. Patients who are immunosuppressed (see Chapter 22, Myelosuppression) should avoid foods or well water that may contain unsafe

TABLE 30–2 ■ Suggested Interventions for Selected Nutrition-Related Symptoms

Symptom	Suggested Interventions
Anorexia	• Eat small, frequent meals, even if not hungry. • Eat high-protein foods (e.g., milk, eggs, cheese, peanut butter, and nuts). • Eat calorie-dense foods (e.g., ice cream, whole milk, cheese, cheesecake, dried fruit). • Add nonfat dry milk, ice cream, or egg substitute to cooking, baking, and beverages. • Add dried fruit to muffins, rolls, cereals. • Drink acidic beverages, e.g., lemonade. • Serve foods attractively and vary odors and textures. • Try a small glass of wine before meals to stimulate appetite, if the physician approves. • Limit fluids when eating solid food to leave room for solid food. • Clean mouth after each meal. • Keep easy-to-prepare or prepared snacks and meals on hand.
Constipation	• Eat high-fiber foods, e.g., whole-grain cereals, bran, raw fruits, dates, prunes, vegetables, dried fruits, and raisins. • Avoid cheese and refined grain products. • Drink a lot of fluids (e.g., 8–10 glasses per day). • Exercise and walk as much as possible.
Diarrhea	• Drink a lot of liquids at room temperature; ginger ale is often tolerated well. • Avoid foods that contain fat or roughage or cause gas or cramps. • Eat foods high in potassium (e.g., bananas, apricots without skin, baked potatoes, broccoli, saltwater fish, asparagus, mushrooms). • Eat food high in calories and protein.
Difficulty swallowing (dysphagia, esophagitis)	• Eat small, frequent meals of foods that are soft, moist, and easy to swallow. • Gargle and swallow an analgesic (e.g., liquid Xylocaine) before meals. • Avoid hard or dry foods (e.g., crackers, nuts, seeds, popcorn, potato chips, pretzels). • Drink beverages that are of thick consistency to avoid aspiration. • Room-temperature foods are often easier to swallow. • Avoid spices, e.g., pepper, chili powder, nutmeg, curry, and cloves. • Put cold compress on throat for 30 minutes before eating. • Avoid tobacco and alcohol.

(continued)

TABLE 30–2 ■ Suggested Interventions for Selected Nutrition-Related Symptoms—*Continued*

Symptom	Interventions
Dry mouth (xerostomia)	• Drink liquids frequently—up to 3 quarts per day. • Suck on ice chips/cubes. • Clean mouth and teeth frequently. • Eat soft, bland foods with high liquid content. • Avoid hot, spicy, or acidic foods. • Avoid tobacco and alcohol. • Sip beverages between bites of food during meals.
Early satiety	• Eat slowly. • Eat small, frequent meals, increasing sweet or starchy foods and low-fat protein foods. • Avoid fatty, fried, and greasy foods; gas-forming foods; carbonated beverages; chewing gum; and milk.
Mouth sores (mucositis, stomatitis)	• Drink liquids to keep mouth moist (e.g., lukewarm tea, Kool-Aid and liquid gelatin). • Avoid very hot and very cold foods and beverages. • Eat bland, cool, soft foods (e.g., custard, yogurt, gelatin, soups, eggs). • Avoid acidic and spicy foods, alcohol, and tobacco products. • Drink soft food from a cup or through a straw if using a fork or spoon is uncomfortable.
Nausea/vomiting	• Eat small, frequent snacks or meals; sweet or salty foods may be tolerated better (e.g., Gatorade, broth). • Rest after meals. • Avoid hot foods; cold foods may be better tolerated. • Avoid greasy foods that take longer to leave the stomach. • If vomiting occurs, eat potassium-rich foods, e.g., bananas, tomatoes, oranges). • Eat slowly. • Chew food well for easier digestion. • Avoid cooking if food odors are nauseating.
Stomach upset/ irritation	• Eat bland foods, e.g., milk products, ice cream, custards, puddings, soft-boiled eggs, cooked cereal. • Avoid alcohol and caffeine.
Taste and smell changes/food aversions	• Avoid eating favorite foods within a day or two of chemotherapy until you know whether or not food aversions are experienced. • Eat alternative foods that taste good and are high in protein. • Prepare foods that look good and smell appetizing. • Use seasonings to improve flavor and aroma of food (e.g., lemon juice, herbs, marinades).

Source: Adapted from Dodd, M.J. (1996). *Managing the side effects of chemotherapy and radiation therapy* (3rd ed.). San Francisco: Regents, University of California

amounts of pathogenic microorganisms. Good practices include washing hands before meals and meal preparation; washing fruits and vegetables thoroughly; avoiding raw meat, fish, poultry, and eggs; cooking foods to proper temperatures; thoroughly cleaning all surfaces and utensils used for food preparation; storing foods below 40°F; avoiding foods that may be contaminated when eating out (e.g., salad bars and sushi); and having well water tested for purity.

Recovery from Treatment

The nutritional goals during recovery from treatment are to return to a healthy diet and to achieve a healthy weight. Many patients with cancer can expect to be cured or have years of disease-free survival, so a lifestyle that promotes health is important (see Chapter 36, Cancer Survivorship). A healthy diet should focus on the recommendations of the United States Department of Agriculture (USDA) Food Pyramid and the American Cancer Society's Guidelines for Diet, Nutrition, and Physical Activity for Cancer Prevention listed in Table 30–3. If an individual cannot achieve a healthy diet based on USDA recommendations, a multivitamin-mineral supplement of the one-a-day variety is recommended. Consultation with a dietitian can be very helpful in finding ways to deal with persistent nutritional problems resulting from cancer treatment (e.g., dry mouth) and to achieve a healthy diet.

■ Living with Advanced Cancer

Effectively managing nutritional symptoms during advanced cancer (see Unit VI) is important to well-being and quality of life. Food choices and eating patterns may need to be adapted based on the symptoms experienced, such as pain, anorexia, or constipation. For individuals with anorexia and weight loss, some medications (e.g., megestrol acetate) may enhance appetite and sense of well-being; however, body composition does not improve. In addition, there is a possible benefit from nonsteroidal anti-inflammatory agents and omega-3 fatty acid oral supplements in improving nutritional status, body weight, and functional status in patients with advanced cancer.

■ Conclusion

Cancer-related nutritional problems are complex and challenging. Ongoing assessment and intervention with patients and their families is often necessary to achieve desired outcomes. It is also important to

TABLE 30-3 ■ American Cancer Society Guidelines on Nutrition and Physical Activity for Cancer Prevention

Eat a variety of healthful foods, with an emphasis on plant sources.

- Eat five or more servings of a variety of vegetables and fruits each day.
- Choose whole grains in preference to processed (refined) grains and sugars.
- Limit consumption of red meats, especially those high in fat and processed.
- Choose foods that help maintain a healthful weight.

Adopt a physically active lifestyle.

- Adults: engage in at least moderate activity for 30 minutes or more on 5 or more days of the week; 45 minutes or more of moderate to vigorous activity on 5 or more days per week may further enhance reductions in the risk of breast and colon cancer.
- Children and adolescents: engage in at least 60 minutes per day of moderate to vigorous physical activity at least 5 days per week.

Maintain a healthful weight throughout life.

- Balance caloric intake with physical activity.
- Lose weight if currently overweight or obese.

If you drink alcoholic beverages, limit consumption.

Source: Byers, T., Nestle, M., McTiernan, A., Doyle, C., Currie-Williams, A., Gansler, T., & Thun, M. (2002). American Cancer Guidelines on Nutrition and Physical Activity for Cancer Prevention: Reducing risk of cancer with healthy food choices and physical activity. *CA: A Cancer Journal for Clinicians, 52,* 92–119. Reprinted with permission.

remember that stable, or gained, weight is not the only desirable outcome. Improved functional status, sense of well-being, and quality of life are also important outcomes to patients and their families. These should be evaluated along with nutrition-related symptoms and weight change.

■ Resources

Treatment Guidelines:

- Byers, T., Nestle, M., McTiernan, A., Doyle, C., Currie-Williams, A., Gansler, T., & Thun, M. (2002). American Cancer Guidelines on Nutrition and Physical Activity for Cancer Prevention: Reducing risk of cancer with healthy food choices and physical activity. *CA: A Cancer Journal for Clinicians, 52,* 92–119.

Publications:

- American Cancer Society (2004). *Eating well, staying well: During and after cancer.* Atlanta, GA: Author.
- American Cancer Society. *Nutrition for the person with cancer: A guide for patients and families* (publication no. 00-Rev. 08/02-200M-No. 9410-HCP). For a free copy, call 800-ACS-2345.
- National Cancer Institute *Eating hints for cancer patients* (NIH publication no. 91-2079). For a free copy, call 800-4-CANCER.
- Weihofen, D., & Marino, C. (1998) *The cancer survival cookbook.* John Wiley & Sons.

Professional Organizations and Web Sites:

- The American Cancer Society provides free information on specific cancers, symptom management, coping, alternative and complementary therapies, diet and nutrition, and a variety of cancer-related topics: 800-ACS-2345 or *www.cancer.org*
- The American Dietetic Association offers nutritional information and tells how to find a registered dietitian: *www.eatright.org*
- National Cancer Institute provides nutritional information for people with cancer and for health professionals: *www.cancer.gov/cancerinformation*

Bibliography

Brown, J. K. (2002). A systematic review of the evidence on symptom management of cancer-related anorexia and cachexia. *Oncology Nursing Forum, 29,* 517–530.

Brown, J. K., Byers, T., Doyle, C., et al. (2003). Nutrition and physical activity during and after cancer treatment: An American Cancer Society guide for informed choices. *CA: A Cancer Journal for Clinicians, 53,* 268–291.

Brown, J. K., Feng, J. Y., & Knapp, T. R. (2002). Is self-reported height or arm span a more accurate alternative measure of height? *Clinical Nursing Research, 11,* 417–432.

Cunningham, R. S., & Bell, R. (2000). Nutrition in cancer: An overview. *Seminars in Oncology Nursing, 16,* 90–98.

McCarthy, D. O. (2003). Rethinking nutritional support for persons with cancer cachexia. *Biological Research in Nursing, 5,* 3–17.

Griffin-Brown, J. (2000). Diagnostic evaluation, classification, and staging. In C. H. Yarbro, M. H. Frogge, M. Goodman, & S. L. Groenwald (Eds.), *Cancer nursing: principles and practice* (pp. 214–239). Boston: Jones & Bartlett.

CHAPTER

31

Skin and Hair Changes

Linda Casey

The effects on the skin of radiation therapy and chemotherapy used in cancer treatment can be dramatic. Health care providers are challenged to decide how to minimize the effects and how to manage the complications of treatment. This chapter focuses on these complications and strategies to manage them creatively.

■ Skin

The skin is the largest organ of the body, receiving approximately one third of the output of oxygenated blood from the heart. It is composed of three layers: the epidermis; a tough, durable but porous dermis; and a lipid-rich, deep layer of subcutaneous tissue. The primary purpose of the epidermis is to form a resistant, permeable barrier between the individual and the environment. The dermis provides strength, elasticity, and nourishment to the epidermis as well as protection of deeper structures from injury. It contains lymphatics, connective and nerve tissue, hair follicles, and sweat glands and regulates body temperature and assists with wound healing. The interface between the epidermis and the dermis acts as a barrier to the movement of inflammatory and neoplastic cells between the two sections. The subcutaneous tissue is composed primarily of adipose tissue that serves as a cushion to physical trauma, an insulator for temperature regulation, and an energy reservoir.

The skin has many functions, including an interactive system of immunologic elements that contribute to immunologic defense. Intact skin is the first line of defense against bacteria, foreign substances, physical trauma, heat, and ultraviolet rays. If the skin is weakened for any reason, permeability to detrimental effects from the environment is increased. Because the skin is visible to others, it is involved in how we communicate. Feelings and emotions as well as individual body image are all involved with, and partially displayed by, the skin. Appendages of the skin are hair, nails, apocrine and eccrine sweat glands, and sebaceous glands.

Assessment

The purpose of a skin assessment is to determine the severity of skin alteration and to establish a baseline assessment for future comparison. The frequency of assessments varies with the patient's condition and needs. Daily skin assessments are recommended in acute-care settings, and weekly assessments should be performed in outpatient, home care, or long-term settings. Skin should be assessed for color, drainage, odor, and presence of sloughing, necrosis, or infection. Patients should be asked questions about the presence of pain or pruritus. Risk factors for skin changes include current cancer therapy, previous cancer therapy, and preexisting conditions that may affect care, such as diabetes and peripheral vascular disease.

Skin Changes with Radiation Therapy

The skin-sparing capabilities of newer megavoltage, high-energy equipment and sophisticated treatment planning methods have reduced the incidence of severe tissue complications once associated with radiation therapy (see Chapter 8, Radiation Therapy). However, certain acute and late side effects of radiation therapy occur and, in some instances, are expected and unavoidable. Skin cells, because of their rapid rate of turnover and little differentiation, are relatively radiosensitive. Damage from radiation is apparent within weeks to months of the first exposure. Risk of damage is limited to the skin within the field irradiated. Acute effects of radiation are those that occur within 6 months of exposure. Late effects occur 6 months to years after exposure to radiation. Acute effects of radiation are usually considered temporary because the normal cells are often capable of repair. Late radiation effects are usually permanent and may become more severe as time passes. The severity of acute and late effects is dependent on the dose of radiation, the time over which the total dose was delivered, and the volume of tissue irradiated. The presence and the severity of acute radiation skin reactions may predict late effects of radiation. However, late skin effects, such as tissue fibrosis or necrosis, can occur independently of acute reactions.

TABLE 31–1 ■ Acute Effects of Radiation on the Skin

Effect	Dose	Onset
Epilation	300 cGy	17–21 days after exposure
Erythema	600 cGy	A few days to a few weeks
Dry desquamation	< 1500 cGy	2–6 weeks
Moist desquamation	2000–5000 cGy	2–6 weeks
Hyperpigmentation	1000 cGy	2–3 weeks
Pruritus	2000–2800 cGy	2–3 weeks

Side effects of radiation on the skin, both acute and late, are local and are confined to the actual tissue irradiated. Reactions include erythema, dry desquamation, pruritus, hyperpigmentation, and moist desquamation (Table 31–1). Not all patients experience all degrees of skin reactions. However, many experience several categories of reactions simultaneously.

Several factors influence the degree, onset, and duration of acute radiation skin reactions. These include age, nutritional status, anatomic site being irradiated (increased reactions in the axilla, groin, and skin folds and around stomas or wounds), concomitant or prior chemotherapy, and the equipment used to deliver the radiation. A higher radiation dose given over a shorter time to a larger volume results in more severe acute skin reactions.

The Role of the Nurse Nurses perform an important role in managing and minimizing the effects of radiation on the skin. In addition to skin assessment, they are responsible for patient education and management of skin reactions. Assessment of the skin in the radiation treatment field is necessary before the initiation of radiation to determine the condition of the skin and the presence of any factors that may increase the sensitivity to treatment. Surgical scars; edema; wounds; prior skin disorders, such as psoriasis; and stomas can influence the timing and choice of interventions in caring for the skin. Medical conditions that affect healing and medications (including past and present chemotherapy), as well as age, nutrition, and knowledge of the individual's treatment plan enhance the nurse's ability to identify those at greater risk for acute skin reactions to radiation therapy.

Once treatment is initiated, skin should be assessed at least weekly during treatment, 1–2 weeks after treatment is complete, and at each follow-up visit. In addition to scheduled skin assessment, consistent,

TABLE 31–2 ■ RTOG Acute and Late Radiation Morbidity Scoring Criteria

Score	Acute	Late
0	No change over baseline	None
1	Follicular, faint or dull erythema, epilation, dry desquamation, decreased sweating	Slight atrophy, pigmentation change, some hair loss
2	Tender or bright erythema, patchy moist desquamation, moderate edema	Patchy atrophy, moderate telangiectasia, total hair loss
3	Confluent, moist desquamation other than in skin folds, pitting edema	Marked atrophy, gross telangiectasia
4	Ulceration	Ulceration, hemorrhage, necrosis
5		Death directly related to radiation late effect

Key: RTOG = Radiation Therapy Oncology Group.

objective documentation is required. Several grading scales are available to provide an objective method for categorizing skin changes. The most commonly used system is from the Radiation Therapy Oncology Group (Table 31–2).

Patient education regarding anticipated skin reactions (acute and late), time frame for occurrence, onset and duration, as well as self-care guidelines promotes optimal outcomes. Table 31–3 gives information for the patient about skin care. Skin care recommendations are often institution specific and must be reinforced as treatment progresses.

Interventions for skin reactions to radiation therapy are based on knowledge of wound healing. Goals include promoting comfort and healing as well as preventing infection and fluid loss. A clean, moist environment encourages epitheliazation in areas of desquamation. Table 31–4 outlines common approaches to acute skin reactions caused by radiation therapy.

Late radiation skin reactions may include photosensitivity, hyperpigmentation, atrophy, telangiectasia, tissue fibrosis, ulceration, or necrosis. Fortunately, these reactions are not common and vary in severity. However, pain may accompany some of these late skin reactions and should be assessed and managed. Nonsteroidal anti-inflammatory agents are often used in this setting. Opioids may be necessary to manage pain in severe reactions. The goals of treatment are to promote comfort and healing as well as to prevent infection and fluid

TABLE 31–3 ■ Information for the Care of Irradiated Skin

- Skin in the treatment area may become sensitive and should be cared for differently during treatment and healing.
- Do NOT remove temporary marks. Small tattoos that are permanent and will not wash off delineate the field of radiation.
- Skin may become red, dry, itchy, or sore. Let the staff know if this occurs.
- You may lose hair in the treatment area.
- Wash skin in the treatment area gently with a mild soap and warm water. Do not scrub the treatment area. Pat the skin dry. Do not rub or scratch the skin.
- Avoid shaving cream and aftershave in the treatment area. Use an electric razor.
- Protect the treatment area from the sun. If sun is unavoidable, use sun block with an SPF of 15 or greater.
- Do not use tape in the treatment area.
- Avoid heating pads or ice packs in the treatment area.
- Wear loose clothing, preferably cotton, over the treatment area.
- Use only skin products in the treatment area that are recommended or approved by the radiation staff.

Key: SPF = sun protection factor.

TABLE 31–4 ■ Interventions for Irradiated Skin Changes

Reaction	Care
Erythema	Use skin care lotions, creams, gels or ointments without menthol, fragrance, or other irritants. Some centers use 1% hydrocortisone.
Dry desquamation	Use skin care lotions the same as for erythema. Some centers use cornstarch in dry areas.
Moist desquamation	Use hydrogel, hydrocolloid, or polyurethane film. Use silver sulfadiazine. Clean with normal saline, wound cleanser or 1/3-strength hydrogen peroxide.

loss. Care is individualized, based on assessment of the severity and the type of reaction.

Skin Changes with Chemotherapy

Chemotherapeutic agents can cause changes in the skin (see Chapter 7, Chemotherapy). Different agents have different effects. Individuals also have different reactions to similar treatment regimens. Pre-existing medical conditions and prior radiation therapy influence skin reactions to chemotherapy.

Skin effects from chemotherapy may include hyperpigmentation, cutaneous hypersensitivity, photosensitivity, pruritus, and alopecia. Hair loss is the most common skin reaction and may be the most distressing.

The Role of the Nurse

Nursing skin care with chemotherapy focuses on environment and administration of therapeutics. Routine skin assessment is important because breaks in skin integrity pose potential threats as a point of entry for infection. Assess skin for dryness, pruritus, cracking, fissures, rash, alopecia, hyperpigmentation and hypersensitivity.

Dry skin may be from chemotherapy, dehydration or aging and can lead to itching, cracking and fissure formation. Adequate hydration promotes healthy skin. To promote skin integrity chemotherapy patients should drink 3000ml of fluid each day and maintain a balanced nutritional intake with adequate protein, iron and zinc. Medicated baths, emollients and anesthetic creams may be useful. Corticosteroids or antihistamines can help manage excessive itching. Mild body soap is recommended. Perfumes, starch-based powders and deodorants should be avoided. Any break in skin integrity should be assessed for interventions to prevent infection. Antifungals or antibiotics may be used to treat chemotherapy skin reactions if indicated. Cool room temperature and room humidity of 30%-40% helps minimize dryness and itching.

Sunscreen with a skin protection factor (SPF) of 15 or greater are recommended. However, the greater the SPF the greater the chance of skin irritation. Sunscreen should be applied 15-30 minutes before sun exposure and reapplied as often as needed. Protective clothing, such as long sleeves and trousers, decreases exposure to the sun. Patients should avoid tanning beds and exposure to the sun between 10a.m. and 3p.m. when the harmful rays are most intense.

Patient education of skin care during and after chemotherapy is a key factor in patient care. Education can help prevent or minimize skin effects from treatment.

Pruritus

Pruritus (itching) is an unpleasant sensation in the skin that can be tickling or tormenting. It elicits the desire to scratch, which may temporarily relieve the symptom. However, scratching may also damage the skin, causing erythema, papules, and excoriation. When this occurs, the protective barrier is compromised and the individual is at risk for infection.

Pruritus with Cancer Treatment Itching is a common complaint of patients undergoing radiation therapy. A radiation dose of 2000–2800 cGy damages the sebaceous glands, causing dry skin and leads to itching. The skin in the irradiated field must be protected from friction and additional irritation. Nails should be cut short. Lotions or creams approved by the treatment team can decrease dryness. The patient must avoid sun exposure and application of drying chemicals (e.g., harsh soap) to the affected area.

Pruritus may also be associated with chemotherapy. Drug reactions, nonmalignant diseases, and stress can also cause itching. It may be local or generalized and causes varying degrees of discomfort, depending on the severity. Severe itching can decrease quality of life by preventing sleep, interfering with concentration, and increasing psychological stress.

The Role of the Nurse Management of pruritus focuses on prevention of dry skin as well as comfort and relief measures. Skin that is nongreasy and slightly dry itches less than very dry skin. Table 31–5 outlines patient instructions to prevent dry skin and manage itching. In addition, pharmacologic agents can be prescribed in an attempt to alleviate itching. Topical corticosteroids, astringents, and moisturizing agents are used. Systemic treatment may include histamines, cimetidine, cholestyramine, and doxepin have been tried with mixed success.

Overall, pruritus is an unpleasant sensation that elicits the desire to scratch. Treatment should focus on prevention, maintenance of skin integrity, pharmacologic intervention, and methods to maintain comfort.

TABLE 31–5 ■ Prevention of Skin Dryness

- Bathe in warm, not hot, water.
- Bath should be between 10 and 20 minutes long.
- Use oil or cream recommended by the care team after a bath.
- Avoid perfumes, deodorants, cosmetics, and starch-based powders.
- Avoid oil or petroleum-based products in skin folds.
- Avoid wool or synthetic fabrics.
- Use mild laundry detergent and bath soap.
- Use loose-fitting clothing.
- Stay in cool, ventilated environment with humidity of 30%–40%.
- Keep nails trimmed short.
- Maintain good nutrition and fluid intake.
- Wear mittens and/or socks at night if needed.
- Apply warmth or cool to area for relief.

■ Hair

The function of the hair is both physical and psychological. Physically, the hair protects the surface of the skin, enhances tactile senses, and provides temperature regulation by conserving body heat. Scalp hair decreases exposure of the scalp to ultraviolet rays and minimizes loss of body heat from the head. Eyelashes and hair lining the nose and ears act as filters to dust and airborne contaminants. Hair contributes significantly to body image and is associated with secondary sexual characteristics. It has a cosmetic value as an adornment. How the hair is groomed and styled makes a statement about one's self-image and identity in both males and females. Cancer therapy can significantly change body hair in ways that affect an individual both physically and psychologically.

Hair Changes with Radiation Therapy

Hair loss associated with radiation therapy is a local phenomenon. It occurs only in the radiation treatment field and may be partial or total, depending on the sensitivity of the hair follicles, the total dose of radiation, and the dose per fraction.

Radiation-induced alopecia follows a predictable pattern. Hair thinning begins 2–3 weeks from the initiation of treatment at a dose of 25–30 Gy. Hair loss continues for the next 2–3 weeks, with almost total or total loss after 45–55 Gy. Regrowth usually occurs 8–9 weeks after treatment. The growth rate, texture, and color of hair may be different than it was before the radiation therapy. If alopecia persists for longer than 6 months, the likelihood that hair will regrow diminishes. Hair and scalp care should be initiated at the onset of treatment. This can minimize scalp irritation and may slow hair loss.

Hair Changes with Chemotherapy

Alopecia is the most noticeable cutaneous side effect of chemotherapy (see Chapter 7, Chemotherapy). Although it is not life threatening, it is frequently very distressing. Chemotherapy potentially effects total body hair, not just hair in the local treatment field, as occurs in radiation therapy. Scalp hair is affected first; however, with multiple exposures to chemotherapy, hair in the axillae, eyebrows, and pubic area may be lost. Higher doses of chemotherapy, or more potent epilators, influence the rate and the extent of hair loss. Table 31–6 provides a list of some chemotherapeutic agents and their potential to produce alopecia.

Chemotherapy induced alopecia occurs rapidly and usually starts 2–3 weeks after the initiation of chemotherapy. Hair loss is usually

TABLE 31-6 ■ Chemotherapy Agents' Potential to Produce Hair Loss

High Potential		
Cyclophosphamide	Etoposide	Paclitaxel
Daunorubicin	Ifosfamide	Taxotere
Doxorubicin		
Moderate Potential		
Cisplatin	Methotrexate	Vinblastine
Dactinomycin	Mithramycin	Vincristine
5-Fluorouracil	Mitomycin	Vindesine
Idarubicin	Mitoxantrone	Vinorelbine
Mechlorethamine	Topotecan	
Low to No Potential		
Bleomycin	Dacarbazine	6-Mercaptopurine
Busulfan	Gemcitabine	Procarbazine
Carboplatin	Irinotecan	Suramin
Carmustine	L-Asparaginase	6-Thioguanine
Chlorambucil	Lomustine	Thiotepa
Cytosine arabinoside	Melphalan	

asymptomatic. If temporary and mild scalp irritation occur, a mild analgesic may be used.

Fortunately, hair loss with chemotherapy is temporary and reversible. Regrowth usually begins 4–6 weeks after discontinuation of epilating drugs. Complete regrowth may take 1–2 years. As hair grows back, there may be alterations in pigment, texture, or type (straight or curly), just as occurs with radiation treatment.

The Role of the Nurse

Body image and sexuality are closely associated with hair (see Chapter 33, Sexuality). The loss of one's hair can be devastating emotionally. These patients require additional psychological support. Patient information about the timing, extent, and duration of hair loss is crucial. They must be given the opportunity to discuss their feelings, choose wigs, and so on.

Obtaining a scalp prosthesis (wig or hairpiece) before hair is lost is strongly recommended. This serves several purposes, including decreasing anxiety and more realistically matching the individual's hair color and style. Patients are encouraged to contact third-party payers because many insurance carriers provide coverage for a "cranial therapeutic prosthesis for treatment-induced alopecia." A prescription or a letter may be necessary to obtain reimbursement. Synthetic material or real hair wigs are available. Both look natural. The American Cancer Society publishes a "tlc" catalog (as well as a web site) offering hats, wigs, and specialized products. Some local offices of the American Cancer Society may offer a selection of hair prostheses.

If hair loss is anticipated, cutting the hair short can make the loss less noticeable or less bothersome. However, if only a portion of the hair will be lost, within a field of radiation, a longer style may provide better camouflage. Once patchy hair loss is significant, shaving the head allows hair to grow in at the same length. This permits patients to give up hair prostheses more quickly. Use of a mild protein-based shampoo with conditioner, avoiding daily shampooing, allowing hair to air dry, and grooming with wide-toothed combs help delay or minimize hair loss.

The "Look Good . . . Feel Better" program offered by the American Cancer Society assists women in finding workable solutions to hair loss, skin care, and cosmetic concerns. This program, developed with the Cosmetology, Toiletry and Fragrance Association and the National Cosmetology Association, teaches women techniques to restore their self-image and cope with appearance-related side effects. Coping mechanisms are boosted through improved appearance, positive attitudes, and positive feelings.

■ Nails

Rarely are fingernails or toenails included in radiation treatment fields. However, radiation therapy to the nails can result in decreased growth rates and development of ridges when they attempt to grow. Patient education and awareness are the main interventions.

Chemotherapy often causes changes in the fingernails and toenails, and the type of reaction is dependent on the drugs used. Hyperpigmentation begins at the base of the nail and is more common in African Americans. If chemotherapy continues, darkening of the nails evens out. Some chemotherapeutic agents cause partial separation of the nail plate. The nail changes are temporary and resolve after the end of the treatment.

■ Conclusion

Skin and hair changes frequently occur during cancer treatment. The challenge is to prevent or minimize the reaction and assist the individual with management of the symptoms. Nurses can use many interventions with ease and autonomy. Patient education regarding the possible symptoms and the ways that the patient can modify his care is vital to managing skin changes.

■ Resources

American Cancer Society: *www.cancer.org* or 800-ACS-2345

- "tlc," or Tender Loving Care, is a "magalog" (magazine/catalog) that combines helpful articles and information with products for women coping with cancer or any cancer treatment that causes hair loss. To request a copy of "tlc," call 800-850-9445 or visit "tlc" online at *www.tlccatalog.org*
- The Look Good . . . Feel Better program is a community-based, free, national service that teaches female cancer patients beauty techniques to help restore their appearance and self-image during chemotherapy and radiation treatments. For more information, call 800-395-LOOK or visit the Look Good . . . Feel Better web site at *www.lookgoodfeelbetter.org*
- Patient Information on chemotherapy and radiation-related hair loss: *www.cancer.org/docroot/MIT/content/MIT_7_2X_Hair_Loss.asp*
- Patient information on changes in skin color due to chemotherapy and radiation *http://www.cancer.org/docroot/MIT/content/MIT_7_2X_Skin_Color_Changes.asp?* National Cancer Institute: 800-4-CANCER or *www.cancer.gov*
- Fact sheet describing pruritus, its causes, and treatment. Separate versions available for patients and health care professionals at: *www.nci.nih.gov/cancerinfo/pdq/supportivecare/pruritus/*

Bibliography

Bord, M. A., McCray, N. D., & Shaffer, S. (1991). Alteration in comfort: Pruritus. In J. C. McNalley, E. T. Somerville, C. Miaskowski, & M. Rostad (Eds.), *Guidelines for oncology nursing practice* (pp. 143-147). Philadelphia: W. B. Saunders.

Goodman, M., Hilderly, L. J., & Purl, S. (1997). Integumentary and mucous membrane alterations. In S. L. Groenwald, M. Goodman, & C. H. Yarbro (Eds.), *Cancer nursing principles and practice* (4th ed., pp.768–822). Boston: Jones & Bartlett.

Haisfield-Wolfe, M. E., & Rund, C. (2000). A nursing protocol for the management of perineal-rectal skin alterations. *Clinical Journal of Oncology Nursing, 4,* 15–21

Maher, K. E. (2000). Radiation therapy: Toxicities and management. In C. H. Yarbro, M. H. Frogge, M. Goodman, & S. L. Groenwald (Eds.), *Cancer nursing principles and practice* (5th ed., pp. 323–351). Boston: Jones & Bartlett.

McNally, J. C., & Strohl, R. A. (1991). Skin integrity, impairment of, related to radiation therapy. In J. C. McNalley, E. T. Somerville, C. Miaskowski, & M. Rostad (Eds.), *Guidelines for oncology nursing practice* (pp. 236–240). Philadelphia: W. B. Saunders.

Reeves, D. (1999). Alopecia. In C. H. Yarbro, M. H. Frogge, & M. Goodman (Eds.), *Cancer symptom management* (pp. 275–284). Boston: Jones & Bartlett.

Seiz, A. M., & Yarbro, C. H. (1999). Pruritus. In C. H. Yarbro, M. H. Frogge, & M. Goodman (Eds.), *Cancer symptom management* (pp. 328–343). Boston: Jones & Bartlett.

CHAPTER

32

Oncologic Emergencies

Keri Hockett

Oncologic emergencies are structural and/or metabolic conditions that can be life-threatening or that seriously affect a patient's physical functioning and quality of life. These emergent situations can result from the disease process or from unintended side effects of cancer treatment. Early recognition, thorough nursing assessment, evaluation, and immediate intervention can significantly alter the course and improve the patient's outcome. Nursing education of patients and their caregivers may prevent these situations altogether or may minimize their intensity and/or duration.

Oncologic emergencies can be divided into two distinct categories: structural emergencies and metabolic emergencies. Structural emergencies are most often recognized and diagnosed by physical assessment, clinical findings, and imaging studies. Metabolic emergencies are more often confirmed by physical assessment, clinical findings, and laboratory values. Learning the risk factors, symptoms, and cardinal signs associated with oncologic emergencies enables the nurse to implement a plan of care that provides the physical, emotional, and psychosocial care and support necessary for recovery, and perhaps prevention, of future occurrences.

■ Structural Oncologic Emergencies

Superior Vena Cava Syndrome

Superior vena cava syndrome (SVCS) (Table 32–1) occurs when blood flow return to the right side of the heart is obstructed. The superior

TABLE 32–1 ■ Superior Vena Cava Syndrome

Possible causes:
- Tumor encroachment
- Compression by lymph nodes
- Fibrin sheaths or clots from a central venous catheter

Possible symptoms:
- Shortness of breath
- Dyspnea
- Periorbital edema
- Neck vein distention
- Development of collateral circulation
- Lightheadedness
- Headache
- Fullness in the ears
- Vocal hoarseness
- Nonproductive cough

Nursing care:
- Maintain oxygenation.
- Minimize activity.
- Provide calm environment.
- Strict intake and output monitoring.
- Administer diuretics as ordered.
- Educate patient about early recognition of signs and symptoms and reporting them.

vena cava is a soft vessel with low pressure. Reduced superior vena cava flow results in venous congestion and decreased cardiac output. Untreated, congestive heart failure may occur. Cancer-related causes of compression include direct extension of a tumor, enlarged lymph nodes from lung cancer, lymphoma, or metastasis or from fibrin sheaths or clots formed along a central venous catheter. The development of SVCS may have a slow onset, or it can develop rather quickly, depending on the cause and the degree of compression.

Symptoms of SVCS include shortness of breath, which may be mild or may progress to severe dyspnea. Edema, particularly periorbital edema, is evident, but it may be present anywhere on the arms, trunk, face, neck, and even the scalp. Weight gain may occur. Neck vein distention may be evident, and collateral circulation may form if the SVCS develops over a period of time. This appears as superficial veins on the chest and arms that may be distended. The patient experiencing

SVCS may complain of lightheadedness, headache, fullness in the ears, anxiety related to air hunger, and vocal hoarseness; a nonproductive cough may also be present.

The diagnosis of SVCS is made through either chest x-ray study or computed tomographic (CT) scan. Treatment is aimed at treating the underlying cause. If a tumor or lymph nodes are compressing the superior vena cava, then either surgical decompression or treatment with chemotherapy or radiation therapy should occur. The choice of treatment depends on the pathology of the cancer. Some tumors are very sensitive to radiation, and so relief may occur through a course of radiation therapy over 2 or 3 days. Certain types of lung cancer may respond better to chemotherapy or a combination of chemotherapy and radiation therapy.

If a fibrin sheath or clot from a central venous line is the cause of the SCVS, then thrombolysis of the clot with tissue plasminogen activator and heparin may be used, thus dissolving the clot and possibly sparing the catheter. Dye-enhanced imaging studies may be performed to assess the integrity of the central venous catheter and to check for clot formation. It may sometimes be necessary to remove the central venous line.

Nursing assessment consists of baseline vital signs, oxygenation status, cardiopulmonary function, assessment of edema, absence or presence of cyanosis, and any evidence of collateral circulation. Nursing care consists of actions to maintain oxygenation, perfusion, and cardiopulmonary function. The patient should be placed in a position that minimizes dyspnea. Oxygen is usually ordered. The patient usually experiences some degree of anxiety when severe dyspnea is present. A calm environment and minimal activity have been found to contribute to reducing anxiety. Diuretics may be used. Careful recording of intake and output is essential. The patient should not be overhydrated; this may aggravate the SVCS. If the central line is the suspected cause, all fluids through that line should be stopped and restarted with the use of another access site. No additional peripheral intravenous (IV) lines should be started in the upper extremities.

Patients usually recover quickly from SCVS after appropriate intervention and treatment. SVCS can recur in advanced or progressive disease. Preparation for home care should address early recognition of signs and symptoms of SVCS and when to report these to the health care provider. Patients with central lines may go home receiving anticoagulant therapy. If a central line is in place, assessment and education about proper maintenance, including proper flushing technique, should take place. Patients and caregivers should be taught about administration, side effects, and follow-up laboratory and physician appointments.

Spinal Cord Compression

Spinal cord compression (SCC) (Table 32–2) occurs when blood flow to the spinal cord tissue is compressed or impinged on by tumor or metastasis to the spine. This condition can result in irreversible paralysis if it is not recognized and treated immediately. SCC can result from primary tumors arising in the spinal column, such as astrocytomas and meningiomas. Most spinal cord compressions occur in the epidural area and are the result of bony metastasis, most often from breast, lung, and prostate cancer. Patients with multiple myeloma are also at risk.

Symptoms of SCC include pain, especially back pain. Back pain is often the presenting symptom of SCC. The patient may experience motor weakness that becomes evident when he or she attempts to get out of a chair or navigate a step. Sensory disturbances may be experienced as numbness or paresthesias, loss of sense of position, loss of sensation of temperature, and loss of sensation of deep pressure. In addition, the patient with SCC may experience autonomic disturbance in the form of bowel and bladder symptoms. This can range from difficulty initiating urination or defecation to complete loss of sphincter control.

Diagnosis of SCC is made by imaging studies. Plain-film x-ray study may demonstrate vertebral fracture and collapse at the site of compression. Magnetic resonance imaging (MRI) is commonly used to

TABLE 32–2 ■ Spinal Cord Compression

Possible causes:

- Compression by tumor
- Compression by bone metastasis
- Compression due to vertebral fracture from disease

Possible symptoms:

- Pain—especially in the back or legs
- Sensory disturbances—paresthesia, loss of temperature sensation, loss of deep pressure sensation; loss of sense of position
- Bowel and/or bladder incontinence

Nursing care:

- Pain assessment.
- Assess safety of patient environment.
- Assess and monitor skin integrity.
- Prepare for diagnostic imaging studies, especially magnetic resonance imaging.
- Administer steroids/anti-inflammatory drugs as ordered and monitor response.

diagnose SCC; it has become the standard of care for diagnosing SCC because it is noninvasive and provides better visualization of masses. When MRI is not available, myelography with computed tomography may be used.

The usual treatment for SCC is steroids with radiation therapy. Dexamethasone has been the drug of choice to relieve pain and reduce edema of the spinal cord. This may be given when SCC is suspected, even before the diagnosis is confirmed. Dexamethasone is given intravenously as a bolus dose, then every several hours, usually at a lower dose. Radiation therapy to the site of compression, as well as to the vertebrae above and below the site, is the treatment of choice. Surgical decompression may be used, particularly if there has been previous radiation therapy to the area of the compression. Laminectomy or vertebral reconstruction may also be performed. Chemotherapy may be used to treat SCC in situations in which the tumor is extremely chemosensitive.

Nursing care for the patient with suspected or actual SCC is focused on assessment and recognizing that SCC may be occurring. Immediate intervention is required. Communication among the multidisciplinary team is essential. All those involved in the care of the patient must understand the urgency of the situation. Imaging studies must be performed "stat," and dexamethasone must be given immediately. Consultants such as radiation oncologists and surgeons must be informed of the actual, or potential, diagnosis of SCC. The patient should be prepared to undergo imaging studies, including MRI. In a closed MRI, some patients may require a mild anxiolytic drug to allay claustrophobia. Additional nursing interventions include assessing and medicating the patient for pain and evaluating the safety of the environment to prevent injury from motor weakness and alterations in mobility. Preservation of skin integrity should also be in the plan of care. Loss of bowel and/or bladder function and loss of motor function present difficult challenges.

Recovery from SCC depends on the amount of tumor involvement before the compression. Most of those patients, who were ambulatory before treatment, remain so after treatment. Ongoing assessment of the skin at home is essential. Physical therapy may be required. The goal of the postdischarge recovery plan is to regain motor skills and bladder and bowel retraining, if necessary. The amount of home nursing care required depends on the degree of residual disease present.

Additional SCC may be avoided by controlling additional spinal metastasis. This can be achieved by the administration of bisphosphonates on an outpatient basis. Nurses should teach patients about the use, side effects, and schedule of these drugs.

Cardiac Tamponade

Cardiac tamponade (Table 32–3) is the result of pericardial effusion and loss of compensatory mechanisms. Excess fluid accumulates in the pericardial sac, putting pressure on the heart chambers, thereby reducing their ability to fill and pump a sufficient volume of blood. The patient becomes hemodynamically unstable, and if the condition is left untreated, cardiovascular collapse and death occur. Pericardial effusion is highly associated with lymphoma, lung cancer, and breast cancer. Other cancers cause cardiac tamponade through direct extension of tumor into cardiac structures. Radiation therapy to the pericardium is also a risk factor.

TABLE 32–3 ■ Cardiac Tamponade

Possible causes:

Pericardial effusion with loss of compensation due to:

- Direct tumor extension into pericardium
- Radiation to the pericardium
- Tumor growing within the pericardium

Possible symptoms:

Increased resting heart rate
Narrowing pulse pressure
Paradoxical pulse
Hypoxia
Anxiety
Chest pain
Dyspnea
Cough
Venous jugular distention

Nursing care:

Maintain oxygenation.
Provide calm environment.
Monitor vital signs, especially blood pressure.
Monitor for paradoxical pulse (drop in systolic blood pressure >10 mm Hg on inspiration).
Assess respirations—lung sounds, respiratory rate, and use of accessory muscles.
Monitor arterial blood gases.
Assess heart sounds.
Educate patient and prepare for diagnostic tests.

Echocardiogram is the test usually performed to confirm the diagnosis of cardiac tamponade. If confirmed, CT scan or MRI may also be used. Plain-film x-ray study is not usually diagnostic but may be suggestive of the condition by showing an enlarged heart. Laboratory evaluation usually consists of arterial blood gas values. These may indicate respiratory alkalosis by increased pH and decreased partial pressure of arterial carbon dioxide.

Treatment of cardiac tamponade consists of pericardiocentesis under ultrasound guidance to relieve pressure and improve filling. Cytologic examination of the removed fluid determines whether cancer cells are present. Pericardiocentesis with instillation of a sclerosing agent may be performed to prevent recurrence of the pericardial effusion. Sclerosing agents include various chemotherapy agents, such as bleomycin, mitomycin, cisplatin, and doxycycline. Pericardial window is a surgical procedure that involves removal of a piece of the pericardium, thereby allowing reaccumulated fluid to escape. Chemotherapy and radiation therapy are also used to prevent recurrent cardiac tamponade by treating the underlying cause.

Signs and symptoms of cardiac tamponade are related to the degree and the duration of the pericardial effusion. These include decreased cardiac output, manifested by increased resting heart rate and narrowing pulse pressure. A cardinal sign of cardiac tamponade is paradoxical pulse. This is a decrease in systolic arterial blood pressure of greater than 10 mm Hg on inspiration. Other symptoms include anxiety related to hypoxia, chest pain, severe dyspnea, cough, peripheral edema, and venous jugular distention. Decreased heart sounds are also evident. As cardiac tamponade progresses, shock may ensue.

Nursing care for the patient with cardiac tamponade includes actions to maintain cardiopulmonary function, oxygenation, and perfusion. The patient is positioned for ease of respiration and oxygen is administered. Cardiopulmonary assessment includes vital signs, including blood pressure, and assessing for paradoxical pulse. Pulmonary assessment includes respiratory rate and use of accessory muscles to breathe, monitoring of arterial blood gases, and heart and lung sounds. Electrocardiographic changes are nonspecific in cardiac tamponade, although pressure from fluid accumulation in the pericardial space can cause low-voltage QRS complexes. The nurse should educate and prepare the patient for diagnostic and therapeutic procedures, and provide a calm environment to decrease anxiety.

Home care of the patient who has experienced cardiac tamponade includes cardiopulmonary assessment and education of the patient and caregiver about the signs and symptoms of recurring tamponade. If the patient had a pericardial window, the surgical site should be assessed. Pain assessment and management should be included in the plan of care.

Increased Intracranial Pressure

Increased intracranial pressure (ICP) occurs when pressure within the cranial vault exceeds all compensatory mechanisms (Table 32–4). The normal cranial vault contains brain tissue, cerebrospinal fluid and blood volume. There is a fixed pressure in the vault: normally, 0–15 mm Hg. A phenomenon called *autoregulation* occurs when blood vessels dilate and constrict to maintain this pressure, even when arterial blood pressure is fluctuating. However, when the arterial pressure is too low or too high, this autoregulation can fail and vault pressure becomes subject to changes in arterial blood pressure.

When significant changes occur in brain tissue mass, as with enlarging brain tumors, the increase in brain mass is compensated for by decreases in cerebrospinal fluid, or blood volume, or both. Smaller volume changes over time are more easily compensated for than rapid or larger changes. Tumor location also plays a role in the severity of in-

TABLE 32–4 ■ Increased Intracranial Pressure

Possible causes:

- Change in brain tissue mass due to tumor
- Obstruction of ventricles due to tumor encroachment

Possible symptoms:

- Headache
- Altered level of consciousness
- Restlessness and agitation
- Personality changes
- Vomiting, possible projectile
- Papilledema
- Motor changes
- Widening pulse pressure—as systolic blood pressure (BP) increases, diastolic BP decreases
- Decorticate or decerebrate posturing in advanced cases

Nursing care:

- Administer steroids as ordered.
- Monitor intake and output.
- Perform neurologic checks, including vital signs, pupil assessment, and level of consciousness.
- Keep head of bed elevated.
- Prevent hyperextension of head and neck.
- Prevent/minimize Valsalva maneuver by suppressing coughing, vomiting, avoiding bending over.

creased ICP. A tumor obstructing the ventricles and its flow may cause a higher increase in ICP than a larger tumor in the front of the brain. When compensatory mechanisms have been exhausted, increased ICP occurs and herniation of brain tissue can lead to severe neurologic damage and death.

Diagnosis of increased ICP is usually made by MRI or CT imaging studies, with MRI being the preferred study. In some cases, positron emission tomography may be performed. Lumbar puncture may also be used to obtain fluid to determine the presence of cancer cells in the cerebrospinal fluid.

Signs and symptoms of increased ICP include headache, altered level of consciousness, restlessness, agitation, personality changes, and vomiting that may be projectile and not necessarily accompanied by nausea. Clinical assessment findings include pupil changes, papilledema, and sensory changes. Motor changes, such as hemiparesis, may also occur. A widening pulse pressure may also occur. In advanced cases of increased ICP, bradycardia, abnormal respiration, and decorticate and decerebrate posturing may occur. In decorticate posturing, the arms are flexed and the legs are extended. In decerebrate posturing, all extremities are extended.

Surgery is the primary treatment for increased ICP. Debulking the tumor mass relieves pressure and provides tissue for a definitive pathological diagnosis. If the tumor cannot be entirely resected, debulking as much as possible may provide significant relief from increased pressure and may alleviate symptoms. Radiation therapy and stereotactic radiosurgery are also used, depending on the pathology. For the most part, chemotherapy has been largely ineffective because of the inability to cross the blood-brain barrier. Some agents, such as BCNU (carmustine) and CCNU (lomustine) are able to cross this barrier. A newer delivery method for chemotherapy is by wafers containing the drugs that are placed in the resected tumor bed at the time of surgery. These wafers gradually release the drug at the tumor site.

Nursing care is aimed at early recognition of ICP and immediate intervention. Steroids are administered to restore disturbances in the blood-brain barrier that have caused fluid leak from the loss of plasma proteins. Osmotic diuretics, such as mannitol, are also given. Careful intake and output recording should be maintained. Neurology checks are performed frequently. The head of the bed should be elevated to promote venous drainage. Coughing, sneezing, bending over, and performing Valsalva maneuver should all be avoided because they increase ICP. The head and neck should not be hyperextended to avoid obstructing venous drainage. The patient with increased ICP should not change position without careful nursing assistance.

Home care of the patient who has experienced increased ICP as a result of a malignant condition may be focused on surgical recovery and may be dealing with the side effects of cranial irradiation. If there are physical or mental deficits as a result of the increased ICP or the mass that caused it, then physical and/or occupational rehabilitation may assist in improving quality of life.

■ Metabolic Oncologic Emergencies

Disseminated Intravascular Coagulation

Disseminated intravascular coagulation (DIC) (Table 32–5) is an abnormal condition in which hemorrhage and clotting occur at the same time. Treatment must be aimed at correcting the underlying cause of the DIC. In DIC, normal coagulation is disrupted. Clots form in the microvasculature, and in an attempt to dissolve these clots, there is consumption of clotting factors and hemorrhage ensues and becomes uncontrollable. The clots that form in the microvasculature impair perfusion of the organ or organs involved, and tissue damage and ischemia occur.

Leukemia, especially acute promyelocytic leukemia, is highly associated with DIC. Solid tumors, infections, and septic shock can also trigger DIC. In the patient with cancer, DIC can be triggered by hemolytic transfusion reaction or by massive transfusion.

There is no one diagnostic test for DIC. Laboratory values reflect abnormal coagulation. The platelet count is decreased. The prothrombin time and the activated partial thromboplastin time are prolonged. Fibrin degradation products, also called fibrin split products, are elevated. Results for the D-dimer test, a test for a substance formed in response to fibrin degradation, is positive.

Correction of DIC with restoration of normal coagulation is aimed at treating the underlying cause: the infection or the leukemia or solid tumor. If the DIC is not corrected, hemorrhage and death can occur.

Blood component therapy with platelets, fresh frozen plasma, and cryoprecipitates, which are rich in clotting factors, are used to assist with restoring normal coagulation. Heparin may be given to prevent further clot formation and subsequent tissue ischemia.

Signs and symptoms of DIC include cyanosis of fingertips, toes, and lips, development of petechiae, spontaneous gum bleeding, and nosebleeds. There may be oozing from IV and vascular access device sites, and from surgical sites or wounds. Stool may be guaiac positive, and urine may reveal microscopic or gross hematuria.

TABLE 32-5 ■ Disseminated Intravascular Coagulation

Possible causes:
- Leukemia, especially promyelocytic leukemia
- Sepsis
- Transfusions
- Solid tumors

Lab results with DIC:
- Platelet count—decreased
- PT—increased
- APTT—increased
- Fibrin degradation products—increased
- D-dimer test—positive

Symptoms of DIC:
- Cyanosis of fingertips, lips
- Petechiae, spontaneous gum bleeding, nose bleeds
- Oozing from wounds and puncture sites
- Guaiac-positive stool
- Microscopic or gross hematuria

Nursing care:
- Administer blood products as ordered.
- Administer heparin as ordered.
- Monitor lab results.
- Avoid/minimize punctures for IVs, lab tests.
- Assess neurologic status.
- Use only electric razors.
- Gentle mouth care only—no toothpicks or floss.
- Do not remove crusted scabs.

Key: DIC = disseminated intravascular coagulation; IV = intravenous line; PT = prothrombin time; APTT = activated partial thromboplastin time.

Nursing care consists of administration of heparin and blood products and monitoring laboratory values. The patient should be protected from further injury by avoiding additional IV sites. Pressure should be applied to any puncture site. The patient should be instructed to use only electric razors. Mouth care should be very gentle, using soft bristles, no toothpicks, or floss. Overinflation of the blood pressure cuff may cause a hematoma. Neurologic and gastrointestinal status should be monitored for signs of covert bleeding, and dressings should be weighed to estimate blood loss. Constant oozing and blood loss can be very distressing to the patient and family. The nurse should explain all procedures and provide a calm environment. Extensive patient education and constant reinforcement of information about injury precautions are necessary.

Septic Shock

Septic shock (Table 32–6) is a physical response to overwhelming infection, leading to hemodynamic instability. The source of the infection may be bacterial, viral, or fungal. Immediate identification of the organism, followed by appropriate treatment, is essential to achieving a favorable outcome. Patients with cancer are especially vulnerable to infection. Diseases such as leukemia impair the immune system. Many treatments for various types of cancer often kill healthy immune system cells in the course of destroying the cancer cells (see Chapters 7 [Chemotherapy] and 21 [Other Cancers]). Either way, the patient is left with a severely compromised ability to fight infection. In septic shock, overwhelming infection produces endotoxins, which trigger hemodynamic responses of fever, tachycardia, and severe hypotension. This hypotension may not respond to fluid challenge, and if it is left untreated, vascular collapse and death can occur.

TABLE 32–6 ■ Septic Shock

Possible causes:

- Bacterial, viral, or fungal infection
- Recent myelosuppressive therapy such as chemotherapy, radiation, biotherapy, or a combination

Possible symptoms:

- Fever, chills, malaise
- Restlessness, agitation
- Confusion
- Cyanosis
- Hypothermia
- Hemodynamic instability

Nursing care:

- Obtain cultures of blood, urine, sputum and wounds as soon as possible.
- Begin antimicrobial therapy as ordered as soon as cultures are obtained.
- Maintain oxygenation. Assess level of consciousness.
- Administer vasopressor drugs as ordered for hemodynamic stability.

The diagnosis of septic shock is based on clinical assessment findings. Blood, urine, sputum, and wound cultures are performed, but in up to 30% of cases, no organism is identified.

Signs and symptoms of septic shock include fever, chills, and malaise with tachycardia, hypotension, and decreased cardiac output. The patient may be agitated, restless, or confused. The skin may be cool, and cyanosis may be present. The white count may be elevated. Oncology patients who have acute leukemia or who have undergone recent myelosuppressive therapy may have a markedly low white count, placing them at greater risk. Treatment is aimed at stabilizing the patient and treating the source infection. Blood cultures should be performed from peripheral as well as central venous lines. Urine, sputum, and wound cultures should be obtained, and antimicrobial therapy should be started as soon as possible. Oxygen is administered as ordered, and intubation and mechanical ventilation may be necessary if hemodynamic instability progresses. Fluid resuscitation and vasopressor drugs may be necessary. Hydration and nutrition requirements should be assessed at this time.

Nursing care consists of actions to maintain oxygenation, perfusion, and hemodynamic stability. The nurse should administer fluids and vasopressor drugs and assesses vital signs frequently for response to treatment. Septic shock may lead to the need for intubation and mechanical ventilation.

Clarification and communication about implementing advanced directives may become necessary. Patients may have an advanced directive that states "no intubation" when the condition is terminal. Septic shock has a high mortality rate, but it is not viewed as a terminal condition. Therefore, patients and caregivers may need more information about the condition and the prognosis.

Hypercalcemia

Hypercalcemia of malignancy (HCM) (Table 32–7) is defined as a serum calcium level greater than 11 mg/dL. It is seen most often in patients with breast, lung, squamous cell head and neck cancer, and multiple myeloma. HCM is a result of metastatic lesions that disrupt the normal process of bone remodeling. Excess calcium is released into the serum and is cleared by the kidney. Elevated serum calcium levels challenge the kidney's ability to excrete the calcium. Polyuria occurs, causing dehydration that leads to resorption of calcium into the kidney, thus elevating the serum concentration. In the presence of a low serum albumin level, the serum calcium level is actually higher than the reported level. This is due to the fact that there is less albumin for

TABLE 32–7 ■ Hypercalcemia

Possible causes:
- Breast cancer
- Lung cancer
- Squamous cell cancer
- Multiple myeloma
- Lytic bone lesions
- Bone metastasis

Possible symptoms:
- Elevated serum calcium
- Polyuria, progressing to oliguria
- Dehydration
- Anorexia
- Vomiting
- Constipation
- EKG changes
- Muscle weakness

Nursing care:
- Monitor serum calcium level and calculate corrected calcium value.
- Administer loop diuretics as ordered.
- Monitor intake and output.
- Administer IV hydration as ordered.
- Assess safety of environment to prevent injury.
- Assess GI system for constipation, nausea, and vomiting.
- Perform active and passive range of motion.
- Perform neurologic checks to assess for impaired cognition.

Key: EKG = electrocardiographic; GI = gastrointestinal; IV = intravenous.

calcium to bind to, making it available in the serum. A formula to calculate the corrected calcium value is:

(4.0 mg/dL – reported serum albumin) × 0.8 mg/dL + reported serum calcium = corrected calcium

For example, if patient has a serum albumin level of 2.8 and a reported calcium level of 13:

$4.0 - 2.8 = 1.2$

$1.2 \times 0.8 = 0.96$

$0.96 + 13 = 13.9$ = corrected calcium level

Signs and symptoms of hypercalcemia include polyuria that would progress to oliguria if HCM is left untreated. Anorexia, nausea and vomiting, and constipation are gastrointestinal manifestations. Altered level of consciousness, muscle weakness, and electrocardiographic changes may also occur.

Diagnosis of HCM is established by an elevated serum calcium laboratory value, corrected for the low albumin level. Blood urea nitrogen and creatinine values are used to assess impact on kidney function. Clinical findings are correlated with degree of HCM.

Treatment of HCM is aimed at increasing excretion of calcium and adequately hydrating the patient. Saline diuresis is essential to restore normal hydration and facilitate excretion of excess calcium. A loop diuretic may also be used once fluid balance is achieved. The current drugs of choice to treat HCM are the bisphosphonates. These drugs correct serum calcium levels within 48 hours and are effective for several weeks. These drugs are given prophylactically to patients who are at high risk for HCM.

Nursing management involves the administration of intravenous fluids, strict recording of intake and output, and monitoring of laboratory values for response to treatment. Preventing injury is a high priority. Impaired cognition and motor skills place a patient at risk for injury. The nurse should assess the safety of the patient's environment and teach the patient and caregiver about their level of activity and risk. Immobility increases hypercalcemia. If the patient is confined to bed, active and passive range of motion should be performed. The nurse should assess for nausea, vomiting, and constipation. Instituting a bowel regimen may be necessary. The patient and caregiver should be taught about adequate fluid intake, diet, and signs and symptoms of HCM that must be reported.

Tumor Lysis Syndrome

Tumor lysis syndrome (TLS) (Table 32–8) occurs when there is massive tumor cell destruction in response to cancer treatment, usually chemotherapy. The intracellular contents of these cells are released into the serum and contain large amounts of potassium, phosphorus, and uric acid. This leads to high serum concentrations of these elements. This severe electrolyte imbalance can lead to renal failure due to the formation of uric acid crystals in the tubules. Abnormal potassium and calcium levels may also cause life-threatening arrhythmias. Patients with leukemia and lymphoma are at a higher risk for developing TLS.

Diagnosis is made by evaluation of laboratory values. These usually document hyperkalemia, hyperphosphatemia, increased uric acid,

TABLE 32–8 ▪ Tumor Lysis Syndrome

Possible causes:

Leukemia recently treated
Lymphoma recently treated

Possible symptoms:

Increased uric acid levels
Increased serum potassium
Increased serum phosphorus
Renal failure
Arrhythmias

Nursing care:

Monitor renal function—perform strict intake and output measurement.
Monitor electrolyte levels.
Administer IV hydration as ordered.
Administer Kayexalate as ordered for increased potassium.
Administer allopurinol as ordered.
Monitor for joint pain, twitching, muscle cramps.

Key: IV = intravenous.

and hypocalcemia. Blood urea nitrogen and creatinine concentrations may be elevated if renal impairment is occurring.

Treatment is aimed at prevention. Tumor lysis syndrome is one of the more preventable oncologic emergencies. Knowing that the patient has a type of cancer associated with increased risk for TLS allows for preventive treatment, including adequate hydration and administration of allopurinol. If the patient does develop TLS, then IV hydration is required. Kayexalate may be given to correct hyperkalemia. Allopurinol is also given, and the calcium level is monitored and corrected, if severely abnormal.

Nursing care of the patient with TLS includes patient and caregiver education about the importance of hydration and of taking the allopurinol. The patient should be taught to report muscle cramps, twitches or spasms, joint pain or swelling, and any nausea, vomiting, or diarrhea. Careful intake and output recording should be undertaken. Laboratory results should be monitored for response to interventions. Home care of the patient with, or at risk for, TLS involves assessment of the patient's knowledge base of signs and symptoms to report, when to take allopurinol, how much fluid to consume, and when to return for follow-up laboratory testing.

TABLE 32–9 ▪ Syndrome of Inappropriate Antidiuretic Hormone

Possible causes:

- Recent surgery
- Morphine administration
- Small cell lung cancer
- Vinca alkaloid administration

Possible symptoms:

- Hyponatremia
- Weight gain without edema
- Headache
- Seizures
- Coma
- Decreased plasma osmolality

Nursing care:

- Perform strict intake and output measurement.
- Ensure fluid restriction as ordered.
- Monitor level of consciousness.
- Administer hypertonic saline as ordered.

Syndrome of Inappropriate Antidiuretic Hormone

The syndrome of inappropriate antidiuretic hormone (SIADH) (Table 32–9) is an excess secretion of the antidiuretic hormone vasopressin. This overexcretion causes excess water to be retained, resulting in water intoxication. Excess water in the intracellular space results in extreme dilution of the normal sodium concentration, causing hyponatremia. In response to the concentration gradient, extracellular water moves into the intracellular compartment, further worsening the problem and leading to cerebral edema, that, if untreated, could result in death. A normal serum sodium level is 135–145 mEq/L. Severe hyponatremia is defined as less than 100 mEq/L. Seizures, coma, and death can occur if the hyponatremia is not corrected. Plasma osmolality is decreased. Blood urea nitrogen and creatinine concentrations may be decreased. The patient experiences weight gain without edema. SIADH is highly associated with small-cell lung cancer. It can also be triggered by vincristine and vinblastine therapy, and by the administration of morphine, a drug commonly used in the treatment of cancer-related pain. Diagnosis of SIADH is made by blood tests confirming hyponatremia.

Treatment is aimed at correcting the underlying cause. This involves treating the malignancy or withdrawing the suspected offending agent. Fluid restriction is the treatment for moderate SIADH—usually 800–1000 ml per 24-hour period. This figure should include fluid from all sources, such as IV fluids and the fluids contained in medications, such as IV piggybacks. Severe SIADH may be treated with 3% hypertonic saline infused slowly. The antibiotic demeclocycline may be used to counteract the effect of vasopressin and initiate diuresis.

Nursing management includes careful recording of intake and output and daily weight. Blood test results should be monitored for response to treatment. The patient and caregiver should be educated about the need for fluid restriction and how to space out fluid allotment. The patient should be assessed frequently for, and instructed to report, headache, altered level of consciousness, muscle weakness or cramps, and decreased urine output.

■ Conclusion

Oncologic emergencies are life-threatening conditions that occur as a result of disease or treatment. By knowing the risk factors for these diseases, nurses can teach patients and families strategies that can significantly alter the course of these conditions. Accurate and early assessment and recognition of these conditions and prompt nursing interventions can alter their course and maintain and promote, good quality of life for the patient with cancer.

■ Resources

Spinal Cord Compression:
The Merck manual of diagnosis and therapy www.merck.com/mrkshared/mmanual/section14/chapter182/182b.jsp
Syndrome of Inappropriate Antidiuretic Hormone (SIADH):
Emedicine:
www.emedicine.com/emerg/topic784.htm
Cardiac Tamponade:
Emedicine:
www.emedicine.com/emerg/topic412.htm

Bibliography

Belford, K. (2000). Central nervous system cancers. In Yarbro, C., Frogge, M., Goodman, M., & Groenwald, S. (Eds), *Cancer nursing* (pp. 1048–1096). Boston. Jones & Bartlett.

Bitran, J. (2000.) *Expert guide to oncology* (pp.47–83). Philadelphia: American College of Physicians.

Flounders, J., & Ott, B. (2003). Oncology emergency modules: Spinal cord compression. *Oncology Nursing Forum Online Exclusive, 30. http://www.ons.org/xp6/ONS/Library.xml/ONS_Publications.xml/ONF.xml/ONF2003/ FebJan03/Members_Only/Flounders_article.xml* Viewed October 15, 2003.

Flounders, J. (2003). Cardiovascular emergencies: Pericardial effusion and cardiac tamponade. *Oncology Nursing Forum Online Exclusive, 30. http://www.ons.org/xp6/ONS/Library.xml/ONS_Publications.xml/ONF.xml/ONF2003/MarchApril03/Members_Only/Flounders_article.xml* Viewed October 15, 2003.

Flounders, J. (2003). Syndrome of inappropriate antidiuretic hormone. *Oncology Nursing Forum Online Exclusive, 30. http://www.ons.org/xp6/ONS/Library.xml/ONS_Publications.xml/ONF.xml/ONF2003/MayJune03/Flounders_article.xml* Viewed October 15, 2003.

Flounders, J. (2003). Oncology Emergency Modules: Superior Vena Cava Syndrome. *Oncology Nursing Forum Online Exclusive, 30. http://www.ons.org/xp6/ONS/Library.xml/ONS_Publications.xml/ONF.xml/ONF2003/JulyAug03/Members_Only/Flounders_article.xml* Viewed October 15, 2003.

Sitton, E. (2000). Superior vena cava syndrome. In Yarbro, C., Frogge, M., Goodman, M., & Groenwald, S. (Eds), *Cancer nursing* (pp. 900–912). Boston: Jones & Bartlett.

CHAPTER

33

Sexuality

Margaret Barton-Burke

As cancer survival rates improve, issues concerning quality of life receive increased attention. One area of quality of life affected by cancer and its treatment modalities is sexuality. Sexuality is a comprehensive term encompassing an integration of physical, psychological, and social dimensions of sexual beings in ways that are enriching and enhance personality, communication, and love. Sexuality involves more than the sex act and reproduction. It encompasses who and what we are as a man or woman, how we get that way, how we feel about it, and how we deal with each other about it. Sexuality consists of sexual drive, sexual activities, intimacy and physical closeness, expressions of maleness and femaleness, and gender identity. Influencing factors include societal norms, religious background, and culture, as well as health and illness. Research suggests that from 20% to 90% of cancer patients experience sexual problems, either as a consequence of the disease itself or as a side effect of treatment.

Cancer and its treatments alter sexual function. Sexual dysfunction occurs when the tumor involves the sex or reproductive organs, requiring surgical procedures such as vaginectomy, prostatectomy, or penectomy. Chemotherapy, radiation therapy, and biotherapy contribute to sexual dysfunction by altering ovarian or testicular function. Infertility may become an issue for both men and women. Changes in body image from a mastectomy or an ostomy, along with consequent distraction or preoccupation with bodily functions, may make the patient unable to relax and enjoy sex. Pain, fatigue, weight gain, and nausea and vomiting may reduce sexual drive and desire, and alopecia can make a patient feel less sexually attractive. The masculinizing or feminizing effects of treatments alter one's libido. Treatment side effects contribute to psychological reactions and changes in social roles. Cancer-related weakness and depression may be associated with a decrease in sexual drive. Medications may affect sexual functioning or responsiveness. Table 33–1 (which begins on page 470) identifies the manifold effects that various cancers have on a patient's sexual function.

■ Barriers to Assessment

Barriers to intervention appear to stem from implicit assumptions about sexuality on the part of both the patient and the nurse. It is a topic that is often not discussed. Obtaining a sexual history or asking clear questions about sexual functioning before and after diagnosis and treatment conveys a willingness to discuss this subject. Incorporating basic questions into the review of systems can introduce the topic and serve as a starting point for more detailed inquiry. The following questions may eliminate discomfort on the part of the nurse or the patient: "Has your surgery (radiation therapy, chemotherapy, or biotherapy) changed the way you see yourself as a man (woman)?" Or, "Has cancer or its treatment affected your sexual function?" Affirmative answers to either question suggest that specific details can be offered.

A subtle bias pervades the manner in which sexual assessments are conducted. There is a presumption that the person with cancer has a sexual partner who is a member of the opposite sex. Questions like, "Do you have a boyfriend or girlfriend?" "Are you married or single?" do not necessarily reveal information about one's sexuality. Single individuals may be highly active sexually and may be more concerned about changes in sexuality and sexual function than their married counterparts. Bias can be minimized by asking open-ended questions, such as "Tell me about who you live with," "Tell me about the importance of sex and/or sexuality in your life," and "Are you sexually active, with men, women or both?" Knowing patients' sexual orientation is not as important as assessing for changes in patients' usual sexual practices. Nonjudgmental inquiries about sexual behavior can help minimize the bias of an assessment and make the patient feel more comfortable revealing information about his or her sexuality.

■ The Role of the Nurse

Interventions should focus on nurse-patient communication. Patients report that they would like to discuss sexual issues with their health care provider but are reluctant to do so. The key to successful communication about sexuality and sexual problems is to give patients permission to discuss their concerns openly in a safe environment. The PLISSIT model, Table 33–2, presents one such intervention.

This model offers four levels for intervention, depending on the nurse's comfort level with the subject matter. It is recommended that discussions of potential sexual problems begin at the time of diagnosis, with the clinician letting patients know that they have permission to discuss the subject whenever necessary. Because the sexual partner plays a pivotal role in sexual recovery after cancer treatment, it is recommended that partners be included when the problem is assessed and in subsequent discussions on the subject. Additional information for male and female patients with cancer can be found in the bibliography and resources sections.

Fertility is an important aspect of treatment, especially for individuals who have not had children. Strategies to conserve fertility are often used and are highly dependent on the type of cancer and the available treatment. Cryopreservation, through the use of sperm banks, is a strategy used to preserve fertility in men. Similar approaches to preserve ovarian tissue, with subsequent reimplantation, are on the horizon for women. A history of cancer, changes in appearance and body image, as well as uncertainty about fertility all contribute to a cancer survivor's sexual function. Specific suggestions and information may help patients understand their options when treatment is over and life resumes.

■ Conclusion

Issues related to sexuality and sexual function may arise at any time during the disease trajectory. It is important to remember is that problems with sexual function are not caused by cancer and its treatments alone. These problems may be exacerbated by them, and, subsequently,

TABLE 33–1 ■ Effects of Cancer on Sexuality, Sexual Function, Fertility, Partners, and Clinical Implications

Site	Dysfunction: Physical	Dysfunction: Psychological	Effect on Fertility
Cervix	Treatment of in situ with cone biopsy will not cause dysfunction. Radical hysterectomy shortens the vagina ⅓ to ½; this may be appreciable but usually is not.	Sometimes	No, with cone biopsy for in situ stages; yes, with hysterectomy and/or XRT.
Uterus	Total abdominal hysterectomy with pelvic node dissection usually causes no dysfunction. XRT to the pelvis causes thickening of the vagina if this is included in the fields.	Sometimes	Yes, with either XRT or surgery.
Ovary	In premenopausal women, bilateral oophorectomy results in menopausal symptoms.	Sometimes	Yes (except with cases of unilateral oophorectomy).
Vulva	Simple vulvectomy can result in introital stenosis. Radical vulvectomy includes removal of the clitoris.	Usually	No, patient is often postmenopausal.
Breast	The absence of foreplay using nipple stimulation for arousal may cause some difficulties.	Usually	Dependent on treatment used.

TABLE 33–1 ■ Effects of Cancer on Sexuality, Sexual Function, Fertility, Partners, and Clinical Implications

Impact on Partner	Comments	Implications for Clinical Practice
Sometimes partner may feel that one can "catch cancer" or be affected by its treatment, especially XRT.	XRT to the pelvis causes thickening of the vagina and may cause stenosis and/or fistula formation and dyspareunia.	Deep pelvic thrusts may be painful, and sexual positions may have to be modified to avoid discomfort. Polyglycol-based or water-soluble lubricants on a woman's thighs, which are then adducted during intercourse, can create the sensation of a deep vagina. Alternative position: vaginal penetration from behind between closely adducted thighs. Vaginal dilators or frequent intercourse may prevent stenosis. Polyglycol-based, water-soluble lubricants are recommended.
Sometimes.	Due to lack of literature on female sexual response, it is difficult to determine differences between physical and psychological dysfunction.	Menopausal changes of sudden onset in previously asymptomatic women include vaginal dryness and hot flashes. Polyglycol-based and water-soluble vaginal lubricants are suggested.
Sometimes.	Dyspareunia can occur. Germ cell ovarian tumors usually occur in one ovary. An oophorectomy of the affected ovary should maintain fertility by preserving the uterus and other ovary.	If premenopausal, treatment of menopausal changes including vaginal dryness and hot flashes. Vaginal lubrication is recommended. Chemotherapy may cause alopecia, nausea, vomiting, and fatigue, minimizing desire for sexual intercourse.
Usually.	Radical vulvectomy can cause a decrease in ROM of lower extremities.	Postoperative perineal numbness may impair arousal. After clitorectomy, there may be a decrease in or absence of orgasms. Need to relearn how to reach orgasm. Intercourse may be painful.
Usually.	If oophorectomy and hormonal manipulations are used, this can affect all aspects of sexuality.	Chemotherapeutic agents may cause ovarian failure with hot flashes and vaginal dryness. Polyglycol-based, water-soluble vaginal lubricants should be used. Mastectomy.

TABLE 33–1 ■ Effects of Cancer on Sexuality, Sexual Function, Fertility, Partners, and Clinical Implications—*Continued*

Site	Dysfunction: Physical	Dysfunction: Psychological	Effect on Fertility
Prostate	Total prostatectomy results in impotence. Simple prostatectomy usually results in retrograde ejaculation. Decreased ability to have an erection appears to be age dependent.	Usually	Usually
Testicular	Nerve damage due to retroperitoneal lymph node dissection usually results in retrograde ejaculation and can cause impotence.	Usually	Sometimes, if unilateral; always, if bilateral. Suggest use of sperm bank before chemotherapy and retroperitoneal lymph node dissection.
Bladder	Local—seldom: in males, radical cystectomy involves removal of bladder, urethra, and	Usually	Always with XRT; this cancer is most common in older males.

TABLE 33-1 ■ Effects of Cancer on Sexuality, Sexual Function, Fertility, Partners, and Clinical Implications—*Continued*

Impact on Partner	Comments	Implications for Clinical Practice
		prosthesis and lingerie may conceal the surgical site. Alternative positions for intercourse may be suggested to keep breast or scar out of sight. To prevent unrealistic expectations after breast reconstruction, a drawing or photograph of how the new breast might look should be shown before the reconstruction.
Usually.	Bilateral orchiectomy or hormonal manipulations can result in erectile failures and ejaculation difficulties. If estrogen treatment is initiated, gynecomastia may result.	At biopsy: erectile difficulties, erectile failure, complete loss or reduced amount of seminal fluid. After surgery: erectile difficulties, retrograde ejaculation. With systemic therapy: malaise, weight loss, anemia, and pain. Impotence treatment: intracavernosal injections of prostaglandin El, papaverine, and phentolamine; vacuum erection devices; vascular surgery; penile implants, either semirigid or inflatable.
Usually.	Hormonal aberration (especially decrease in androgen) causes a decrease in libido and may cause impotence, retarded ejaculation, and decrease in sexual responsiveness.	Retroperitoneal lymphadenectomy has a significant negative impact on sexual functioning and fertility due to difficulty with ejaculation. Reduced semen volume may occur from radiation scatter to the prostate and seminal vesicles. Higher radiation doses may cause greater erectile and orgasmic difficulties. Impotence treatment: intracavernosal injections of prostaglandin El, papaverine, and phentolamine; vacuum erection devices; vascular surgery; penile implants, either semirigid or inflatable.
Usually.	The development of continent urostomies has made the use of the ostomy bag	In females: there is limited research. Bladder cancer in women has similar sequelae to gynecologic cancers receiving an anterior pelvic

TABLE 33-1 ■ Effects of Cancer on Sexuality, Sexual Function, Fertility, Partners, and Clinical Implications—*Continued*

Site	Dysfunction: Physical	Dysfunction: Psychological	Effect on Fertility
	prostate; therefore, he is impotent. Ability to have an erection appears to be age dependent. In females, cystectomy usually includes urethra, uterus, and anterior vagina.		
Colon/rectum	Usually; nerve damage in males negatively affects erectile ability.	Usually; especially with formation of an ostomy.	None; except with XRT and Chemotherapy.
Hodgkin's lymphoma/ non-Hodgkin's lymphoma	The disease process and the effects of the therapy may decrease sexual drive and ability.	Sometimes	Yes, with XRT to the pelvis without shielding of the gonads; chemotherapy will decrease sperm and ova maturation.
Leukemia	The disease process and associated blood counts with chemotherapy may affect ability to have an erection.	Sometimes	Chemotherapy affects sperm count and ova maturation; but they may rebound after cessation of treatment.

TABLE 33-1 ■ Effects of Cancer on Sexuality, Sexual Function, Fertility, Partners, and Clinical Implications—*Continued*

Impact on Partner	Comments	Implications for Clinical Practice
	unnecessary in many cases. Wearing a cummerbund, decorative stoma covering or underwear with a crotch cut out may help.	exenteration with a narrow vagina. Dyspareunia resulting from vaginal tightness and lack of lubrication. In males: inadequate or brief erections can occur in almost all men. Orgasm, if experienced, is less intense and without ejaculation.
Sometimes.	Women sometimes have a hysterectomy with the operative procedure. With ostomies and external collection devices, specific suggestions about emptying appliances before engaging in sex can relieve anxiety about leaks and odors.	Anterior resection is a surgical procedure with better sexual outcomes than abdominoperineal resection. Women report more positive sexual outcomes than men, regardless of the surgical procedure. Dyspareunia may be present. Men report some perineal pain or phantom rectal pain.
Usually.	Patients on chemotherapy alone should be using some form of contraception. The effects of chemotherapy on sperm counts and ova maturation are not totally understood. Extensive fatigue often diminishes sex drive and function.	Most frequent sequelae include poor body image and decreased sexual drive and satisfaction. Further research is needed to sort out multiple variables and their influence on sexuality in Hodgkin's and non-Hodgkin's' lymphoma survivors.
Usually.	Patients on chemotherapy alone should be using some form of contraception. The effects of chemotherapy on sperm counts and ova maturation are not totally understood.	Most frequent sequelae include poor body image and decreased sexual drive and satisfaction. Further research is needed to sort out multiple variables and their influence on sexuality in leukemia survivors.

TABLE 33–1 ■ Effects of Cancer on Sexuality, Sexual Function, Fertility, Partners, and Clinical Implications—*Continued*

Site	Dysfunction: Physical	Dysfunction: Psychological	Effect on Fertility

Note: Chemotherapy, radiation therapy, and analgesics are all associated with generalized feelings of malaise. This can have a profound effect on feelings of self-image, self-worth, and sexuality and libido.

All these factors should be taken into consideration when assessing the sexual needs and/or problems of cancer patients and their families.

Key: XRT = radiation therapy; ROM = range of motion.

TABLE 33–2 ■ The PLISSIT Model

(P) Permission:	Give *permission* to be sexual when undergoing or recovering from treatment or when living with the disease.
(LI) Limited Information:	Provide factual *information* about the effects of the disease and treatment on sexuality, sexual function, and fertility. Basic information about sexual function may be necessary. Common areas of concern may be the capacity for continued performance (e.g., full erections, ejaculation, orgasm), fertility, or possible interferences such as pain and fatigue.
(SS) Specific Suggestions:	Provide *specific strategies* for managing sexual activity. Examples include setting the context for sex so that it is optimal for comfort and arousal (e.g., choosing times when rested, emptying urinary pouches), ways to decrease discomfort or conserve energy (e.g., different coital positions), or activities in lieu of intercourse (e.g., body massage, masturbation).
(IT) Itensive Therapy:	Refer to *sexual therapy* or *psychotherapy* to manage sexual dysfunctions, permanent sexual disabilities, distress from the sexual changes, or marital distress. Such problems require mental health professionals who are experienced in many intervention strategies.

Source: Adapted from Annon, J. (1974). *The behavioral treatment of sexual problems.* I. Honolulu: Kapiolani Health Services; Andersen, B. L., & Lamb, M. A. (1995). Sexuality and cancer. In G. P. Murphy, W. Lawrence, & R. E. Lenhard (Eds.), *American Cancer Society textbook of clinical oncology* (2nd ed., pp. 699-713). Atlanta, GA: American Cancer Society.

TABLE 33-1 ■ Effects of Cancer on Sexuality, Sexual Function, Fertility, Partners, and Clinical Implications—*Continued*

Impact on Partner	Comments	Implications for Clinical Practice
	Extensive fatigue often diminishes sex drive and function.	

Source: Adapted from Andersen, B. L, & Lamb, M. L. (1995). Sexuality and cancer. In G. P. Murphy, W. Lawrence, & R. E. Lenhard (Eds.), *American Cancer Society textbook of clinical oncology* (2nd ed., pp. 699–713). Atlanta, GA: American Cancer Society; Lamb, M. L, & Woods, N. F. (1981). Sexuality and the cancer patient. *Cancer Nursing, 4,* 138–139; Halfin, V., Morgantaler, A., Barton Burke, M., & Goldstein, I. (1996). Sexuality and cancer. In R. Osteen (Ed.), *Cancer manual.* Framingham, MA: American Cancer Society; Ganz, P. A.., Litwin, M. S., & Meyerowitz, B. E. (2001). Sexual problems. In V. T. DeVita, S. Hellman, & S. A. Rosenberg (Ed.), *Cancer: Principles & practice of oncology* (Books @ Ovid, Section 56.3). Philadelphia: Lippincott Williams & Wilkins.

sexual function may cease because of lack of information and communication. Understanding the disease, the organs involved, the treatment used, and the long-term effects of disease makes the nurse better able to inform patients about what to expect after their experience with cancer. The nurse is pivotal in supporting patients and their partners, while being able to suggest resources such as support group and printed material, related to various aspects of sexuality and sexual health.

■ Resources

American Cancer Society: 800-ACS-2345 or *http://www.cancer.org*

- Sexuality for Men and Their Partners: *http://www.cancer.org/docroot/MIT/MIT_7_1x_SexualityforMenandTheirPartners.asp*
- Sexuality for Women and Their Partners: *http://www.cancer.org/docroot/MIT/MIT_7_1x_SexualityforWomenandTheirPartners.asp*
- Sexuality & Cancer—for the woman with cancer (pamphlet)
- Sexuality & Cancer—for the man with cancer (pamphlet)

National Cancer Institute: 800-4-CANCER or *www.cancer.gov*

- Sexuality and Reproductive Issues (PQD) (Patient) (also available in Spanish): *http://www.cancer.gov/cancerinfo/pdq/supportivecare/sexuality/patient*
- Sexuality and Reproductive Issues (PQD) (Health Professionals) (also available in Spanish): *http://www.cancer.gov/cancerinfo/pdq/supportivecare/sexuality/healthprofessional*
- Facing Forward Series: Life After Cancer Treatment: *http://www.cancer.gov/cancerinfo/life-after-treatment*

Bibliography

Gallo-Silver, L. (2000). The sexual rehabilitation of person with cancer. *Cancer Practice, 8,* 10–15.

Jenkins, M. & Ashley, J. (2002). Sex and the oncology patient: Discussing sexual dysfunction helps the patient optimize quality of life. *American Journal of Nursing, 102*(suppl.), 13–15.

Potter, J. E. (2002). Do ask, do tell. *Annals of Internal Medicine, 137,* 341–343.

Shell, J. A. (2002). Evidence-based practice for symptom management in adults with cancer: sexual dysfunction. *Oncology Nursing Forum, 29,* 2002.

Simkin, R. (1998). Not all your patients are straight. *Canadian Medical Association Journal, 159,* 370–375.

Wilmoth, M. C. (1998). Sexuality resources for cancer professionals and their patients. *Cancer Practice, 6,* 346–348.

Wilmoth, M. C. & Bruner, D. W. (2002). Integrating sexuality into cancer nursing practice. *Oncology Nursing Patient Treatment and Support, 9,* 1–14.

CHAPTER

34

Pediatric Symptoms and Responses

Katherine Patterson Kelly

Mary C. Hooke

With their healthy organ systems, children and adolescents tolerate the acute effects of high-dose chemotherapy better than their adult counterparts. However, their growing organ systems are vulnerable to the acute and late effects of cancer treatment. All body systems can be affected by chemotherapy and radiation therapy. Children with cancer are at risk for potentially life-threatening complications regardless of their diagnosis or treatment. Medical emergencies can happen quickly. Supportive care must be carefully individualized. Medication dosage and fluids are based on the child's weight and body surface area. Nurses must monitor laboratory and test results closely because the normal ranges for these tests are developmentally derived. Expert family-centered nursing care is needed to minimize complications, facilitate positive patient outcomes, and support the growth and development of the child and family. In this chapter, common treatment- and disease-related symptoms and strategies that nurses can use to help patients who experience these symptoms are described.

■ Myelosuppression

Children with cancer typically receive intensive multimodal therapy to treat their disease. This is partly because they rarely have comorbid chronic illnesses that could limit the intensity of their treatment. Even so, children commonly experience moderate-to-severe bone marrow suppression secondary to the high-dose chemotherapy used to treat childhood malignancies. Bone marrow suppression, or *myelosuppression,* occurs as a result of the disease (marrow replacement by malignant cells) or treatment (cytotoxic effect of rapidly dividing hematopoietic cells) (see Chapter 22, Myelosuppression). Bone marrow suppression is the most common dose-limiting toxicity for most pediatric cancer therapies. It results in decreased levels of red blood cells (RBCs), white blood cells, and platelets and occurs most commonly 10–14 days after each course of chemotherapy. Managing the effects of myelosuppression takes priority over managing other symptoms in pediatric oncology. Pediatric oncology nurses report that teaching patients and their parents about how to monitor the patients' blood counts and how to initiate protective behaviors is their most common nursing care activity.

Anemia

Anemia is defined as a reduction in the red cell mass or the blood hemoglobin concentration. Anemic children experience symptoms such as irritability, lethargy, fatigue, headache, and dizziness. Physical findings may include pallor, tachycardia, hypotension, and a mild systolic ejection flow murmur. Treatment strategies include providing adequate rest and RBC transfusions as needed. Indication for RBC transfusion varies between treatment centers, but they most often occur when the hemoglobin decreases to < 7 g/dl or if the child experiences severe symptoms. Transfusion doses for children are calculated based on body weight. The standard infusion volume is 10–15 ml/kg of irradiated, leukocyte-depleted RBCs. For small children weighing less than 30–40 kg, infusion rates are typically 5 m/kg/hr or less, to diminish the likelihood of volume overload. Erythropoietin is an effective treatment for most anemic children and adolescents but requires 4–8 weeks to induce a hematopoietic response and may be refused by the child or family if they have to administer it subcutaneously.

Thrombocytopenia

Defined as an abnormally small number of platelets in the circulating blood, thrombocytopenia presents a potentially serious safety concern in young children. Children who have platelet counts of less than 75,000–100,000/mm^3 are at risk for increased bleeding if they are injured. Spontaneous bleeding can occur with platelet counts of less than 5,000–10,000/mm^3. Children most commonly have bruising, petechiae, epistaxis, and mucosal bleeding during periods of thrombocytopenia. The child's urine, stool, and emesis must be monitored for obvious or occult blood.

Controversy exists about the indications for platelet transfusion. Many pediatric oncology clinicians administer transfusions to children prophylactically who have platelet counts of less than 10,000–20,000/mm^3, especially if the child presents an injury risk. An active toddler, a child with infection and fever, or a child requiring invasive procedures, such as lumbar puncture and bone marrow aspiration, poses a significant risk for bleeding during periods of thrombocytopenia. Care must be taken to avoid volume overload when a child requires both RBC and platelet transfusions on the same day.

Neutropenia

Neutropenia, a decrease in the number of segmented and banded neutrophils, presents the most life-threatening risk for children with cancer. Neutropenia is calculated by multiplying the percentage of segmented and banded neutrophils by the total white blood count (% segs + % bands x white blood count (WBC)) and is reported as an absolute neutrophil count. Children who are neutropenic are at risk for life-threatening bacterial, fungal, or viral infections.

Because children with cancer often experience neutropenia, any fever (temperature ≥ 38.5 °C or 101.5 °F) is considered life-threatening until proven otherwise. When a child develops fever, an immediate physical examination, blood count, and blood cultures are needed. The child is examined carefully for any signs or symptoms of infection. If the absolute neutrophil count is less than 500, the child is admitted to the hospital for broad-spectrum antibiotics. Figure 34–1 depicts the typical treatment for a pediatric cancer patient with fever.

Children may require treatment with granulocyte colony-stimulating factor (G-CSF) to stimulate bone marrow production of neutrophils and to reduce the length and the severity of neutropenia. These treatments can be stressful for young children because the granulocyte colony-stimulating factor is a daily subcutaneous injection. Newer, long-acting preparations of granulocyte colony-stimulating factor have promise for reducing the pain of these treatments, but these have not yet been fully evaluated in young children.

In addition to neutropenia, children with cancer are at risk for infection because of cellular and humoral immunosuppression. For this reason, routine childhood immunizations are held during therapy and for 6–12 months after treatment ends. Influenza immunizations are recommended for the child and immediate family members to prevent

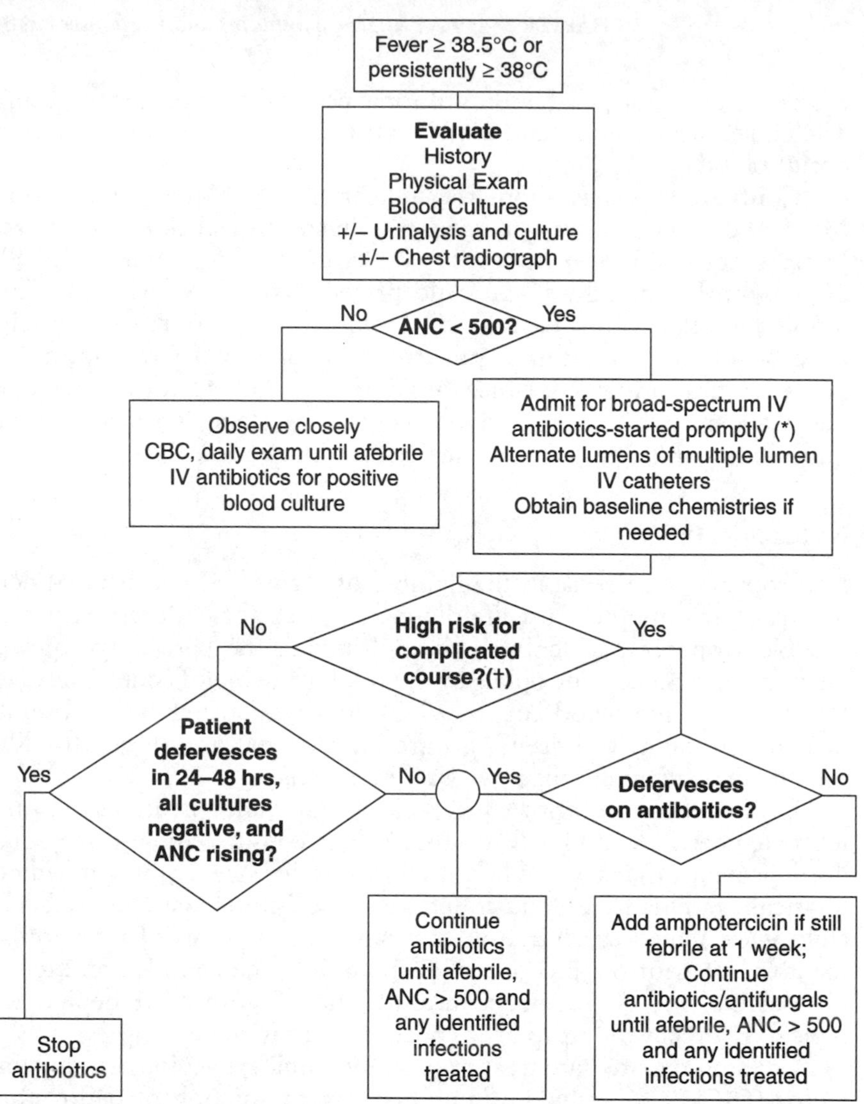

(*) If patient lives far from pediatric oncology center, may admit locally with daily follow-up with primary oncologist. If fever persists > 3 days, recommend transfer to pediatric oncology center.

(†) Hypotension, uncontrolled cancer (e.g., leukemia in induction, unresponsive or metastatic cancer), impaired organ function, or mental status changes.

FIGURE 34–1 ■ Algorithm for Oncology Patient with Fever.

Key: ANC = absolute neutrophil count; CBC = complete blood count; IV = intravenous.

Source: Reprinted from Kline N. E. (2002). Prevention and treatment of infections. In C. R. Baggott, K. P. Kelly, D. Fochtman, & G. V. Foley (Eds.), *Nursing care of children and adolescents with cancer* (3rd ed., p. 269). Philadelphia: W. B. Saunders. Copyright (2002) by W. B. Saunders, with permission from Elsevier.

severe infection. Children often require prophylactic treatment for *Pneumocystis carinii* pneumonia throughout therapy.

The most important care consideration for children with bone marrow suppression is preventing severe complications by close monitoring and early intervention. The nurse obtains frequent CBCs and reports results to parents and patients, along with instructions for patient safety as listed in Table 34–1.

Children with cancer often have central venous catheters to facilitate the delivery of chemotherapy, as well as blood products, intravenous fluids, nutritional support, and intravenous antibiotics. The presence of a central venous catheter places the child at added risk for the development of infection. Nurses must use meticulous central line care to prevent serious complications. Care for the pediatric central venous catheter is adapted from adult standards to meet the needs of this special population. The nurse must provide developmentally appropriate comfort care to reduce the child's distress when these catheters are used.

Children and adolescents are quick studies in learning the care and management of their central venous catheter. Nursing care strategies for accessing implanted venous access devices or central line dressing changes often include inviting the child to participate in accessing his or her implanted venous access device or in changing the central line dressing by helping cleanse the site, holding supplies, or pushing the syringe plunger to flush the catheter. Nurses caring for the child or adolescent with a central venous catheter should ask the patient and family about the child's preferred level of involvement and coping strategies so that these can be supported. Table 34–2 outlines nursing care recommendations designed to prevent complications related to the use of central venous catheters in children with cancer.

Fatigue

Bone marrow suppression contributes significantly to fatigue in children with cancer. Children report cancer treatment, myelosuppression, side effects, fever, and pain, as well as trying to do too many activities, as causes of their fatigue. Changes in sleep patterns, especially staff interruptions during hospitalizations, also contribute to fatigue in children. Adolescents add worry and fears to the causes of fatigue. Parents and staff report waiting and inadequate nutrition to be factors that contribute to fatigue in children and adolescents.

In addition to correcting physiologic causes of fatigue, such as anemia, pain, dehydration, and malnutrition, treatment for fatigue must target the child's reported causes of fatigue. Differentiating depression

TABLE 34–1 ■ A Basic Format that Can Be Used in Teaching Parents About Blood Counts

Red Blood Cells		
Purpose	**Normal Values**	**Special Care for Low Values**
• Give energy to the body. • Provide color to the skin. • Carry oxygen to all parts of the body.	Normal 13.5–17.0 g/ Adequate/Acceptable > 7–8 g/d Transfusion < 7 gm/d	• Transfusion may be necessary. • Watch for increasing fatigue, headache, dizziness, pallor (particularly in conjunctiva and lips) and irritability. • Provide rest between periods of activity.

Platelets		
Purpose	**Normal Values**	**Special Care for Low Values**
• Prevent bleeding. • Promote clotting.	Normal 150,000-450,000/mm³ Adequate/Acceptable 50,000-100,000/mm³ Transfusion Often Needed <10,000–20,000/mm³ –	• Transfusion may be necessary. • Provide for safety in activity when platelets low-avoid activities that can cause injury when platelet count below. 50,000–100,000/mm³ • Clean teeth with soft toothbrush, gauze, or washcloth. • Wear a helmet when bike riding. • Avoid contact sports. • Shave with an electric razor only. • Avoid sexual intercourse. • Know how to stop nosebleed or profuse bleeding. • Watch for gum bleeding or bleeding from other sources. • Prevent perirectal injury by maintaining soft stools, avoiding rectal temperatures, enemas, or suppositories. • Avoid medications containing ibuprofen or aspirin and Pepto Bismol.

TABLE 34-1 ■ A Basic Format that Can Be Used in Teaching Parents About Blood Counts—*Continued*

White Blood Cells		
Purpose	**Normal Values**	**Special Care for Low Values**
• Fight infection. • Neutrophils are type of WBC that fight bacterial infections. • Neutrophils are also called segs & bands, polys, stabs, or granulocytes.	Normal 4,500–11,500/mm^3 Adequate/ ANC >1,000/mm^3 Watch ANC < 500/mm^3	• Learn how to calculate an ANC; know your child's current ANC level. • Calling for fevers (T >/= 38.5)-single most important activity to prevent severe complications from low ANC; children are admitted with fever for IV antibiotics if ANC. < 500/mm^3 children can die within 12–24 hours of an untreated bacterial or fungal blood infection. • Do not give acetaminophen for fevers unless you have talked with the oncology team; may use for pain after checking temperature and level is below 100°F (one dose only). • Good handwashing is essential. • Avoid ill contacts. • Monitor the skin for signs of infection. • Call if the child has chills especially after flushing IV or becomes extremely fatigued or has other significant change in condition. • Avoid rectal temperatures, enemas, and suppositories.

Source: Reprinted from Panzarella, C., et al. (2002) Management of disease and treatment-related complications. In C. R. Baggott, K. P. Kelly, D. Fochtman, & G. V. Foley (Eds.), *Nursing care of children and adolescents with cancer* (3rd ed., p. 281). Philadelphia: W. B. Saunders. Copyright (2002) by W. B. Saunders, with permission from Elsevier.

TABLE 34-2 ■ Adapting Central Line Care to the Pediatric Patient

Central Line Care Component	Pediatric/Adolescent Considerations
1. Preventing infection	1a. For children over 2 months of age: disinfect skin with 2% chlorhexidine-based preparation before accessing port or during central line dressing changes. 1b. For children less than 2 months of age: disinfect skin with 70% alcohol or 10% providine-iodine. 1c. Transparent dressing may be changed weekly and as necessary when soiled or loose. 1d. Do not submerge catheter or port needle under water during bathing. Catheter or port needle may be protected with an impermeable cover during showering.
2. Preventing thrombotic occlusion	2a. Concentrations of 1–10 units/ml should be used for flushing catheter of pediatric patients. 2b. Volumes are based on central catheter internal lumen volume. • Broviac/ Hickman: 2–5 ml • Implemented port: 5 ml
3. Treating thrombotic occlusion	3a. Alteplase is a thrombolytic agent used to dissolve thrombus that is occluding catheter. 3b. Dose is based on internal volume of catheter, with a dose maximum of 2 mg/2ml. Dose of 0.5 mg/0.5ml can be used in neonates and children with Broviac 4.2-French catheter or smaller. 3c. Dwell time for Alteplase is 30–120 minutes.
4. Protecting central line or port needle from accidental removal	4. Prevent tension on catheter or port needle by applying tape tab to IV tubing and securing the tape tab to patient's clothing with a safety pin. Tension on the tubing is then absorbed at this point rather than the catheter site.
5. Providing comfort care for implemented port access	5. Topical analgesics (EMLA or ELA-Max) access are applied 30–60 minutes before procedure following manufacturer's instructions.

Source: Data from Wallace, J. D. (in press). Central venous access. In N. Kline. (Ed.), *Essentials of pediatric oncology nursing: A core curriculum* (2nd ed., publication still in process). Glenview, IL: Association of Pediatric Oncology Nurses; Hooke, C. (2000). Recombinant tissue plasminogen activator for central venous access device occlusion. *Journal of Pediatric Oncology Nursing, 17,* 174–178; Intravenous Nurses Society (2002). *Policies and procedure for infusion nursing* (2nd ed.). Cambridge, MA: ; Intravenous Nurses Society, (2000). Infusion Nursing Standards of Practice. *Journal of Intravenous Nursing, 23,* S1–S87. O'Grady N. P. (2002), Guidelines for the prevention of intravascular catheter-related infections. *Infection Control and Hospital Epidemiology, 23,* 759–769.

from fatigue and noting the child's activity patterns are also important. Children and parents identify naps; distractions, including visitors and fun activities; and sleep medications as helpful self-care strategies. Nurses can support these efforts by encouraging adequate rest and nutrition, providing distraction activities during treatment and hospitalization, minimizing sleep interruptions during hospitalizations, and encouraging participation in usual activities as tolerated. Creative solutions, such as attending half versus whole school days, can promote normalization while decreasing the child's fatigue.

■ Pain

Childhood cancer pain arises from the disease, treatment, or procedures needed to deliver therapy and monitor the disease. Treatment-related pain dominates other forms of childhood cancer pain. Treatment of pain in the child with cancer is similar to the therapeutic approach used with adult cancer patients (see Chapter 23, Cancer Pain).

Treatment of pain in children with cancer has multiple challenges, including assessment accuracy and staff and parent fears related to opioid medications. Ongoing assessment of pain combined with around-the-clock analgesic administration is the standard of care for cancer pain treatment.

Because pain is a subjective experience, optimal pain assessment includes a self-report. When asked in a developmentally sensitive manner, children as young as 3–4 years of age can provide information about their pain. When the child is too young to communicate, assessment techniques depend on parent and/or nurse proxy assessments using behavioral scales. Table 34–3 provides a description of the most widely used pain rating scales for children.

Treatment of disease and treatment-related pain recommendations follow the World Health Organization analgesic ladder. Adjuvant agents and complementary health practices may be useful in treating childhood cancer pain. Because children are especially susceptible to distraction and play as methods of pain relief, it is helpful to combine these strategies with appropriate pharmacologic measures to maximize pain relief.

Painful medical procedures present a unique problem in pediatrics. Uncontrolled treatment-related pain causes severe distress in young children. As a result, pediatric oncology clinicians pay particular attention to preventing procedure-related pain. Children benefit from both psychological and pharmacologic methods. Table 34–4 summarizes common techniques used in pediatric procedural pain control.

TABLE 34-3 ■ Pain Rating Scales for Children

Rating Scale	Age Range	Description
Wong-Baker Faces Scale (self)	3–8 years	Simple cartoon faces represent levels of pain.
Oucher (self)	3–12 years	Photographic scale of children in different levels of pain. The child points to the face that best represents his or her current level of pain. Available in a variety of ethnic variations. Includes a 100-point vertical scale for use by older children.
Poker chip tool (self)	4–13 years	Four poker chips represent pieces of hurt, from a little hurt to as much hurt as you could ever have.
Color scale (self)	4–10	The child ranks colors to represent pain intensity and then uses the colors to draw his or her pain on a body outline representing both location and intensity of pain.
CRIES (proxy)	6–12 months	Acronym for 5 physiologic and behavioral indicators of pain (**C**rying, ***R***equires O2 for saturation > 95%, ***I***ncreased vital signs (heart rate and blood pressure), ***E***xpression, ***S***leeplessness).
OPS (proxy)	12 months –3 years	Five indicators include blood pressure, crying, movement, agitation, verbal evaluation or body language (if preverbal or unable to communicate).
PIPPS (proxy)	Preterm and term neonates	Seven indicators include physiologic, behavioral, and contextual measures.

Source: Data from Norden, J., Hannalah, R., Getson, P., O'Donnell, R., Kelliher, G., & Walker, N. (1991). Concurrent validation of an Objective Pain Scale for infants and children. *Anesthesiology, 75,* A934; Patterson, K. L. (1992). Pain in the pediatric oncology patient. *Journal of Pediatric Oncology Nursing, 9,* 119–130; Sentivany-Collins, S. (2002). Treatment of pain. In C. R. Baggott, K. P. Kelly, D. Fochtman, & G. V. Foley (Eds.), *Nursing care of children and adolescents with cancer* (3rd ed., pp.319–333). Philadelphia: W. B. Saunders Company.

It is important to note the dosing requirements for analgesics in children. Calculation errors in small children can produce significant toxicity. Table 34–4 summarizes the childhood dose recommendations used for common opioid and adjuvant pain control agents. Pediatric cancer patients often report that the fear of pain is greater than the fear related to the cancer diagnosis. Therefore, clinicians must strive to ensure that the knowledge and resources for safe and effective pain control are made available to all children with cancer, their families, and the members of their health care team.

TABLE 34-4 ■ Pain Control Methods for Children

Physiologic Drug	Equianalgesic Doses (mg/kg)	Onset (minutes) Duration (hours)	Comments
Codeine (PO)	0.5–1	30–60 min. 3–4 hrs.	Often used with acetaminophen.
Oxycodone (PO)	0.1	30–60 3–4	Less nausea than codeine; sustained-release preparation available.
Morphine (IV, SC, IM, PO)	0.1 (IV/SC/IM) 0.6 (PO)	5–10 (IV); 30–60 (PO) 3–4	Sustained-release preparation available.
Hydromorphone (IV, SC, PO)	0.015 (IV/SC) 0.075 (PO)	5–10 (IV); 30-60 (PO) 3–4	
Meperidine	1 (IV)	5–10 (IV)	Not recommended for PO use because it is not well absorbed. Not recommended for long-term use because it causes seizures.
Fentanyl (IV)	0.001 (IV)	3–8 (IV) 0.5–1	Rapid IV administration causes chest wall rigidity; transdermal preparation is available.

Psychological Strategy	Description
Providing information	Giving child specific information about the procedure, including what the child will see and feel.
Breathing	Helping child take slow deep breaths during the procedure. Using blowing toys (bubbles, pinwheels) can help child implement this strategy. The child is told to blow away the pain.
Distraction	Teaching child to shift point of focus away from the procedure. Use of engaging activities, e.g., video games or pop-up books, is useful.
Relaxation	Teaching child to relax muscle groups of the body
Imagery	Helping child visualize positive, distracting images e.g., going to the beach, riding a bicycle. Uses as many senses as possible to create a pleasant image.
Hypnosis	Combining deep relaxation and shift of focus to produce a trance state. Guided only by qualified, trained professional.

Key: IM = intramuscular; IV = intravenous; PO = oral; SC = subcutaneous.

Source: Data from Deshpande, J. K., & Tobias, J. D. (1996). *The pediatric pain handbook.* 7St. Louis: Mosby; Patterson, K. L. (1992). Pain in the pediatric oncology patient. *Journal of Pediatric Oncology Nursing, 9,* 119–130; Sentivany-Collins, S. (2002). Treatment of pain. In C. R. Baggott, K. P. Kelly, D. Fochtman, & G. V. Foley (Eds.), *Nursing care of children and adolescents with cancer* (3rd ed., pp. 319–333). Philadelphia: W. B. Saunders Company.

■ Malnutrition

Children with cancer can develop malnutrition secondary to uncontrolled nausea and vomiting, taste alterations, oral mucositis, pain, and psychosocial responses to the disease and treatment. Children can develop food aversions when oral medications are "hidden" in favorite foods or when children associate those foods with the adverse effects of emetogenic chemotherapy. Additionally, young children often exert control over what goes into their mouths when all other control has been removed from them during the course of treatment.

Stable weight is not an acceptable nutritional standard in young children. Lack of weight gain in young children is a signal of impending malnutrition. The child's growth must be tracked on standardized growth charts to ensure adequate monitoring and interpretation of nutritional status. Typically, a weight reduction of two percentiles on the growth chart, or a 10% or greater weight loss, mandates prompt nutritional intervention. Nutritional interventions used in children mirror those used in adult cancer patients, as discussed in Chapter 30 (Anorexia and Weight Loss). Table 34–5 summarizes important age-based nutritional requirements for children.

TABLE 34–5 ■ Pediatric Nutritional Requirements

Nutritional Parameter	Calculation of Daily Requirement		
Fluid	1st 10 kg		100 ml/kg/day
	2nd 10 kg		50 ml/kg/day
	each additional kg		20 ml/kg/day
Calories	Infants 0–1 yr		100 kcal/kg/day
	Children	1–3 yr	100 kcal/kg/day
		4–6 yr	90 kcal/kg/day
		7–10 yr	70 kcal/kg/day
		11–14 yr	55 (boys) 47 (girls) kcal/kg/day
		15–18 yr	45 (boys) 40 (girls) kcal/kg/day
Protein	Age:	0–1 yr	2–3 g/kg/day
		1–7 yr	55–90 g/kg/day
		> 7 yr	55–75 g/kg/day

Source: Data from Gunn, V. L., & Nechyba, C. (2002). *The Harriet Lane handbook: A manual for pediatric house officers.* Philadelphia: Mosby.

Fluid and electrolyte balance are also critical aspects of the response to cancer therapy in children. Children can quickly become over- or underhydrated. Their growing bodies need adequate protein and calorie intake to ensure growth. Children with cancer who are undernourished are more prone to treatment complications, such as neutropenia and infections.

Nurses play a major role in the preventing and managing malnutrition in children with cancer. Nurses must monitor weight, intake and output, and fluid/electrolyte balance. Aggressive management of other gastrointestinal complications, such as nausea and vomiting, mucositis, and taste alterations, can help prevent nutritional complications in young children. Parent and child education emphasizes the importance of oral hygiene, home management of nausea and vomiting, and the link between nutrition and clinical outcomes. The need for nutritional supplementation is introduced, not as a treatment for failure to maintain weight, but as a means to promote greater treatment tolerance and thus greater potential for positive therapeutic outcomes.

■ Psychosocial Responses in the Child and Family

Children and adolescents undergoing treatment for cancer face challenges to normal growth and development. Side effects of cancer therapy such as fatigue, pain, mucositis, immobility, and changes in appearance can interfere with normal developmental experiences. Isolation and hospitalization separate the child and adolescent from family, school, and peer experiences that are important to the developing child and adolescent. The child's and adolescent's increasing desire for autonomy and independence are challenged by treatment-related increased dependency and loss of control. These patients, as well as their families, need the support of the health care team to foster healthy development at a time when it can be impeded. Table 34–6 describes the major tasks of each developmental task of each stage and the nursing assessments and interventions designed to support appropriate development and coping skills.

The child's or adolescent's responses to the stress of the cancer experience may include withdrawal, regression, anxiety, and sadness. The nurse assesses these normal reactions and provides support and consistent care to the child or adolescent and their family. Resources to help the nurse assist patients and families in developing effective coping strategies include the psychosocial team of child life specialists, social workers, and psychologists. Despite the extreme rarity of severe depression, suicidal ideation, and/or psychosis in this population, these

TABLE 34–6 ■ Developmental Care of the Pediatric Oncology Patient

Developmental Stage	Developmental Tasks/ Significant Relationships	Nursing Assessment and Interventions
Infants (Birth to 1 year)	• Developing trust in parents and caregivers. • Developing body image and sense of self: uses oral route as source of exploration and pleasure. • Developing attachment to mother and father.	• Support bonding and interplay between infant and parent(s). • Provide sensorimotor experiences. • Encourage sucking and oral intake. • Provide comforting touch. • Provide consistent caregivers and establish routines with cares.
Toddlers (1–3 years)	• Developing sense of independence and self-mastery. • Developing sense of cause and effect and language skills. • Exploratory in behavior. • Egocentric in thought, play, and behavior. • Parents are of primary importance; developing parallel play with peers.	• Interview parents about toddlers' routines, patterns, fears, security objects, and comfort measures and incorporate into cares with consistent caregivers. • Encourage independence by providing appropriate choices. • Encourage mobility and exploration, even if in wagon or stroller. • Provide safe environment for play. • Provide simple explanations immediately before experience; doesn't yet understand cause and effect relationships.
Preschoolers (4–6 years)	• Developing sense of mastery over physical skills. • Developing ability to think and verbalize their mental processes. • Utilizing magical thinking. • Becoming aware of changes in appearance and sexual identity. • Working through anxieties and fears through play. • Parents continue to be of primary importance; peers and other significant adults from preschool also important.	• Interview parents about preschooler's routines, patterns, fears, security objects, and comfort measures and incorporate into cares with consistent caregivers. • Assess understanding of disease and its treatment and cares. • Encourage mastery of self-care skills and support independence. • Provide opportunities for stimulating play in safe boundaries.

TABLE 34-6 ■ Developmental Care of the Pediatric Oncology Patient—*Continued*

Developmental Stage	Developmental Tasks/ Significant Relationships	Nursing Assessment and Interventions
		• Provide simple explanations about experiences and treatment a short time before they occur.
School-aged children (7–12 years)	• Developing proficiency at accomplishing skills; becoming increasingly independent. • Goal is to answer "What can I do?" • Concrete thinkers; are able to inductively reason and understand reversibility. • Peer relationships becoming important. • Self-esteem linked to competence at performing tasks, including mastery at school. • Parents, peers, and school staff are important.	• Assess level of knowledge and information needs about disease and its treatment. • Support child's sense of mastery; encourage play, hobbies, school-work, and socialization. • Foster normalcy through supporting routines and being as flexible as possible. • Support peer relationships. • Prepare for procedure by explaining sensations that will be felt and how they will occur, and explain behavior that is expected and strategies for self-control. • Praise any sign of helpful behavior and positive coping. • Encourage involvement in cares; allow some control over aspects of care. • Encourage self-care activities.
Adolescents (13–18 years)	• Developing own identify, values, and independence. • Goal is to answer, "Who am I?" • Capable of abstract thought, able to reason and conceptualize beyond their actual experience. • Peer acceptance is of key importance; fear rejection by peers. • Body-image is important as is privacy; physical changes impact sense of self-esteem. • Discovering and processing sexual identity.	• Assess level of knowledge and information needs about disease and its treatment. • Support teenager's independence in answering questions and making decisions. • Encourage parents to allow teen autonomy to learn about disease and its management. • Assess symptom distress caused by disease and its treatment and respond with aggressive symptom management.

(continued)

TABLE 34-6 ▪ Developmental Care of the Pediatric Oncology Patient—*Continued*

Developmental Stage	Developmental Tasks/ Significant Relationships	Nursing Assessment and Interventions
	• Developing sexual attraction in 1:1 relationships that include opposite sex or may be to same sex. • Beginning to consider characteristics important in a life partner. • Peers are most important relationships as well as parents, family, and adult role models.	• Foster normalcy through supporting routines and being flexible as possible. • Support positive peer relationships. • Use adult approaches to support and teach. • Promote positive coping utilizing procedural preparation, relaxation, and imagery. • Encourage involvement in care; allow as much control as possible over aspects of care. • Encourage self-care activities. • Utilize appropriate humor in interactions. • Assess educational needs regarding sexuality and level of activity through confidential discussions without parent present. • Provide information about birth control, safety precautions, and sexual functioning as relates to cancer therapy in private interaction. • Provide privacy in cares and when peers visiting.

Source: Data from Hinds, P. S., Quargnenti, A. G., Wentz, T. J. (1992). Measuring symptom distress in adolescents with cancer. *Journal of Pediatric Oncology Nursing, 9,* 84–86; Hooke, C. (Section Ed.), (in press). Psychosocial issues. In N. Kline (Ed.), *Essentials of pediatric oncology nursing: A core curriculum* (2nd ed). Glenview, IL: Association of Pediatric Oncology Nurses; Walker, C. L., Wells, L., M., Heiney, S. P., Hymovich, D. P. (2002). Family-centered psychosocial care. In C. R. Baggott, K. P. Kelly, D. Fochtman, & G. V. Foley (Eds.), *Nursing care of children and adolescents with cancer* (3rd ed., pp. 365–390). Philadelphia: W. B. Saunders.

represent emergent situations that warrant immediate intervention. Referral for psychiatric treatment can be coordinated through the pediatric cancer center.

■ Conclusion

Fortunately, most children who have cancer enjoy a favorable prognosis and long-term survival. Improved survival mandates that close attention be paid to symptom management for children with cancer throughout therapy to promote quality of life during and after therapy. A child's growth and development cannot be interrupted during cancer therapy without long-term consequences. Because childhood cancer is rare, extensive studies of pediatric cancer symptom management are not common. Therefore, pediatric cancer specialists apply findings from symptom management research in the adult cancer patients to children. More research is needed to document optimal symptom management strategies for children. Clinicians must work closely with the health care providers from the child's community to ensure continuity of care and promotion of the child's growth and development. Nurses provide critical links between the treatment center and the child's community through care coordination, communication, and patient and family education.

■ Resources

- American Brain Tumor Association: *www.abta.org/*
- American Cancer Society: *www.cancer.org*
- Association of Pediatric Oncology Nurses: *www.apon.org*
- Cancer Source Kids: *www.cancersourcekids.com/*
- Cancervive, Inc.: *www.cancervive.org*
- Caring Bridge: *www.caringbridge.org/*
- Children's Oncology Group: *www.childrensoncologygroup.org/*
- Leukemia and Lymphoma Society of America: *www.leukemia.org*
- National Childhood Cancer Foundation: *www.conquerkidscancer.org/*
- National Cancer Institute Cancer Information: *www.nci.nih.gov/cancerinfo/*
- National Cancer Institute Clinical Trials: *www.nci.nih.gov/clinicaltrials/*

- STARBRIGHT Pediatric Network: *www.starbright.org/*
- Teens Living with Cancer: *www.teenslivingwithcancer.org/*

Bibliography

Baggott, C. R., Kelly, K. P., Fochtman, D., & Foley, G. V. (Eds.) (2002). *Nursing care of children and adolescents with cancer* (3rd ed.). Philadelphia: W. B. Saunders.

Hockenberry-Eaton, M., Hinds, P. S., Alcoser, P., et al. (1998). Fatigue in children and adolescents with cancer. *Journal of Pediatric Oncology Nursing, 15,* 172–182.

Kline, N. (Ed.) (in press). *Essentials of Pediatric Oncology Nursing: A core curriculum (2nd* ed.). Glenview IL.: Association of Pediatric Oncology Nurses.

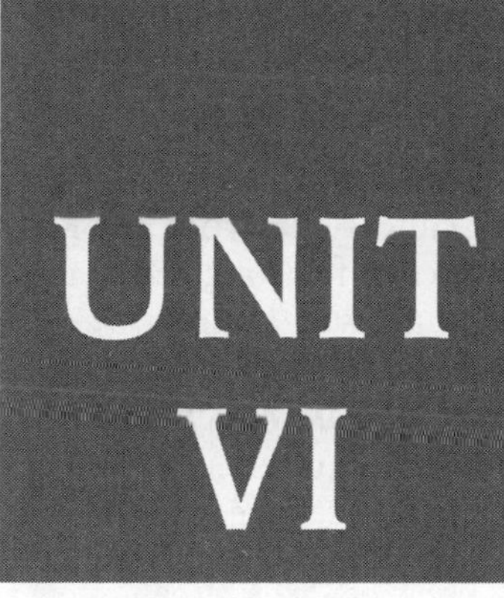

UNIT VI

Cancer Care Continuum

Andrea M. Denicoff

Nurses have an impact on the cancer continuum, from primary prevention, screening and early detection, diagnosis, treatment, survivorship, recurrence and progression, through the end-of-life, by helping to reduce the burden of cancer. Nurses play a key role across the entire continuum, through interventions such as health promotion and education, psychosocial support, and direct care.

Family members are an integral part of the cancer experience. The nurse's role includes helping the patient with cancer by gathering and sharing information, aiding in decision making, and giving the necessary emotional support. Health professionals should consider a patient's family in a broad sense, as those people with a significant interest and role in the patient's life, and the nurse should clarify with each patient who makes up his or her family.

As cancer has been transforming into a chronic illness for many patients, the need to include family members in the plan of care has become more important. Cancer has become a curable disease for many more patients. Rapid advances in cancer research have lead to improved cancer therapies and improved early detection and screening strategies; thus, the numbers of people living with and surviving cancer will rise.

As the population of cancer survivors has grown, the need to better understand, prevent, and care for long-term and late effects of cancer and its treatment has also grown. *Long-term* or *persistent effects* refer to any side effects that began during treatment and continue after the end of treatment. In contrast, *late effects* appear months to years after the completion of treatment. Late effects refer specifically to toxicities unrecognized at the end of cancer treatment that emerge later because of growth, development, or aging. It is critical that we incorporate cancer survivorship research findings in practice and use effective surveillance methods for both physiologic and psychosocial sequelae of cancer. Detecting late effects early and intervening early can decrease the severity of these effects. Many survivors are at greater risk for developing second malignancies. Regular surveillance in this population serves two purposes: to diagnose a late effect early and to diagnose a second cancer early.

Previous definitions of palliative care have focused on care at the end of life. Recognizing the importance of providing symptom management and other aspects of palliative care much earlier has lead to expansion of the definition (Figure VI-1). The current definition from the World Health Organization (2002) states that palliative care should begin at the time of a cancer diagnosis and currently defines palliative care as "An approach which improves the quality of life of patients and their families facing the problem associated with life-threatening illness, through the prevention and relief of suffering by means of early identification and impeccable assessment and treatment of pain and other problems, physical, psychosocial and spiritual."

Palliative care uses a team approach to address the needs of patients and their families. It begins early in the course of illness, in conjunction with other therapies that are intended to prolong life, such as chemotherapy and radiation therapy, and may positively influence the course of illness.

Nurses, as essential members of the health care team, provide care to individuals and their families throughout the cancer experience. We will continue to play a key role in reducing the burden of cancer by initiating palliative care strategies early. Providing high-quality care for patients as they deal with the physical symptoms of cancer and its treatment, and the psychological, social, spiritual and existential crises it produces along the entire cancer trajectory, will lead to improving the quality of lives for people with cancer and their families.

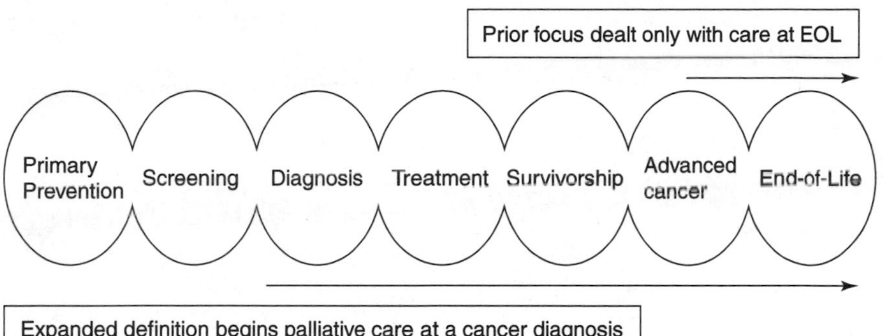

FIGURE VI–1 ■ Palliative Care along the Cancer Continuum.

CHAPTER

35

Psychosocial-Spiritual Responses to Cancer and Treatment: Living with Cancer

Michelle Rhiner

Shirley Otis-Green

Neal E. Slatkin

She arrived to the clinic, visibly exhausted and uncomfortable from the long drive. Pain was only one of her symptoms that needed attention today. As usual, she minimized her shortness of breath, saying that it would pass, that it was only because of a car ride without air conditioning. Her husband accompanied her as he always did. He is a rock, her source of strength, and she reciprocates his caring. She is protective of him, as he is of her. I'm conscious that she tries to limit the time they are away from their shop, so much so that she's willing to limit her access to care, shielding precious time for him to complete orders, the only thing that is keeping a roof over their heads, albeit hidden behind the factory walls.

Each year, 1.3 million persons are diagnosed with cancer, and an additional 9 million individuals are living as cancer survivors. Cancer survivors (here defined as anyone with cancer, from the time of diagnosis through death) face numerous psychosocial and spiritual challenges throughout the continuum of care (see Chapter 36, Cancer Survivorship). Receiving a diagnosis of cancer is an invitation to consider the possibility of one's own mortality, and it elicits a spiritual and existential crisis for many. Patients and their families are challenged to cope with an array of emotions that can, at times, seem overwhelming. Caregivers are instrumental in assisting those living with the impact of cancer. This chapter offers an overview of some of the more common psychosocial and spiritual concerns of the patient, the family caregiver, and the health care professional. Not surprisingly, there may be strong emotional responses to concerns such as limited access to cancer specialists and treatment options, denial of life and health insurance, financial instability (which continues long after the diagnosis and treatment), discrimination in the work place, psychological stressors, strain on personal relationships, and the profound fear of recurrence and death.

"Who would have thought that I would be celebrating my 48th birthday after being diagnosed with lung cancer 8 years ago? But I know that things are getting worse. I know because of the pain and because I can no longer use my hand to write or draw. I am told that I should have a port placed for better pain relief, but I'm afraid that means the beginning of the end, and although I will have to walk that road eventually, for now, I can make do with the medications given to me for the pain. I feel badly for Den, he tries so hard to give me everything I need, but we can't afford the new medications that you recommend—perhaps that's why the pain is still so severe . . . You want us to see the other team members, but every time I come to the hospital, it's extra miles on an old car and time away from the shop, which means even less money for basics, such as food and medication."

■ Impact of Cancer on the Patient

The diagnosis of cancer remains a "death sentence" in the minds of many, even though the 5-year survival rate for all cancers combined is greater than 60%. Fear of pain, disfigurement, loss of function, loss of control, and financial insecurity can be manifested by symptoms of depression, anxiety, hopelessness, fear and panic disorders. The incidence and the severity of these various negative sequelae have a considerable impact on the quality of a person's life. How the patient adapts to the rigors of treatment, the requisite follow-up appointments, and the impact of chronic illness depends on many factors, including his or her general coping strategies, problem-solving abilities, communication skills, resiliency, flexibility, hope, level of family support, ability to maintain a seminormal routine, and tolerance of ambiguity.

Unless the patient is asked specific questions regarding his or her economic status, emotional responses, coping strategies, social support network, and activities of daily living, the health care professional is not able to understand the true impact that cancer and its treatment is having on the patient and his or her family unit. The gathering of such information is vital to strengthening the patient's abilities and motivations to adhere to the prescribed cancer treatment. Early involvement of an integrated and interdisciplinary team consisting of physicians, nurses, clinical social workers, chaplains, psychologists, and rehabilitation professionals is the approach most likely to elicit, from the patient and family, the kinds of diverse biologic, psychosocial, and spiritual information that is so essential for developing a comprehensive plan of care. The nurse plays a vital role in the coordination of these efforts by continuously educating other members of the team on the sometimes day-to-day changes in the patient's condition and thereby maintaining optimal team involvement.

The symptoms of cancer, like cancer itself, evoke dramatic responses from those people whose life it affects. Pain is sometimes present at the time of diagnosis, is exacerbated by treatment, and increases with the progression of the disease. Because uncontrolled pain is associated with poor outcomes in most medical situations, especially cancer, the association of pain with apprehensions about death is not surprising. Pain, when persistent and increasing, only strengthens this association (see Chapter 23, Cancer Pain). Patients and families often attempt to deny the presence of pain because of its potentially ominous meanings. Only through vigorous educational efforts, focusing on the multiple meanings of pain can the barriers to adequate pain recognition and management be lowered. Education is therefore a vital component of pain and symptom management. Through education, the patient is empowered and is able to regain some sense of control in what may otherwise appear to be an uncontrollable situation. The patient who is empowered can communicate more effectively with his or her physician about such important issues as diagnosis, treatment options, and symptom management. This enhanced collaboration with the health care team increases the likelihood that the patient's needs will be recognized and met (see Unit V for additional information).

The "pain" reported by patients with cancer is not only physical but often psychological and spiritual. Psychological issues such as depression and anxiety must also be identified and treated (see Chapter 27, Anxiety and Depression in the Oncology Setting) Anxiety is common in patients with cancer, is associated with a decrease in quality of life, and may be manifested by insomnia, sexual dysfunction and decreased sexual desire. Untreated depression or anxiety may result in patients' inappropriately using prescribed analgesics in an attempt to relieve psychological distress.

The emotional reactions of the patient and family (e.g., anxiety, fear, depression) to the cancer at its different stages are qualitatively similar. In the terminal phase of the patient's illness, the caregiver's emotional reactions to stress and the impending loss of a loved one may even be more extreme than those of the patient. Some factors that affect caregiver adjustment to increasing emotional demands are (a) the patient's stage of illness and prognosis, (b) the magnitude of physical and emotional caregiving demands, (c) the patient's duration of illness, (d) the site or sites of cancer involvement, (e) the intensity and side effects of ongoing cancer treatment, (f) the patient's own coping mechanisms and levels of stress, and (g) the quality of the caregiver's and patient's pre-morbid relationships.

Caregivers have numerous concerns about their loved one's pain, including the potential for pain to worsen over time. Pain can be so dramatic and distressing that caregivers question their ability to care for this symptom in the home setting. Family members' concerns about poor pain relief are often counterbalanced by concerns about the possibility of drug addiction, respiratory depression, or drug tolerance to opiate analgesics. They may therefore undermedicate the patient, even as they worry about poor pain relief. It is vital that the health care team address these myths and misconceptions if good symptom management is to be achieved.

Symptom management becomes increasingly complex with the use of multiple medications, and complex dosing schedules. The variety of drug delivery systems may include oral, transdermal, transmucosal, intraintestinal (via gastrostomy or other feeding tube), subcutaneous, or intraspinal routes of delivery and the technology to support some of these methods. Family members who manage pain for the person with cancer need to routinely assess the pain, decide on the amount and type of medication to be administered, and sometimes determine how often medication is taken. Finally, family members must contend with the fact that worsening pain often does represent a worsening of the tumor, and they must avoid falling into the trap of attempting to deny the severity of the pain as a means of attempting to deny disease progression. Given the complexities facing family caregivers, the importance of providing adequate education and support cannot be overemphasized.

Fear of cancer recurrence is present for many patients, even for years after apparently successful cancer treatment. Despite long-term survival, severe anxiety may be manifested before routine diagnostic scans or with the appearance of even benign symptoms, such as a cough or cold. Talking with a mental health professional about these fears allows the individual to gain useful strategies in managing stress or anxiety during these follow-up evaluations.

The recurrence of cancer often heralds the transition of the patient from one who is on a curative treatment track to someone whose primary goal is maintaining some quality of life and symptom management (see Chapter 37, End of Life). At these times, efforts to provide effective palliative care need to take at least as much precedence as those directed at tumor control. This transition marks not only the beginning of more intensive physical and psychosocial symptom management, but often, an ending of the life the person once knew. Making the transition from someone who has cancer to one who is "dying from cancer" may once again require a team approach. The team's goals are to identify and help resolve, if possible, any conflicts that may be present within the family structure and to help all concerned in coming to an acceptance of that which cannot be changed.

Survivorship is defined as beginning at time of cancer diagnosis and ending with death. Throughout this trajectory, patients often experience what is described as a "roller coaster" of emotions (see Chapter 36, Cancer Survivorship). Davies (2001) described the transition away from hopes of cure to "fading away" as characterized by seven dimensions (Table 35–1). One of the many jobs of the nurse is to assist the patient in finding meaning in both the highs and the lows. This allows the patient to better respond to the situation at hand, and in those with clearly advanced disease, to better prepare for the final stages of life.

TABLE 35–1 ■ Dimensions of the Transition Away from Hopes of Cure

1. *Redefining,* making the switch from "that was then, this is now."
2. *Burdening,* concern by the patient of putting additional stress and work on the caregiver.
3. *Struggling* with paradox, the paradox is that although the patient is living, he or she is dying and although hopeful for a cure, knows that he or she will not be.
4. *Contending* with change, all aspects of a patient's daily life changes.
5. *Searching* for meaning, a journey inward to seek greater understanding.
6. *Living* day to day, "carpe diem."
7. *Preparing* for death, concrete actions that would have benefit in the future.

Source: Adapted from Davies, B. (2001). Supporting families in palliative care. In B. Rolling Ferrell, & N. Coyle, (Ed.), *Textbook of palliative nursing* (pp. 363–373). New York: Oxford University Press.

Impact of Cancer on the Family Caregiver

He has had his own serious health problems. Today, as he accompanies her to the clinic, it appears that he is the one who is in need of care. "The pain has been awful. We have been awake all night. The only thing I can do for her now is to make certain she has the medications she needs."

The impact of the cancer diagnosis resonates within not only the patient but also the entire family. Caregivers reflect the stressful events in the home. One has only to look at the family caregiver at times to determine how well things are being managed at home. Although the caregiver does not experience the physical symptoms of the patient, the suffering the caregiver experiences is based on several other factors, such as prior pain experiences, cultural milieu, relationship to the patient, and the meaning the caregiver ascribes to the patient's symptoms. The impact of the patient's symptoms on the caregiver and the latter's interpretation of these symptoms can be manifested by the caregiver's own struggles with anger, anxiety, depression, and existential suffering. The caregiver burden refers not only to the physical demands placed on caregivers but also to emotional burdens. The cancer experience is therefore a shared experience, the emotional and physical demands being somewhat different for patient and the caregiver, but distressing all the same.

The home may be the setting for cancer care, even if the caregiver is physically, emotionally, or financially challenged to do so. Family caregiving requires adjustments in daily schedules, imposes financial burdens, and causes the individual members to re-evaluate their relationships. With advances in cancer treatment, extended survival times have led to caregiving demands that may continue for years. These changes can profoundly affect roles and relationships, ranging from financial responsibilities to matters of intimacy.

Family members adjust to a loved one's chronic illness with highly individualized coping styles. Examples include a tendency to minimize the seriousness of the situation through inappropriate humor, obstruction of information received, intellectualization with a de-emphasis of emotions, or repeated questioning. With each member having their own style, conflicts may develop. These conflicts may interfere with care and may increase the level of distress for all concerned. Some families avoid such conflicts by formally, or more commonly, informally, designating members to specific roles, such as information gatherer, emotional "rock," and logistical expert.

If the family is resilient, an adaptation to the patient's various treatment-related role changes, physical alterations, and emotional changes occurs. Over time, a semistable transition may be made from the precancer family state to a new family identity.

All of this may be dealt a severe shock when the cancer progresses or recurs. A return to family disruption and helplessness may result. Communication between the health care team and patients may become increasingly guarded as they realize that their cancer may not be controlled by medical intervention. Depression, denial, and withdrawal from family may result as patients face their own imminent mortality. During this phase, the family experiences uncertainty about the future, as well as anticipatory grief, fear, and anger, as they come to terms with the unpredictability of the disease and the increasingly limited treatment options. Spiritual and existential concerns may take on increased importance.

The terminal phase is marked by an increasing loss of independence and an increasing dependence on the family. The patient's withdrawal from family that began in the relapse phase may continue, causing the family to feel rejected and unable to comfort the patient. The family's concerns may now be focused on the management of side effects, the patient's decreased mobility, issues relating to impending death, and the increasing emotional demands on family members (see Chapter 37, End of Life).

Family caregivers have important needs that change throughout the trajectory of a patient's illness. Seeking information about the disease and treatment options is replaced, as the cancer progresses, by the need to learn about the management of side effects and the need to master caregiving skills demanded by the increasing technology of medical care. These skills range from the maintenance of central catheter lines and ambulatory infusion pumps to wound care. Caregivers must begin to develop coping strategies for fatigue and depression, the patient's and their own, and to look more actively for support from outside of the family to help contend with the spiritual, financial, and emotional demands placed by advancing illness.

■ Impact on Health Professionals

How can a person have so much pain despite the enormous amounts of medications that she is receiving? The disease has spread like wildfire, and all we can do now is listen to the patient's final request to make her comfortable. Funeral plans have been discussed. She is at peace and ready to make the transition. He knows she will be going to a "better place," and yet they have not been apart for even a day in the past 28 years.

Assisting in the care of a person coping with cancer invites the nurse to explore his or her own feelings and attitudes regarding the ultimate meaning of life. Working with those with a life-threatening disease offers ample opportunity to consider the possibility of one's own future demise. Compassion-related fatigue and burnout are common responses to the stress of working with these vulnerable populations. These responses are more often manifested by those who are emotionally and spiritually unprepared to deal with the fact that corporeal life is finite and death a natural consequence of living. In preparation for this work, it is essential to consider one's own attitude toward cancer, spirituality, and death and dying. Attendance at bereavement debriefings and participation in patient memorials are important means through which the health care team members can process the grief that attends loss. Vicarious opportunities for learning, for both the family and the health professional abound. A great deal of satisfaction can be gained from recognizing that acts of kindness and concern are tremendously meaningful for those who are most needy and fragile. These factors also contribute to professional job satisfaction.

We are therefore wise to consider our own coping styles so that we might be aware of our own tendencies to cope in a less than healthy manner. Health care professionals are at increased risk for substance abuse, binge eating, and relationship discord. These tendencies are likelier to occur when the professional feels stressed from exposure to situations where one is less confident in one's competence. Unfortunately, working with persons with life-threatening disease is an area in which many health care professionals feel ill prepared to address. Our professional education has not adequately prepared us for long-term exposure to those who are actively suffering and for whom the only treatments are those aimed at palliating the suffering. Staff members report that colleague support is most valuable to help one cope after the death of a patient. Suitable mentorship in this area may require committed searching. The importance of sharing the joys and sorrows of this work is another reason that professionals are encouraged to develop a team approach to oncology practice. Interdisciplinary palliative care teams are important in alleviating the stress that could quickly become too burdensome to the health professional if it is not shared.

Recognizing personal signs of compassion fatigue is a necessary first step if one is to maintain a healthy balance in this work. It is not unusual for the caring practitioner to experience emotional, spiritual, and physical reactions that mirror those experienced by the patient and family such as (depression, sleeplessness, and anxiety). It is vital that a sense of boundaries and balance is established and limitations are recognized. Nurses should seek information, education, and support to help build competence in providing specialized care. Finally, knowing what allows a nurse to feel refreshed is important in day-to-day stress management. Senior health care professionals often encourage new staff to consider developing their own "mission statements" to use as a professional compass during difficult times.

To further ease the stress associated with grief-work, it is useful to develop additional competence in this area. There are now numerous resources, books, conferences, and training opportunities available to offer professional education in end of life care. Another way to gain exposure and confidence in this work is by cofacilitating a cancer support group with a senior colleague. The benefits of hearing the day-to-day concerns of patients and families who are living and dying with this disease offer professional opportunities to develop assessment and empathy skills that have value in all areas of one's practice.

■ Social Implications

Cancer occurs in people who have their own unique life histories, with attendant failures and successes, and their own unique interpersonal relationships. There are also a variety of cultural, ethnic, and religious variables that need to be considered when one is working with those who are ill. In certain communities, a diagnosis of cancer is still associated with social stigma, isolation, and despair. Disparities in the provision of health care, related to such matters as fluctuations in levels of public support or the ever-changing polices of managed care, can also be exceedingly frustrating. The financial burdens of protracted treatment can be frightening, even for those with the top-of-the-line health insurance. Recent increases in the incidence and severity of violence in health care institutions underscore the need to be aware of the emotional toll that this can take. In order to provide optimal patient care, especially in patients with a disease as complex as cancer, health care professionals must assess and address a variety of psychosocial, cultural, and spiritual variables. This requires discipline, patience, and great sensitivity to the potential for social inequities.

■ Conclusion

A comprehensive assessment should be conducted with each patient that focuses on psychosocial stressors, financial concerns, and spiritual matters necessary in tailoring a treatment plan that is specific to the patient's and the family's needs. An understanding of family dynamics may help avert potentially damaging situations. An experienced nurse, social worker, psychologist, or physician will have several alternative supportive care plans in place before a crisis occurs. Additionally, by fostering communication between the patient, family, and team members, potential conflicts may be averted or minimized.

The patient and family must be helped to refocus their therapeutic goals as medical conditions change. Whether the cancer is progressing, regressing, or stable, a constant refocusing of hope is imperative. The hope for cure or the hope for control of symptoms must be equally valued. Clinicians, as potential patients or family members of patients themselves, know that hope is enduring, although constantly evolving, expansive, and resilient. Health care professionals assist patients to understand that they have the strength to achieve their goals if they call on their previous experience and acknowledge that flexibility, dedication, and compassion are shared attributes.

Those working with oncology patients and their families will at some point quite likely find that the skills that they have developed in the work place will have applicability within their own family or friendship network. We will eventually face the same fears of disability, dependence, deformity, and death encountered daily by our oncology patients. Being open to these vicarious learning opportunities will serve us well when we are the one facing the potential impact of a life-threatening illness. We all benefit from learning to live fully even in the ever-present shadow of death.

■ Acknowledgment

The authors wish to dedicate this chapter to Kat and Den in thankfulness for all that they have taught us.

Resources

Websites and Professional Organizations:

- Cancer Care
  www.cancercare.org
  breastcancer.org
  www.breastcancer.org
- ELNEC: End of Life Nursing Education Consortium: *www.aacn.nche.edu/elnec*
- EPEC: Education for Physicians on End of Life Care: *www.epec.net*
- City of Hope Pain/Palliative Care Resource Center: *www.cityofhope.org/prc/*
- WHO: World Health Organization: *www.who.int/en/*

Publications (available at no cost):

- American Cancer Society: 800-ACS-2345 or *www.cancer.org*
  Talking with your doctor or health care professional
  Listen with your heart
  Caring for the person with cancer at home: A guide after diagnosis
  Advanced cancer: Financial guidance for cancer survivors and their families
  A message of hope
- The National Cancer Institute: 800-4-CANCER or *www.cancer.gov*
  Taking time: Support for people with cancer and the people who care about them
  Facing forward: Life after cancer treatment

Bibliography

Davies, B. (2001). Supporting families in palliative care. In B. Rolling Ferrell, & N. Coyle, (Ed.), *Textbook of palliative nursing* (pp. 363–373). New York: Oxford University Press.

Rolling Ferrell, B. & Coyle, N. (Ed.), 2001 *Textbook of palliative nursing.* New York: Oxford University Press.

Fitchett, G. & Handzo, G. (1998). Spiritual assessment, screening, and intervention. In J. Holland, (Ed.), *Psycho-oncology* (pp. 790–808). New York: Oxford University Press.

Given, B. A., Given, C. W., Kozachik, S. (2001). Family support in advanced cancer. *CA: A Cancer Journal for Clinicians, 51,* 213–231.

CHAPTER

36

Cancer Survivorship

Karen Hassey Dow

Major changes in cancer treatment over the past several decades have resulted in increased survival. At the same time, we are at a unique juncture in our scientific knowledge of late effects among childhood, adolescent, and adult cancer survivors. The aims of this chapter are to:

- Describe cancer survival statistics
- Discuss selected major late effects among childhood and adult survivors
- Discuss survivors' concerns about health promotion and cancer surveillance
- Discuss the nurse's role in supporting and providing resources to cancer survivors

Cancer Survival Statistics

The American Cancer Society estimates that there are almost 9 million cancer survivors in the United States, representing 3.3% of our population. Cancer survivors are living longer now than ever before. About 60% of adults and 77% of children are living 5 years or more after diagnosis. Figure 36–1 shows that 14% of all cancer survivors were diagnosed more than 20 years ago.

The largest groups of survivors were diagnosed with breast, prostate, and colorectal cancers. The improvement in cancer survival rates and the decline in the cancer death rate are related to many

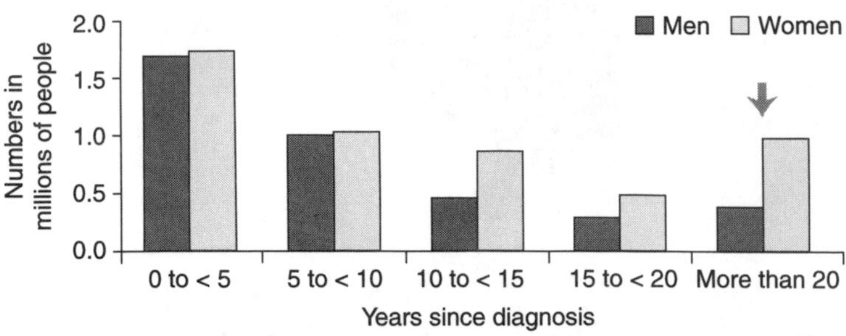

FIGURE 36–1 ■ Comparison of Survival by Gender
Data from: ACS 2003 Statistics Rowland et al., 2001, Simmonds, 2003

factors, including changes in our fundamental understanding about genetics, the translation of basic science results to clinical practice, the decrease in dose-limiting treatment toxicities, the increase in screening and early detection activities, the improvement in rehabilitation and support interventions, and the awareness of the effect of sociocultural factors on survival.

Two important population trends, aging and diversification, are expected to contribute to an increase in cancer burden. Cancer in the elderly is expected to increase because of the aging population. About 60% of cancer survivors are aged 65 or older. The current median age at time of diagnosis is 68 and 67 years, respectively, for male and female cancer survivors. An increasingly diverse population is expected, with Hispanics predicted to make up 25% of the population, and African Americans, Asian Americans, and Native Americans are projected to make up an additional 25% of the population by 2050.

■ Late Effects Affecting Cancer Survivors

Childhood and adult cancer survivors are at risk for late effects (e.g., earlier death, secondary cancers, cognitive dysfunction, cardiac dysfunction, reproductive changes, and psychosocial late effects) of cancer and of cancer treatment. The major late effects are briefly described in the following discussion, and the reader is referred to the references at the end of the chapter for more in-depth discussions of each topic.

Early Death After Treatment

Although childhood and adolescent cancer survivors have excellent prospects for long-term survival and cure, they also face the potential

TABLE 36–1 ■ Secondary Cancers Occurring after Treatment for Hodgkin's Disease

Type of Cancer	Related Implicating Factor
Leukemia	Chemotherapy
Non-Hodgkin's lymphoma	Chemotherapy
Lung cancer	Radiation therapy and smoking after treatment
Breast cancer	Mantle radiation therapy occurring before age 20
Thyroid cancer	Radiation therapy
Sarcomas of the bone and soft tissue	Chemotherapy and radiation therapy combined

for long-term health risks and late effects from cancer treatment. Data from two studies of childhood cancer survivors in the United States and Scandinavia revealed that death among childhood cancer survivors was 10.8 times higher than that of the general population. Causes of death were related to disease recurrence, cardiac toxicity, and pulmonary toxicity.

Second Cancers

Adolescent survivors of Hodgkin's disease are 6.4 times likelier to die earlier than adolescents in the general population as a result of their cancer. Table 36–1 shows the major types of secondary cancers for which adolescent cancer survivors are at increased risk. Hodgkin's disease survivors have a higher risk of lung cancer when they smoke tobacco after treatment ends. In addition, female Hodgkin's disease survivors who underwent mantle radiation therapy (that included their breasts in the treatment field) before the age of 20 have an increased risk of breast cancer.

Cognitive Dysfunction

Cognitive dysfunction has occurred in pediatric, adolescent, and adult cancer survivors (see Chapter 29, Cognitive Impairment). The following discussion focuses on cognitive dysfunction seen in cancer survivors *after* treatment ends. The major factor that increases the risk of cognitive dysfunction is younger age at the time of radiation therapy. It is thought that the developing brain tissue in young children (usually under the age of 2 years) is most susceptible to the effects of radiation. Over time, the pattern of cognitive functioning declines, with pediatric survivors having slower ability to learn new knowledge and develop skills compared with that of healthy peers of the same age. Some childhood cancer survivors may need remedial education and tutoring to help them better learn and retain information.

Cognitive dysfunction has also been seen in adult survivors of breast cancer, lung cancer, lymphoma, and melanoma. The major factors that increase the risk of cognitive dysfunction in the adult is high-dose chemotherapy and duration of chemotherapy. Adult survivors may complain of forgetting easily or having difficulty concentrating on tasks. They may complain of tiring easily, particularly during stressful, mentally focused, tasks. It is helpful to teach them that cognitive changes may occur, and that we are learning more about how to manage these changes. Other helpful suggestions are to divide the mental tasks into segments that can be accomplished with less stress, keep a list or calendar of tasks that need to be accomplished in specific time periods, prioritize tasks that require more comprehension earlier in the day, and make time for restful periods throughout the day.

Cardiac Toxicity

Cardiac toxicity is a late effect that can occur in childhood and adolescent cancer survivors. Factors that increase cardiac risk are anthracycline-based chemotherapy and mediastinal radiation therapy. As a result, these survivors may have marginal cardiac reserve that leads to earlier-onset congestive heart failure. Cardiac toxicity is also a late effect in adults. Factors that increase cardiac risk in adults are anthracycline-based chemotherapy, trastuzumab, and high-dose chemotherapy.

Childhood and adolescent survivors may not express symptoms until they engage in strenuous physical exercise or have conditions, such as pregnancy, that require additional cardiac output. Symptoms include shortness of breath, dyspnea with minimal exertion, and arrhythmias. Survivors are referred for additional cardiac testing and imaging studies (e.g., echocardiogram or multiple-gated acquisition scans) to evaluate the extent of the cardiac dysfunction. Other modalities, such as nuclear medicine scintigraphy and endomyocardial biopsy, may also be needed. However, routine use of imaging studies to monitor asymptomatic survivors is not generally the standard of care.

Reproductive Late Effects

Factors affecting reproductive late effects after treatment are personal, treatment, and timing. Personal factors include the age at which treatment is started. Prepubescent children have more protection against the deleterious effects of chemotherapy compared with older patients (> 35 years). Treatment factors include the type and the extent of chemotherapy, such as alkylating agents, antimetabolites, anthracyclines, and procarbazine, as well as the use of abdominal radiation. Timing of fertility-sparing procedures is critical before cancer therapy is started.

Advances in assistive reproductive technologies are enabling cancer survivors to maintain fertility and have children after treatment. Examples of newer assistive reproductive technologies are embryo cryopreservation and in vitro fertilization. Embryo cryopreservation must be accomplished before treatment.

Cancer survivors often question whether their cancer history may affect their offspring. They may worry that their children may have a higher risk of developing cancer, or that their pregnancy may start a recurrence of their disease. Research findings show no evidence that children born to cancer survivors have a higher incidence of birth defects than the general population. There is evidence, however, that women who received abdominal radiation therapy have a higher risk of having low-birth-weight infants. Unless there is a known inherited susceptibility, children born to cancer survivors are not at higher risk of developing cancer themselves. Moreover, studies do not show that subsequent pregnancy increases the risk of disease recurrence or death. (The reader is referred to Chapter 33 [Sexuality] for a discussion of symptom management for sexuality, fertility, and self-image issues during treatment).

■ Quality of Life

Quality of life issues that are major concerns of long-term cancer survivors include health-promoting activities, such as weight management and smoking cessation; employment and economic issues; and disease surveillance. The reader is referred to Chapter 35 (Psychosocial-Spiritual Responses to Cancer and Treatment: Living with Cancer) for psychosocial issues relating to recurrence and advanced disease.

Health-Promoting Behaviors

Long-term disease-free cancer survivors often express a strong interest in developing and maintaining health-promoting behaviors, such as weight management through physical activity and healthy nutritional choices. They may be highly motivated to participate in smoking cessation programs. Thus, cancer survivors are a highly motivated group that are receptive to health education and prevention activities.

Women with breast cancer who have been treated with chemotherapy often have a weight increase of about 10%–20% during treatment. The weight gained is very difficult to lose after treatment ends. Weight gain became an important concern when a study showed that premenopausal women who gained weight were 1.5 times more likely to experience recurrence and to die of their disease compared with women who gained less weight. Subsequent studies continue to examine the correlation of weight gain and risk of recurrence. Cancer survivors express interest in learning ways to manage weight gain through physical activity and nutrition.

Regarding this issue, the American Cancer Society recently released nutrition and physical activity recommendations for cancer survivors. Although the nutrition and physical activity guidelines established by the society for the prevention of cancer are likely to be beneficial to survivors, the new report has recommendations specifically for cancer survivors. They include the following:

- Physical activity may help even people with advanced cancer by increasing appetite and reducing constipation and fatigue.
- Being overweight can increase the risk of cancer recurrence and may even affect overall survival.
- A standard multivitamin and mineral supplement in amounts equivalent to 100% of the daily value can help survivors meet nutrient needs when it is difficult to eat a healthy diet. Some supplements, like those containing high levels of folic acid or antioxidants, may be harmful during cancer treatment.
- A vegetarian diet has many health-promoting features, but there is no direct evidence that it can prevent cancer recurrence, and survivors who eat a vegetarian diet should take particular care to ensure adequate nutrient intake.
- Alcohol can have positive and negative effects, increasing the risk of new cancers in survivors while reducing the risk of heart disease, so health care providers need to individually tailor advice to cancer survivors.

In general, studies support the combined use of good nutrition and exercise and resistance training. A diet rich in vegetables, fruit, whole grains, and low-fat dairy products combined with exercise to preserve or increase lean muscle mass may help lower disease risk.

Smoking Cessation

Smoking prevention or cessation to reduce tobacco-related cardiac and pulmonary disease is another important area of health promotion for cancer survivors. Unfortunately, many young cancer survivors are not taught the adverse health effects of smoking and the increased risks to themselves of smoking after cancer treatment. Smoking behaviors are related to age at cancer diagnosis and the perception that they are vulnerable to smoking-related illnesses.

Strategies to help patients with cancer quit smoking include assessing smoking status and the survivors' readiness to quit; providing brief, supportive messages consistently over time; offering or referring patients to appropriate resources; and providing continued follow-up. In addition, the Agency for Health Care Policy and Research and the American Cancer Society Smoking Cessation Guidelines (see Chapter 14, Lung Cancer) can be used effectively with cancer survivors.

Return-to-Work Issues

Cancer survivors often return to work and lead full, productive lives after treatment. In most instances, cancer survivors want to return to work because it is an important part of their lives. In some instances, cancer survivors may have long-term disability or dysfunction requiring changes in either employment status or type of employment. Other cancer survivors, with recurrent or advanced disease, may undergo significant changes in their employment situation. Employers may have the mistaken notion that cancer survivors are not able to perform their job responsibilities or may consider survivors a poor risk for promotion. Cancer survivors may need to ask for assistance with work place issues.

The Americans with Disabilities Act (ADA), enacted by Congress in 1990, protects individuals with disabilities, including cancer survivors, from work place discrimination. Organizations having at least 15 employees must comply with ADA guidelines. Table 36–2 lists the questions that individuals must answer to receive protection under ADA.

Most often, cancer survivors return to work with very little job adjustment needed. Flexibility in hours, particularly for follow-up care, may be needed. Cancer survivors must disclose their diagnosis to their employer in order to be protected by the ADA.

TABLE 36–2 ■ Questions Requiring Answers to Receive Protection Under the Americans with Disabilities Act (ADA)

- Are you a disabled person under the ADA?
- Are you qualified for the job?
- Can you perform the essential functions of the job?
- Has your employer provided you with a reasonable accommodation?
- Will your accommodation cause "undue hardship" to the employer?
- Do you create a direct threat to your own or others' health or safety?

The ADA provides protection for cancer survivors when they apply for a job. The ADA prohibits a potential employer from asking questions about an individual's health history or current health status during an interview. Moreover, cancer survivors are not required to disclose a cancer history. However, when a cancer survivor is hired and must undergo a physical examination, it is prudent to disclose one's cancer history.

The Equal Employment Opportunity Commission is the federal agency that investigates discrimination in the workplace. The commission investigates allegations against an employer about perceived discrimination and inappropriate behavior and policies.

■ Cancer Surveillance for Survivors

Currently, no evidence-based guidelines for cancer screening or surveillance of survivors exist. It is known that cancer survivors require lifetime surveillance, but the timing of surveillance and the specific provider (e.g., oncology versus primary care practitioner) are not well defined. We do know some things:

- Childhood and adolescent cancer survivors will need lifelong surveillance.
- Young female survivors of Hodgkin's disease who received mantle radiation therapy are at higher risk of developing breast cancer. Thus, Hodgkin's disease survivors may require initiation of screening at an earlier age than the standard recommendation.
- Despite limited guidance for cancer surveillance in survivors, Table 36–3 lists several suggestions to provide survivors and their families.

■ Conclusion

The growing number of cancer survivors presents tremendous opportunity for clinical practice, education, and research. Cancer survivors are living longer, but long-term survival is tempered by the prospect of late effects. At the same time, cancer survivors are eager to learn ways to improve their health through physical activity and nutrition and to monitor their progress through cancer surveillance.

TABLE 36–3 ■ Suggestions for Cancer Surveillance

- Keep a personal copy of your cancer treatment history.
- Become knowledgeable about the different types of surveillance procedures and their purpose (e.g., timing of follow ups, type of blood studies, tumor markers, x-ray studies, scans, and other tests required).
- Surveillance may occur more frequently within the first 2 years after treatment and then is gradually increased to once a year or less often several years later.
- Maintain regular contact with your oncology team.
- Become familiar with the reimbursement for your particular surveillance procedures.
- Keep track of out of your out-of-pocket expenses.
- Use advocacy resources available on the Internet and through your local organizations.
- Keep current date on cancer treatments and clinical trials relating to your cancer.
- Maintain contact with other individuals who have similar cancer.

■ Resources

Publications

- The article "Nutrition and Physical Activity During and After Cancer Treatment" is available online at *CAonline.AmCancerSoc.org*
- The National Coalition for Cancer Survivorship (NCCS) offers "The Cancer Survival Toolbox," which consists of audiocassettes providing basic guidelines in helping navigate through survivorship and Essential Care Resource Guide. The toolkit and the guide are available free of charge through the NCCS website at *www.canceradvocacy.org*
- NCI publication "Facing Forward: Life after Cancer Treatment" is available at *www.cancer.gov/cancerinfo/life-after-treatment*

Professional Organizations and Websites

- American Cancer Society: 800-ACS-2345 or *www.cancer.org*
- The American Cancer Society's Cancer Survivors Network at *www.cancer.org* or *www.acscsn.org/* provides an opportunity for online survivor discussions and includes a resource library.

- The American Cancer Society program, "Taking Charge of Money Matters," uses a workshop format to address money issues that arise during or after cancer treatment. Taking Charge of Money Matters is an optional course of the *I Can Cope* educational program. Call 800-ACS-2345 for communities where the program is offered.
- Childhood Cancer Survivors: *www.patientcenters.com/survivors/*
- Equal Employment Opportunity Commission: *www.eeoc.gov*
- Lance Armstrong Foundation: *http://www.laf.org/*
- National Cancer Institute Office of Cancer Survivorship: *dccps.nci.nih.gov/ocs/follow.html*
- National Coalition for Cancer Survivorship: 800-828-7866 or *www.canceradvocacy.org*

Bibliography

Brown, J., Byers, T., et al. (2003). Nutrition and physical activity during and after cancer treatment: An American Cancer Society guide for informed choices. *CA: A Cancer Journal for Clinicians, 53,* 268–291.

Ferrell, B. R., & Dow, K. H. (1997). Quality of life among long-term cancer survivors. *Oncology, 11, 565–576.*

Gotay, C. C., & Muraoka, M. Y. (1998). Quality of life in long-term survivors of adult-onset cancers. *Journal of the National Cancer Institute, 90, 656–667.*

Harpham, W. (1998). Long-term survivorship: Late effects. In A. Berger, R. Portenoy, D. Weissman. (Eds.), *Principles and practice of supportive oncology* (pp. 889–297). Philadelphia: Lippincott-Williams & Wilkins.

Messner, C., & Patterson, D. (2001). The challenge of cancer in the workplace. *Cancer Practice, 9,* 50–51.

Varricchio, C. (Ed.). (2001). Cancer survivorship (entire issue). *Seminars in Oncology Nursing, 17*(4), 234–287.

CHAPTER

37

End of Life

Ann O'Mara

Between 1973 and 1999, cancer deaths for all cancer types and races declined by 1.5% in males and 0.6% per year in females. Despite these modest gains, more than 500,000 Americans will die of cancer, and many will experience multiple physical and psychosocial problems that can be severe. Table 37–1 lists the symptoms that terminally ill cancer patients might experience in the last few weeks or days of their lives. Figure 37–1 shows the prevalence of six of the most commonly experienced symptoms in this population. Because most cancer deaths occur in patients older than 60 years, the patients' symptoms are often worsened by other concomitant chronic illness. In addition to the physical and emotional problems faced by the terminally ill patient, family members experience numerous physical, emotional, and economic problems as they face the eventual loss of their loved one. These problems can extend into the bereavement period and can be further exacerbated if the family members are not receiving adequate support, particularly if the patient is dying at home.

In many respects, nursing care of the terminally ill cancer patient is no different than care provided to patients succumbing to other chronic diseases. Ensuring adequate relief of the patient's physical and psychosocial symptoms, helping families and loved ones cope with the impending loss of their family member, and maintaining the dignity of the patient and the family are essential activities of high-quality end-of-life care and cannot be accomplished by nurses alone. Experts in the fields of social work, nutrition, spiritual ministry, pain management, psychiatry, and psychology are indispensable to the care of the terminally ill. Table 37–2 lists recommendations for actions aimed at ensuring high-quality end-of-life

TABLE 37–1 ■ Physical and Psychosocial Symptoms in the Terminally Ill Cancer Patient

- Pain
- Fatigue
- Constipation
- Dyspnea
- Nausea & Vomiting
- Sleep problems
- Depression
- Anxiety
- Confusion
- Restlessness
- Anorexia/Cachexia

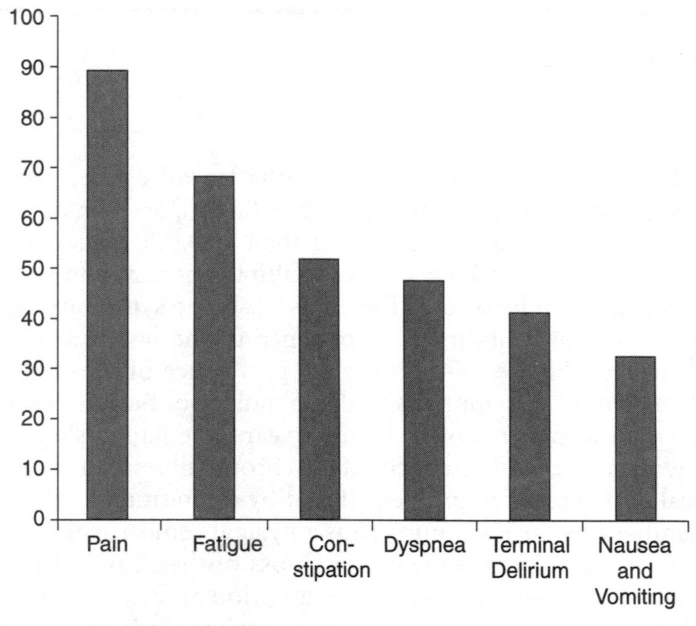

FIGURE 37–1 ■ Prevalence of Physical Symptoms in Advanced Cancer

care. These recommendations have been endorsed by more than 30 professional, scientific, and advocacy organizations.

Using these recommendations as a framework, this chapter describes the management of the more common advanced cancer symptoms that terminally ill cancer patients experience related to pain, fatigue, gastrointestinal problems, respiratory problems, and cognitive failure. Special attention is given to feeding and hydrating terminally ill patients. In addition, the unique challenges that family members face during this period are highlighted, with particular emphasis on nurse-

TABLE 37-2 ■ Recommendations to Ensure High Quality End-of-Life Care

- Alleviate physical and emotional symptoms
- Support the function and autonomy to help the patient maintain his dignity
- Guard against inappropriate aggressive care
- Make time spent at the end of life precious—not merely tolerable—to the patient and family
- Ensure that quality of the patient's life is good despite declining physical health
- Work to minimize the financial burdens that care places on the family
- Educate patients in the length of time insurance companies cover treatment of a terminal illness
- Help the family with bereavement

Adapted from Virani & Sofer, 2003

patient communication principles. Finally, an overview of the importance of hospice in coordinating services and providing support, particularly during the bereavement phase, for family members is included.

■ Physical Symptoms

The management of symptoms at the end of life requires a multidisciplinary approach, using multiple treatment modalities. Often, symptoms experienced during earlier stages of the disease re-emerge at this time, sometimes more severely. Patients, with the support of their families, may opt to participate in cancer treatment clinical trials that can contribute to the symptom experience. Pharmacologic agents are often the treatment of choice for many of the physical symptoms. There is an array of psychosocial and educational interventions that are an integral component to symptom management. Tables 37–3 and 37–4 highlight the commonly recommended pharmacologic and nonpharmacologic interventions for pain, fatigue, constipation, dyspnea, cognitive failure, and nausea and vomiting. The reader is also referred to Unit V: Symptom Management for in-depth discussions of the management of selected symptoms encountered at the end of life.

Pain

Pain, the most frequent symptom at the end of life, has been estimated to occur in more than 80% of terminally ill cancer patients. Pain continues

TABLE 37–3 ■ Pharmacological Agents for Treating Symptoms

Symptom	Pharmacological Agents
Pain	• See WHO Ladder or NCCN guidelines; • NSAIDS & Corticosteroids for bone pain; • Bisphosphonates for metastatic breast and prostate bone pain; • Tricyclic antidepressants, anticonvulsants, local anesthesia for neuropathic pain
Fatigue	• Amphetamines, dexamethesone
Constipation	• Dosing related to opiod dosing; • Senna concentrate and docusate sodium - dosing based on severity of constipation; • Lactulose; • Milk of Magnesia;
Dyspnea	• Morphine – oral, parental, nebulized • Benzodiazepines • Phenothiazines • Cannabinoids
Cognitive Failure (Somnolence, delirium, agitation)	• Haloperidol • Cogentin • Chlorpromazine • If no evidence of pain, discontinue opiods as they may cause restlessness, diaphoresis, and hallucinations
Nausea & Vomiting	• Anticholinergics • Antihistimines • Benzodiazepines • Butyrophenones • Cannabinoids • Corticosteroids • Phenothiazines • 5-H_3 receptor antagonists

to be undertreated. In the patient with advanced cancer, the pain experience may involve somatic, visceral, and neuropathic components. Thus, its management can involve titrating numerous different types of opioid and nonopioid medications to achieve the best results. For example, a patient may be experiencing pain both from bony metastasis and from neurologic involvement. Therefore, treatment would include opioids for the bone pain and anticonvulsant agents for the neuropathic component.

TABLE 37–4 ■ Non-Pharmacological Agents for Treating Symptoms

Symptom	Interventions
Pain	• Teach advantages to around the clock treatment; • Dispell myths of addiction; • Teach and encourage reporting of side effects • Use heat, cold, massage, relaxation, distraction; • Assess for non-adherence
Fatigue	• Obtain equipment to maintain mobility, e.g., walker, wheelchair • Involve occupational and physical therapy to plan efficient, non-fatiguing ADLs
Constipation	• Institute laxative therapies in conjunction with opiods; • Encourage high-fiber diet or bulk laxative containing bran, methylcellulose, psyllium;
Dyspnea	• Teach pursed lip breathing; • Use fan or open window for facial cooling; • Institute frequent mouth care; • Use humidified oxygen • Obtain home humidifiers if oxygen unavailable; • Elevate head of bed
Cognitive Failure (somnolence, delirium, agitation)	• Provide comfortable, familiar surroundings; • Encourage family to touch and hold patient; • Play music if it provides an additional soothing effect
Nausea & Vomiting	• Encourage small, frequent meals at room temperature; • Discourage frying of foods; • Remove unpleasant room odors • Teach progressive muscle relaxation, hypnosis, and systematic desensitization

The first step to ensuring good pain management is to conduct a thorough and consistent assessment (see Chapter 23, Cancer Pain). The terminally ill patient poses several challenges to conducting a thorough assessment. Metastatic disease may have an effect on cognitive functioning, and as a result, the patient's verbal responses may not accurately reflect his or her pain experience. The nurse has to rely on nonverbal cues, such as increased restlessness, moaning, diaphoresis, increased respiratory, and heart rates. The patient's family can be a valuable source of information about the patient's previous experiences with pain.

The nurse plays an important role in helping patients and their families adhere to the analgesic plan of care. Lack of adherence to the prescribed pain medications has been attributed to unrelieved or inadequately treated side effects, such as constipation, negative interactions with clinicians, and strongly held convictions that all medications should be avoided. Individualized information for both the patient and the family can correct these misunderstandings. As soon as patients begin opioid analgesic therapy, they must also be started on a bowel regimen that should include a laxative. Patients need to understand that a variety of opioids exists, and each has different side effects. It may be necessary to try different types before a satisfactory regimen has been achieved. In this terminal stage of the disease, it is important to address myths related to addiction. The nurse, patient, and family must acknowledge that addiction at the end of life is not an issue.

Fatigue

Almost as prevalent as pain, fatigue is often characterized by the terminally ill cancer patient as overwhelming. In addition to its effects on activities of daily living, unrelieved fatigue can have profound effects on the individual's psychological functioning, sleeping patterns, appetite, and pain level (see Chapter 25, Fatigue). The sedating side effects of analgesic opioids and certain cancer treatments, most notably interferon alfa, often contribute to the severity of the fatigue. In early-stage disease, exercise modestly improves fatigue; however, this intervention may not be appropriate for patients with advanced cancer. Instead, a thorough assessment of the patient's environment to identify ways of improving mobility and conserving energy should be the priority. For example, patients may benefit from a walker or wheelchair. Other nonpharmacologic approaches that may be beneficial include behavioral therapies to improve sleep and nutritional support. Several pharmacologic approaches, such as psychostimulants, corticosteroids, and selective antidepressants, are being tested in clinical trials.

Constipation

As stated earlier, the biggest risk factor for developing constipation is opioid use. Other risk factors include immobility; altered nutrition, including inadequate fluid intake; certain chemotherapeutic agents, such as vincristine; other medications, such as calcium channel blockers and iron; and bowel obstruction. Prevention and early reversal are essential to adequate management of constipation (see Chapter 24, Gastrointestinal Symptoms).

When opioid use is the major contributor to the problem, laxative therapy, usually senna, must be started concomitantly with opioid analgesic therapy. As the dosage of opioids increases, so must the dosage of laxatives. If fluid intake is diminished, stool softeners are also added to the regimen to reduce dry, hard stools. Other agents that have been effective are the liquid osmotic laxatives, such as sorbitol and lactulose. Because patients at the end of life are often debilitated and are experiencing decreased peristalsis due to the opioids, they are often unable to consume the large quantities of fluid required with bulk-forming laxatives. They can be at risk for developing intestinal obstruction or impaction.

Oral naloxone, a potent-receptor antagonist, may provide relief in severe opioid-induced constipation. It can reverse constipation without reversing analgesia; however, even in small amounts, it may be sufficient to produce withdrawal symptoms in some patients who have developed a physical dependence on the drug.

Dyspnea

Increasing tumor size from primary lung cancer and lung metastasis are the principal factors contributing to dyspnea in the terminally ill cancer patient (see Chapter 28, Respiratory/Dyspnea). These patients may have other comorbid problems, such as chronic obstructive pulmonary disease and congestive heart failure, which can further exacerbate the problem. Other symptoms, such as pain and fatigue may accompany dyspnea. It is important to distinguish between these overlapping symptoms. The sense of breathlessness can be extremely anxiety producing, and being left alone only worsens these symptoms. The severity of dyspnea seems to increase as patients approach death.

Rehabilitative measures, such as exercise training, that are recommended in early-stage disease are not of benefit to the terminally ill patient. The focus of care should be immediate relief of the feeling of suffocation and the anxiety that often accompanies it. Therapies in which the focus is treatment of the underlying disease without relieving the symptom or therapies that are burdensome should be discontinued. Oxygen, starting at 1 to 3 L/min, may be helpful and should be tried for a short period of time. Patients have found cool air directed against their faces also to be beneficial. Opioids are the mainstay of management of dyspnea and related anxiety. They are often augmented with corticosteroids and benzodiazepines. Opioids and benzodiazepines have been used in the nebulized form with mixed results.

Cognitive Failure

As the disease progresses and the patient approaches death, his or her behavior can range from increasing somnolence to extreme restlessness, agitation, and confusion. The restlessness phase is termed *terminal delirium* and can be an extremely stressful period for the patient's family and caregivers. In addition to disease progression, opioids, anticholinergics, corticosteroids, and antineoplastic drugs can initiate and exacerbate the problem. Adjustment in medication regimens may be the priority to decrease or reverse the delirium. The first step in managing the patient is to create a quiet, safe, and supportive environment. Once the primary cause has been determined, several medications, most notably haloperidol and chlorpromazine, have been found to be very effective in improving the delirium. Special attention must be directed to the family, who will most likely be very distressed by their loved one's behavior. Encouraging the family to speak softly and to touch and hold the patient is vital to the comprehensive care of the patient.

Nausea and Vomiting

Despite the advances in the development of effective agents for the management of chemotherapy-induced nausea and vomiting (see Chapter 24, Gastrointestinal Symptoms), nausea and vomiting in the terminally ill remains a significant problem because its mechanism and pathophysiology are different. Etiologic factors contributing to nausea and vomiting in this population include electrolyte disorders (e.g., hypercalcemia, hyponatremia, uremia), bowel obstruction, brain metastasis, visceral distention, altered taste sensation, and gastric stasis. Choosing the most effective antiemetic depends on the cause or causes of the nausea and vomiting. A combination of several medications may be needed. For example, if the patient is receiving a highly emetic chemotherapeutic agent and is also experiencing nausea and vomiting from brain metastasis, the drug regimen might include a serotonin (5-HT3) receptor, a histamine receptor blocker, and a corticosteroid.

An essential adjunct to the pharmacologic management of nausea and vomiting is the education of the patient and family about appropriate food selection and preparation, ways to create an environment where eating is a pleasant experience, and regular meticulous mouth care. An alcoholic beverage, such as wine, before a meal may help stimulate the appetite and reduce the sensation of nausea.

■ Nutrition in the Terminally Ill

'Tis not the meat, but 'tis the appetite

Makes eating a delight.
(Sir John Suckling, 1609–1642)

Providing food and nutrition to a terminally ill patient raises many questions and concerns for both the family and the health care team.

Eating and drinking are essential to life and are symbolic in all cultures, and when a dying person no longer expresses interest in these activities, our basic intuition is to intervene. Experts in the field of hospice and end-of-life care have provided excellent guidance in helping caregivers understand when and what types of interventions are appropriate. In general, the aim of nutritional support should be guided by the needs and the desires of the terminally ill patient and family caregivers. Ongoing teaching and reinforcing of information about the dying process are essential first steps in implementing the nutritional plan of care.

The dying process appears to set in motion a cascade of physiologic events whereby the patient becomes less interested in, and reliant on, food and hydration. Early satiety is frequently seen in conjunction with anorexia (see Chapter 30, Anorexia and Weight Loss). It is important to differentiate between anorexia related to some underlying remedial cause and anorexia related to dying. When the underlying cause or causes, such as nausea and vomiting, constipation, depression, and pain are corrected, the patient's interest in eating and drinking often returns. In addition, administering certain pharmacologic agents, such as corticosteroids, dronabinol, and metoclopramide, and implementing artificial hydration and nutrition may improve appetite, increase weight gain, and palliate symptoms overall. When no underlying causes can be found, there is some evidence that artificial nutrition and hydration may actually increase patient suffering by increasing fluid in the circulatory, and respiratory systems. This, in turn, can lead to increased dyspnea, nausea and vomiting, and incontinence.

Helping family members understand why their loved one is no longer interested in eating and drinking and how anorexia and weight loss will progress until death is critical to the comprehensive care of the terminally ill. Observations in the hospice setting have shown that the development of anorexia is a gradual process, not a sudden event. Thus, family members need to be taught the subtle signs of decreasing food intake and how to adjust their roles in providing nutrition to the patient. Although patients may experience increasing anorexia and early satiety, their desire to relieve thirst may persist. Offering small sips of drinks and ice chips is often sufficient and can give family caregivers enormous satisfaction. Some patients may actually benefit from a trial of time-limited intravenous fluids if there are no contraindications.

■ The Role of Hospice

Meeting the multiple physical and emotional needs of a terminally ill patient can be both challenging and rewarding. When patients and their family members decide that dying at home is a realistic option, hospice personnel can play an important role in helping the family

TABLE 37–5 ■ Principles of Hospice Care

1. Care involves an interdisciplinary approach to expert medical and nursing care, pain management, and emotional and spiritual support.
2. Family is the unit of care
3. Patient has the right to die pain-free and with dignity
4. Loved ones will receive necessary support
5. Focus is on caring, not curing
6. Care is provided primarily in the home, but can also be provided in free-standing hospice facilities, hospitals, and nursing homes

through this difficult period. The concept of hospice has been in existence for many centuries; however, it is relatively new in America. The US hospice movement first began in Connecticut in 1974 and has expanded to more than 3,200 hospice programs nationwide.

Hospice is not a place, but a concept of how care should be delivered to terminally ill patients and their families. Table 37–5 lists the primary principles of hospice care (National Hospice and Palliative Care Organization, 2000). When hospice care is delivered in the home, an individual must be designated as the primary caregiver. He or she will be making many decisions for the terminally ill patient. The hospice staff make regular visits to assess the patient and caregiver, and they develop a plan of care that focuses on pain management and symptom control.

Hospice care is generally covered under most insurance plans, including Medicare. In order to qualify for the Medicare benefit, the patient must agree to several stipulations, which are outlined in Table 37–6. All services are covered under the benefit, and if the patient lives longer than 6 months, hospice care will continue.

Hospice care does not end with the patient's death, but extends 1 year beyond death in the form of bereavement service to the family. Although grief and bereavement are considered normal responses to the impending and eventual loss of a loved one, patients and families may display a variety of behaviors. Thus, the ongoing assessment of the family is important.

■ Caregiver Burden

The patient's and family's desire to receive care at home, coupled with increasing pressure on hospitals to discharge patients early, have con-

TABLE 37–6 ■ Qualifying for the Hospice Benefit

- Be certified by the doctor and the hospice director as terminally ill and have a life expectancy of six months or less;
- Sign a statement choosing hospice care using the Medicare Hospice Benefit, rather than curative treatment and standard Medicare covered benefits the terminal illness; and
- Enroll in a Medicare-approved hospice program

National Hospice and Palliative Care Organization, 2000

tributed to enormous pressure being placed on family caregivers. They may be ill equipped, lacking knowledge and information as well as economic resources to care adequately for their dying loved ones. Hospice staff can provide many of the essential services required by caregivers, particularly ongoing teaching and support. However, not all terminally ill patients have access to hospice care. Their link to professional support and information may be the discharge nurse or staff nurse.

The role of family caregivers has shifted from custodial care to a complex, multifaceted role that includes symptom management, with all the related equipment to deliver the care, patient advocacy, transport, and management of activities and responsibilities that the patient has foregone because of illness. As the patient approaches death, the caregiver assumes increasing responsibility for administering medications; assisting with mobility, bathing, nutritional support; and providing emotional support. In addition to providing direct hands-on care, family members are required to perform other activities, such as obtaining medications, transporting the patient to appointments, and filing medical bills and reimbursement forms. Findings from numerous studies have shown that inadequate preparation of the family caregiver for these roles and responsibilities can have a profound negative impact that can extend into the bereavement period.

Family caregivers are in need of step-by-step information that is specific and concrete and is reinforced often. Vague or global information may only increase their anxieties and frustrations. Asking family members and patients general questions, such as "Do you have any questions?" is generally not productive. Table 37–7 highlights information that caregivers need when caring for their loved one. However, just as each patient presents with a unique set of physical and psychosocial problems that require varying levels of interventions, each caregiver possesses varying levels of knowledge and skill. Helping caregivers provide appropriate and competent care consists of more than offering specific information; they may also need counseling services

TABLE 37-7 ■ Specific Information Needed by Caregivers

Disease related:
- Treatment options
- Expected trajectory of illness

Symptom management:
- Nonpharmacological approaches
- Administering and titrating medications
- Observing for side effects
- Observing for complications

Keeping Records of Symptoms and Medications
- Maintaining of log of symptom severity, new symptoms

Reporting Untoward Effects and Treatment Effectiveness
- Keeping health care providers phone numbers
- Understanding what to report

Determining Need for Altered Medications

Adapted from: Given et al, 2001

and support groups. Table 37–8 lists the many types of interventions and strategies that may assist caregivers in providing high-quality care.

■ Conclusion

Meeting the physical and emotional needs of terminally ill cancer patients and their families requires expertise and compassion from many disciplines. Nurses must be prepared and know the principles of symptom management and how and when to call on the other team members. Of the many disciplines that are fundamental to good end-of-life care, the hospice movement has been instrumental in providing family and professional caregivers with effective interventions and practical advice on how to ameliorate the pain and suffering that patients with cancer may be experiencing. Hope for a cure is a reasonable expectation in early-stage disease. When the disease progresses, hope must be redefined and redirected to the goal of caring and living for the moment.

TABLE 37-8 ■ Interventions and Strategies in Support of Family Caregivers

Information
- Family Conferences
- Skills Training
- Problem-Solving Strategies
- Caregiver Training
- Books, Videos, CD ROMs, Web Pages
- Help sheets

Psychotherapeutic
- Support Groups
- Psychologists/Counselors
  - Psychiatric referral
- Counseling Sessions
  - Telephone
  - In person

Mobilize Resources
- Support Groups
- Caregiver Classes
- Visiting Nurses
- Chore Services

Reprinted with permission from Given et al., 2001

■ Resources

- National Hospice and Palliative Care Organization: *www.nhpco.org*
- NCI publication "When Cancer Recurs: Meeting the Challenge" is available at *www.cancer.gov*
- ACS publication "Caring for the Person with Cancer at Home" discusses approaching death; it is available free of charge by calling 800-ACS-2345 or by visiting their web site at *www.cancer.org*
- NCCN/ACS Advanced Cancer and Palliative Care Treatment Guidelines for Patients are available by calling 800-ACS-2345 or by visiting their web sites at *www.cancer.org* and *www.nccn.org*

References

Given, B.A., Given, C.W., Kozachik, S. (2001). Family support in advanced cancer. *CA Cancer J Clin, 51,* 213–231.

Komurcu, S., Nelson, K., Walsh, D., et al. (2000). Common symptoms in advanced cancer. *Seminars in Oncology 27,* 24–33.

Lipman, A.G. Lipman, K.C. Jackson III, L.S. Tyler (Ed.) (1999), *Evidence Based Symptom Control in Palliative Care: Systematic Reviews and Validated Clinical Practice Guidelines for 15 Common Problems in Patients with Life Limiting Disease.* Binghampton, NY: Pharmaceutical Products Press.

Nelson, K.A., Walsh, D., Behrens, C., et al. (2000). The dying cancer patient. *Seminars in Oncology 27,* 84–89.

Schwarte, A. (2001). Ethical decisions regarding nutrition and the terminally ill. *Gastroenterology, 24,* 29–33.

Sutton, L.M., Demark-Wahnefried, W., & Clipp, E.C. (2003). Management of terminal cancer in elderly patients. *Lancet Oncol, 4,* 149–157.

Virani, R. & Sofer, W. (2003). Improving the quality of end-of-life care. *AJN, 103,* 52–61.

Walsh, D., Doona, M., Molnar, M., & Lipnickey, V. (2000). Symptom Control in advanced cancer: Important Drugs and Routes of Administration. *Seminars in Oncology 27,* 69–83.

Glossary

Linda H. Yoder
Kathleen M. O'Leary

Ablation Destruction of, as in myeloablation, which refers to destruction of the bone marrow in conjunction with high-dose chemotherapy in preparation for bone marrow transplantation.

Absolute neutrophil count (ANC) The actual count of the neutrophils in the blood.

$$\frac{\text{Total WBC count} \times (\%\ \text{segmented neutrophils} + \text{band neutrophils})}{100} = \text{absolute neutrophil count}$$

Addiction A combination of physical and psychological compulsive and maladaptive dependence on a substance (e.g., alcohol, illicit drugs, nicotine).

Adenocarcinoma A malignant neoplasm of epithelial cells arising from glandular tissue or in which the cancer cells form recognizable glandular structures.

Adjuvant therapy A therapy that aids another, such as chemotherapy after surgery.

Adrenocorticotropic hormone (ACTH) A hormone secreted by the anterior lobe of the pituitary gland that has a stimulating effect on the adrenal cortex.

Age-adjusted incidence/mortality rate A cancer incidence or mortality rate that has been mathematically adjusted to account for the difference in the age distributions of the populations being compared.

Ageism Prejudice or discrimination against a person because of his or her age.

Allogeneic bone marrow transplantation Transplantation of bone marrow from one person (donor) to another person who is of the same tissue type.

Alopecia Lack or loss of hair from skin areas where it is normally present. Results from chemotherapy, radiation therapy, and endocrine disorders. May be transient or permanent, depending on the type of cancer treatment received.

Alpha-fetoprotein (AFP) A protein normally present in high concentrations in the fetal blood but disappears shortly after birth. If it is found in the blood of adults, it could indicate that a hepatocellular carcinoma, teratocarcinoma, or embryonal cell carcinoma is present; tumor marker used as a diagnostic tool and used to monitor response of hepatomas and germ cell tumors to treatment.

Anemia Below-normal concentration of circulating red blood cells or hemoglobin, measured by volume of red blood cells per 100 ml of blood. Symptomatic anemia occurs when the oxygen-carrying demands of the body are not met. Anemia is not a disease; it is a symptom of illness.

Angiogenesis In relation to tumor angiogenesis, the induction of the growth of blood vessels from surrounding tissues into the tumor by a diffusible protein factor released by the tumor cells.

Anorexia Loss of appetite.

Antibody An immunogloblulin produced by B lymphocytes in response to a unique antigen. Each antibody combines with a specific antigen to control or destroy it.

Anticipatory nausea The inclination or desire to vomit because of the sight or odor of a substance that stimulates a mental image of a distressing situation that has occurred previously; occurs in cancer patients as a result of classic operant conditioning from stimuli associated with chemotherapy, most commonly when efforts to control vomiting related to the therapy have been unsuccessful.

Antigen A protein or group of monosaccharide units on the surface of cells that identify each cell as self or foreign. Antigens stimulate an immune response by producing antibodies or other sensitized cells of the immune system, such as T lymphocytes.

Anti-oncogenes Genes that inhibit tumor cell growth. Also referred to as *tumor suppressor genes.*

Aromatase inhibitors A class of drugs that inhibit estrogen production by hindering aromatase activity; used to treat breast cancer.

Astrocytoma A tumor of the brain or central nervous system composed of astrocytes. This tumor is graded according to prognosis: grade I (consists of fibrillary or protoplasmic astrocytes), grade II (astroblastoma), or grades III or IV (glioblastoma multiforme).

Autologous bone marrow transplantation (ABMT) The harvest, cryopreservation, and reinfusion of a patient's own bone marrow. This procedure is used after ablative cancer therapy.

B cells Another term for B lymphocytes (bursa-equivalent lymphocytes). These cells develop from stem cells and are involved in humoral immunity. Mature B cells can independently identify foreign antigens and differentiate into antibody-producing plasma cells (memory cells). Memory cells allow the body to produce antibodies quickly when invaded by the same organism at a later date.

Bence-Jones protein A low-molecular-weight, heat-sensitive protein found in patients with multiple myeloma. The presence of these proteins in the urine may lead to the formation of precipitates in the tubules, resulting in tubular obstruction, foreign body reaction, and tubular degeneration.

Benign Nonmalignant; favorable for recovery.

Biologic response modifiers (BRMs) Agents such a cytokines, vaccines, and monoclonal antibodies that change host-tumor interactions by enhancing the antitumor mechanism of the immune system, thereby modifying the host's own biologic response to a tumor.

Biotherapy The use of agents derived from biologic sources that enhance the immune response or assist in cancer treatment.

Blast crisis A sudden, severe change in the course of chronic myelocytic leukemia in which the clinical picture resembles that seen in acute myelogenous leukemia; that is, the proportion of myloblasts increases.

Blocks Devices used in radiation therapy to prevent radiation beams from striking areas of the body that require shielding from treatment, such as the heart.

Body surface area Calculation of area of body mass expressed in square meters (m^2); determination is usually accomplished with the use of a nomogram (body surface calculator).

Brachytherapy Treatment with ionizing radiation, the source of which may be placed within the body or on the surface of the body.

BRCA1 A breast cancer susceptibility gene; found in a small number of patients with breast cancer and carried by some people who may develop breast cancer later in life; located on chromosome 17; carriers of the *BRCA* gene are estimated to have an 87% cumulative risk of developing breast cancer by age 70 and a 62% risk of developing ovarian cancer by the age of 70.

BRCA2 A breast cancer susceptibility gene found in a small number of patients with breast cancer and carried by some people who may develop breast cancer later in life; located on chromosome 13; like *BRCA1,* it is associated with the breast/ovarian cancer syndrome; *BRCA2* is more commonly associated with male breast cancer.

Breast self-examination (BSE) Visual and manual examination of the breast. A physician should be contacted if any lump in the breast can be felt.

Cachexia A condition of severe malnutrition, emaciation, and debility.

Cancer Malignant neoplastic disease marked by the uncontrolled growth of cells resulting in the invasion of healthy tissues locally or throughout the body. Cancer cells exhibit the properties of invasion and metastasis.

Cancer of unknown primary Inability to isolate the site of origin of cancer cells through diagnostic testing.

Carcinoembryonic antigen (CEA) A glycoprotein found in increased amounts in the blood of patients with cancers of the colon, breast, stomach, lung, pancreas, thyroid, liver, bladder, and cervix. It is also increased in other diseases and in heavy smokers. Used to monitor the effectiveness of treatment for colorectal cancer.

Carcinogen A substance that causes cancer or increases the risk of developing cancer.

Carcinogenesis Process by which cancer occurs.

Carcinoma A malignant growth consisting of epithelial cells that tend to infiltrate surrounding tissues and give rise to metastases.

Basal cell (carcinoma) An epithelial tumor of the skin that seldom metastasizes but has the potential for local invasion and destruction; the most common form of skin cancer.

Carcinoma in situ Neoplastic activity in which the tumor cells have not yet invaded the basement membrane but remain confined to the epithelium of origin; a lesion with all the histologic characteristics of malignancies except invasion; also called *preinvasive carcinoma.*

Squamous cell carcinoma Neoplastic cells arising from the squamous epithelium (e.g., on the skin or in the mouth, esophagus, bronchi, or cervix) and having cuboid cells.

Cardiac tamponade A life-threatening condition in which the heart is compressed by the accumulation of blood or fluid in the pericardium, causing impaired filling of the heart during diastole. May be acute or chronic.

Cell cycle Sequence of steps through which cells grow and replicate. Consists of five phases: *the* G_0 phase, the resting or dormant phase in which cells are out of the cycle, but have the potential to reenter at any time; *the* G_1 phase, in which RNA and protein synthesis occur; *the* G_2 phase, the time after cells complete DNA synthesis and are preparing to enter mitosis; the *S phase,* in which DNA is synthesized; and *the M phase,* which includes the four phases of mitosis.

Cell cycle specific Drugs (chemotherapeutic) that exert their effect during a particular phase of the cell cycle; for example, antimetabolites exert their effect during the S phase by interfering with RNA and DNA synthesis. Most effective against cells when they are rapidly dividing.

Cell cycle nonspecific Drugs that exert their effect on the cell without regard to a particular phase of the cell cycle; for example, antitumor antibiotics interfere with DNA function; they act on both proliferating and nonproliferating cells.

Cell-mediated immunity The mediating activities of T lymphocytes during a specific immune response. Occurs through the T cell–triggered release of lymphokines or through direct T-cell cytotoxicity.

Central nervous system prophylaxis Administration of intrathecal chemotherapy and/or cranial irradiation, designed to eradicate cancer cells that may sequester themselves behind the blood-brain barrier, thus out of reach of most systemic chemotherapy.

Cervical intraepethelial neoplasia (CIN) A classification that demonstrates the continuum of change in the cervical epithelial tissue beginning as a well-differentiated lesion (CIN 1) and progressing to an undifferentiated intraepithelial lesion (CIN 3).

"Chemo-brain" Unclear thought processes ("fuzziness") and short-term memory loss described by patients undergoing chemotherapy; may also include inability to perform higher-level cognitive functions, such as arithmetic.

Chemoembolization Used in cancer treatment to deliver sustained therapeutic levels of a tumorocidal agent by percutaneous introduction of a substance to occlude a vessel.

Chemopreventive agents Drugs, vitamins, or micronutrients used in the prevention of cancer.

Chemotherapy The systemic treatment of illness by medication. The term was first applied to the treatment of infectious diseases, but it is now used primarily in the context of cancer treatment. Also referred to as *antineoplastic drugs.*

Chondrosarcoma A malignant tumor derived from cartilage cells or their precursors.

Choriocarcinoma A malignant neoplasm of trophoblastic cells formed by the abnormal proliferation of the placental epithelium, without the production of chorionic villi.

Citrovorum factor Folinic acid. Also called *leucovorin.* A metabolically active derivative of folic acid used to treat anemia due to folic acid deficiency and as an antidote to folic acid antagonists, such as methotrexate.

Clinical trial Rigorous evaluation to determine the effectiveness and safety of a specific intervention; the procedure by which new cancer treatments are tested in humans.

Cognitive function Includes all aspects of thinking, perceiving, and remembering; the operation of the mind by which an individual becomes aware of objects via thought or perception.

Colony-stimulating factors (CSFs) Soluble protein factors that stimulate division and maturation of bone marrow stem cells. All CSFs are named as a function of the cell most responsive to the factor (e.g., granulocyte-stimulating factor).

Colposcopy The process of examining the vagina and cervix by means of a speculum and a magnifying lens; procedure used for the early detection of malignant changes on the cervix/vaginal cuff.

Complementary and alternative medicine (CAM) A diverse set of systems of prevention, diagnosis, and treatment based on philosophies and techniques other than those used in conventional Western medicine. *Complimentary* medicine is used in addition to conventional Western practice, whereas *alternative* medicine is used instead of conventional Western practice.

Computed tomography A radiologic imaging technique that produces images of "slices" 1 cm thick through a patient's body. Also referred to as *computerized axial tomography, CAT scan,* or *CT scan.*

Conditioning or preparative regimen Doses of chemotherapy and/or total-body irradiation that are lethal to bone marrow and are given in an effort to eradicate the population of tumor cells in the body; commonly used in the treatment of leukemia.

Conformal radiation therapy Optimal targeting of tumor cells with modern linear accelerators to more accurately shape beams that conform more closely to the size and shape of the tumor in order to minimize damage to collateral healthy tissue.

Congenital melanocytic nevus A congenital lesion of the skin that contains melanocytes; usually pigmented.

Conization The removal of a "cone" of tissue as a partial excision, especially of the uterine cervix, with a scalpel or electrocautery. The scalpel technique preserves the histologic elements of the tissue better. Also referred to as *cone biopsy.*

Consolidation chemotherapy A phase of treatment in leukemia consisting of one to three intensive cycles of chemotherapy designed to bring together the gains made during remission-induction therapy. This therapy begins as soon as a complete remission is documented to ensure that any remaining leukemic cells are eradicated; typically, doses of chemotherapy are administered to induce an anticipated marrow hypoplasia, from which the patient recovers within 7–14 days.

Contact inhibition The suppression of cell division and motility caused by close contact with similar cells.

Continent urinary reservoir Also called the *Kock pouch;* a surgical procedure that provides an intra-abdominal pouch that stores urine and has two nipple valves that maintain continence and prevent ureteral reflux.

Cytokines Proteins produced primarily by white blood cells after contact with specific antigens that assist in regulating normal cell growth and function during inflammation and specific immune response; used as biologic response modifiers. These soluble proteins have a variety of activities that may alter the growth and metastasis of cancer cells by enhancing the immune responsiveness of noncancerous cells.

Cytoreduction Decrease in the number of cells, such as in a cancerous tumor after chemotherapy.

Cytoreductive surgery Surgery to reduce the bulk of a malignant tumor. Also known as *debulking.*

Cytotoxic agent An agent capable of specific destructive action on, or lysis of, certain cells; usually used in reference to antineoplastic drugs that selectively kill dividing cells.

Debulking Surgery to reduce tumor size/burden; improves the response to postoperative chemotherapy; also called *cytoreductive surgery.*

Detection Finding or discovering the existence of disease. In relation to cancer, this can occur via screening methods or tests such as mammography, colonoscopy, or prostate-specific antigen blood test.

Diagnosis A concise, technical description of the cause, nature, or manifestations of a condition, situation, or problem.

Diethylstilbestrol (DES) A synthetic nonsteroidal estrogen used in the palliative treatment of prostate and breast cancer; also used for female hypogonadism, prevention of threatened or habitual abortion, suppression of lactation, atrophic vaginitis, and primary ovarian failure.

Differentiated Fully matured cell; ready to perform the specific function unique to its cell type.

Differentiation The act or process of having recognizable, specialized structures and functions; usually refers to a cellular process that causes an increase in morphologic heterogeneity.

Digital rectal examination (DRE) An examination of the rectum performed with the examiner's fingers; used to check the rectum for masses and to ascertain the size of the prostate.

Disseminated intravascular coagulation (DIC) A pathological condition in which coagulation pathways are hyperstimulated, resulting in diffuse rather than localized activation of coagulation factors. Clotting factors are consumed to such a degree that generalized bleeding occurs. It is a secondary complication of a diverse group of hemolytic and neoplastic disorders that in some way activate the intrinsic coagulation sequence.

Ductal carcinoma in situ (DCIS) Carcinoma confined to the epithelium of a duct (as in breast cancer) without invasion of the basement membrane; later invasive growth is presumed to be high.

Duke's staging A system of staging colorectal tumors based on an assessment of the depth of invasion of the carcinoma and the absence or presence of metastasis.

Dumping syndrome A complex reaction resulting from excessive, rapid emptying of the stomach contents into the jejunum of the gastrointestinal tract.

Dyspareunia Painful intercourse experienced by women.

Dysphagia Difficulty swallowing.

Dysplastic nevi Acquired atypical moles that have a greater tendency to be malignant; they differ from normal moles because they are irregular in shape, variably pigmented, larger, and located in unusual places (scalp, buttocks, breasts). Often a precursor to malignant melanoma.

Dyspnea Shortness of breath, difficulty breathing.

Emetogenic An agent or stimulus with the propensity to cause vomiting.

Endoscopic laser therapy Transmission of light beams through thin flexible fibers within a flexible endoscope to deliver treatment in a controlled fashion to a small area; used in the treatment of gastrointestinal and urogenital cancers.

Enteral feeding Nutrition administered directly to the stomach or small intestine.

Epidemiology The science concerned with the study of factors determining and influencing the frequency and distribution of disease, injury, and other health-related events.

Equianalgesic Having equal pain relieving potential; morphine sulfate, 10 mg intramuscularly, is generally used for opioid comparisons.

Estrogen/progesterone receptor status (ER/PR status) The use of a biomarker to determine whether the tumor is sensitive to estrogen and/or progesterone. Tumors lacking estrogen and progesterone receptors are not sensitive to these hormones. Tumors that are estrogen receptor negative but progesterone receptor positive still respond to an antiestrogen such as tamoxifen. In general, tumors that are ER/PR positive are slightly slower growing and have a slightly better prognosis.

Ewing's sarcoma Highly malignant, metastatic, small round-cell, marrow-originating bone cancer seen primarily in children and adolescents.

Extravasation Escape from the blood vessel into the tissue; term used to describe chemotherapeutic agents escaping from a blood vessel into the surrounding tissue, resulting in tissue damage.

FAB morphology The French-American-British classification system, developed in 1976 to describe cellular morphology of the acute leukemias. The purpose of the classification system was to provide a methodical, objective system that could be used in most hematology laboratories.

Familial adenomatous polyposis A hereditary condition marked by many polyps with high malignancy potential lining the intestinal tract, especially the colon; usually begins around the time of puberty.

Fecal occult blood test Testing a stool sample to determine the presence of hidden (occult) blood. This test is indicated when intestinal bleeding is suspected, but the stool does not appear to contain blood on gross examination.

Flexible sigmoidoscopy A procedure using a hollow lighted tube to visually inspect the wall of the rectum and the distal colon.

Flow cytometry A test of tumor tissue to see how fast the tumor cells are reproducing and whether the tumor cells contain a normal or abnormal amount of DNA. This test is used to help predict how aggressive a cancer is likely to be.

Fractions (fractionation) Divisions of the total dose of radiation into small doses given at intervals, usually causing less biologic destruction than the same total dose given at once.

Gene therapy A form of biotherapy that attempts to alter patients' genetic material by introducing nucleic acid sequences into the chromosomes of targeted cells to prevent, mask, or lessen the effects of a genetic disorder or diseased cells in order to alter cellular metabolism, immune response, or reaction to therapeutic agents.

Gestational trophoblastic disease (GTD) A neoplasm that occurs as the result of the excessive proliferation of chorionic epithelium during very early pregnancy; includes benign hyatidiform mole, malignant choriocarcinoma, and chorioadenoma destruens.

Gleason score Used in prostate cancer to determine the tumor grade through microscopic examination of biopsied tissue. A scale of 2—20 is used; the higher the number, the faster the cancer is likely to grow and the likelier it is to spread beyond the prostate.

Glioblastoma multiforme Astrocytoma grade III or IV; a rapidly growing tumor, usually of the cerebral hemispheres, composed of spongioblasts, astroblasts, and astrocytes.

Glioma A tumor composed of neuroglia in any state of development; sometimes extended to include all intrinsic neoplasms of the brain and spinal cord, such as astrocytomas, neurogliomas, and medulloblastomas.

Gonadotropin-releasing hormone (GnRH) A decapeptide hormone of the hypothalamus that stimulates the release of follicle-stimulating hormone and luteinizing hormone from the pituitary gland; used in the differential diagnosis of hypothalamic, pituitary, and gonadal dysfunction.

Grade A qualitative assessment of the differentiation of tumor cells to the extent that tumor cells resemble the normal tissue at that site; expressed in numeric grades of differentiation from most differentiated (grade 1) to least differentiated (grade 3).

Graft-versus-host disease (GVHD) A frequent complication of allogeneic bone marrow transplantation. Immunocompetent T lymphocytes derived from the donor tissue recognize the recipient's tissue as foreign and react to it, producing clinical manifestations that include skin disease ranging from maculopapular eruption to epidermal necrosis; intestinal disease marked by diarrhea, malabsorption, and abdominal pain; veno-occlusive disease; and loss of hair, and heart and joint lesions similar to those occurring in connective tissue disorders.

Granulocytopenia A decrease in white blood cells.

Gray The S1 (Système International d'Unités) unit of absorbed radiation dose, defined as the transfer of 1 joule of energy per kilogram of absorbing material. 1 Gray = 100 rads.

Gynecomastia Abnormally large mammary glands in the male.

Hematopoiesis The formation and development of blood cells, which occurs mainly in the bone marrow.

Hematopoietic growth factors A group of at least seven natural body proteins that regulate the growth, differentiation, and biologic activity of blood cells.

Hematopoietic stem cell transplantation Stem cell/bone marrow transplantation, which includes autologous, allogeneic, syngeneic, and peripheral blood stem cell transplantations.

Her2/neu Epidermal growth factor receptor 2; presence of too much of this protein on the surface of breast cancer cells signifies a more aggressive type of breast cancer; accounts for approximately 25% of all breast cancers.

Hereditary nonpolyposis cancers Types of colorectal cancers that run in families that are not associated with the formation of polyps in the intestinal tract; associated with a specific genetic defect; accounts for only 5% of colon cancers.

Histology Examination of tissue dealing with the minute structure, composition, and function of tissues as seen through a microscope.

Hodgkin's disease A specific type of lymphoma, differing from all other lymphomas in its predictability of spread, microscopic characteristics, and occurrence of extranodal tumors. The presence of the Reed-Sternberg cell is essential to the diagnosis.

Hormone receptor assay A laboratory test used to determine the quantity of autoantibodies to the particular hormone receptor in question; identifies those tumors that are endocrine sensitive. Used commonly in breast and prostate cancer to plan treatment.

Hospice An interdisciplinary program of palliative and supportive care that addresses the physical, spiritual, social, and psychologic needs of terminally ill patients and their families.

Human chorionic gonadotropin (HCG) A glycopeptide hormone produced by the fetal placenta that is thought to maintain the function of the corpus luteum during the first few weeks of pregnancy. It also is present in certain neoplastic conditions; used as a tumor marker in choriocarcinoma and testicular cancer.

Human leukocyte antigen (HLA) The human major histocompatibility complex located on the short arm of chromosome number 6. Transplantations and platelet/leukocyte transfusions are least likely to be rejected by the recipient when the donor and the recipient are HLA identical.

Humoral immunity A response that begins as soon as a substance enters the body and is interpreted as being foreign. Antibodies are released from plasma cells and enter the body fluids, where they can react with the specific antigens for which they were formed. This release of antibodies is stimulated by antigen-specific groups of B lymphocytes.

Hydatiform mole An abnormal pregnancy resulting from a pathological ovum, with proliferation of the epithelial covering of the chorionic villi. It results in a mass of cysts resembling a bunch of grapes. Also called *hydatid mole.*

Hyperalimentation The enteral or parenteral infusion (total parenteral nutrition) of a solution that contains glucose, amino acids, fatty acids, electrolytes, vitamins, and minerals in quantities sufficient to sustain life and provide for needed tissue repair.

Hypercalcemia Excessive quantity of serum calcium. Weakness, confusion, and possible ventricular dysrhythmias are classic symptoms and require immediate intervention.

Hyperplasia Abnormal proliferation of normal cells in normal arrangements in a tissue type.

Hypertrophy Enlargement or overgrowth of an organ or body part due to an increase in size of its constituent cells.

Hyperviscosity syndrome Caused by a high concentration of proteins, resulting in vascular sludging. Found in several hematologic illnesses, such as multiple myeloma (< 5%) and sickle cell disease. Plasmapheresis is the treatment of choice.

Immunophenotype The characterization of cells according to the antigens present on their cell membranes.

Immunotherapy The use of natural and synthetic substances to provide active and passive immunization; the use of immunopotentiators and immunosuppressants; includes replacement of immunocompetent tissue (bone marrow) and infusion of specially treated white blood cells.

Incidence The rate at which a certain event occurs, such as the number of new cases of a specific disease occurring within a specific population or group during a certain time period.

Incidence rate The number of new cases of cancer divided by the number of people in the population during a given period of time (usually 1 year). The results are usually multiplied by 100,000 to express the rate more conveniently.

Induction chemotherapy The initial chemotherapy regimen used in the treatment of leukemia, when the greatest number of leukemic cells are affected. The combination of drugs is designed to cause severe bone marrow depression and the goal of treatment is remission of the disease.

In situ Confined to the site of origin.

Intensity-modulated radiation therapy (IMRT) A newer radiation technique that facilitates shaping the intensity of the radiation beam to allow for more precise dose distribution around the target site.

Interferons Natural glycoproteins released by cells invaded by viruses or certain infectious agents; act as stimulants to noninfected cells, causing them to synthesize another protein with antiviral capabilities. Interferons are divided into three subsets, with each originating from a different cell and having distinctive chemical and biologic properties:

- **Alfa** Produced by leukocytes in response to a viral infection.
- **Beta** Produced by fibroblasts in response to a viral infection.
- **Gamma** Produced by lymphoid cells in culture that are stimulated by a mitogen.

Interleukins A group of multifunctional cytokines produced by lymphoid and nonlymphoid cells that aid in the control of specific immune responses; 15 interleukins have been identified.

Interleukin-2 A glycoprotein produced by helper T cells that is an essential factor in the growth of T cells and the synthesis of T cell–derived cytokines. It is used as an anticancer drug in the treatment of a wide variety of solid tumors.

Intraoperative radiation (IORT) Specialized radiation technique used during surgery to treat cancers deep in the body with large, single doses while avoiding irradiation of normal tissues; it can be used alone or can be given as a boost to fractionated external-beam therapy.

Intraperitoneal implanted port A hollow housing containing a septum over a portal chamber that is connected via a tube of silicone or a polyurethane catheter that is inserted into the peritoneal cavity; peritoneal ports usually have catheters with larger lumens and multiple exit sites to allow for rapid infusion of fluids; usually placed on the lower rib cage but could be in a pocket of the lower abdomen; used to administer intermittent intraperitoneal chemotherapy for colon or ovarian cancer.

Intrathecal chemotherapy Cytotoxic drugs injected into the cerebrospinal fluid, thereby bypassing the blood-brain barrier.

Intravesical chemotherapy Chemotherapy administered via a urinary catheter for the treatment of bladder cancer. The catheter is usually clamped for a period of time and then emptied. This procedure delivers a high local concentration to the tumor area. Patients receiving this therapy require life-long cytoscopic surveillance for recurrent disease.

Invasive mole (chorioadenoma destruens) A form of hydatidiform mole in which molecular chorionic villi penetrate into the myometrium and may invade the parametrium. Hydropic villi may be transported to distant sites, most often the lungs, but they do not grow as metastases.

Leukemia A progressive disease of the blood-forming organs, marked by distorted proliferation and development of leukocytes and their precursors in the blood and bone marrow. It is accompanied by a reduced number of red blood cells, normal white blood cells, and platelets, resulting in anemia, increased susceptibility to infection, and bleeding. Leukemia is classified according to the degree of cell differentiation (acute or chronic) and the cell type—myelogenous or lymphocytic.

Acute lymphocytic leukemia (ALL) Most common type of pediatric leukemia; infiltration and accumulation of immature lymphoblasts occur within the bone marrow, as well as the extramedullary lymphatic tissue, causing painful lymphadenopathy and hepatosplenomegaly.

Acute myelocytic leukemia (AML) Acute leukemia of the myelogenous type; affects mostly middle-aged to elderly individuals.

Acute nonlymphocytic leukemia (ANLL) A broad term referring to all leukemias that are not lymphocytic. This leukemia is characterized by pancytopenia, megablastic bone marrow, nucleated red cells in the peripheral marrow, and refractoriness to treatment, with a short survival time. Most patients have chromosomal abnormalities in marrow cells.

Chronic lymphocytic leukemia (CLL) An adult-onset form of leukemia seen primarily in the elderly; the leukemic cells have T-cell properties, with frequent dermal involvement, lymphadenopathy, hepatosplenomegaly, and a subacute or chronic course. It is associated with human T-cell leukemia-lymphoma virus.

Chronic myelocytic leukemia (CML) Chronic leukemia of the myelogenous type primarily occurring between the ages of 25 and 60 years; the onset is insidious, and the leukocytosis consists of predominantly mature white blood cells.

Hairy-cell leukemia (HCL) An adult leukemia marked by splenomegaly and by an abundance of large, mononuclear, abnormal cells with numerous irregular cytoplasmic projections that give them a flagellated or hairy appearance in the bone marrow, spleen, liver, and peripheral blood.

Leukopheresis Removing white blood cells from the patient; usually used in patients with leukemia when the white blood cell count gets too high. Can be accomplished by continuous-flow cell separators or filtration techniques.

Leukoplakia The development of white, thickened patches on the mucous membranes of the cheeks, gums, or tongue. These patches are considered precancerous and can become malignant. They tend to grow into larger patches, or they may take the form of ulcers. Those in the mouth may cause pain during swallowing, eating, or talking.

Leukostasis Occurs as a result of leukemic blast cells accumulating and invading vessel walls, causing rupture and bleeding.

Limb perfusion Used in the treatment of malignant melanoma; certain chemotherapeutic drugs are instilled into the affected extremity by arterial perfusion. A pump system counteracts the normal arterial pressure, permitting a steady state of infusion, allowing the drugs to have the greatest effect at the disease site. Usually performed after surgical removal of the bulk of the tumor mass.

Lobular cancer in situ (LCIS) Microscopically seen as very small, round cells filling the lobules; studies suggest that LCIS (of the breast) does not grow into cancer but indicates a higher risk of developing cancer.

Luteinizing hormone-releasing hormone (LHRH) agonist Pharmacologic agent that stimulates the pituitary to increase luteinizing hormone (LH), thereby stimulating testosterone production. With continued use, the pituitary stops initiating the production of LH or testosterone. ALHRH agonist may be combined with an antiandrogen (e.g., flutamide) to produce total androgen blockade in the treatment of prostate cancer.

Lymphadenectomy Surgical excision of one or more lymph nodes.

Lymphocyte Any of the mononuclear, nonphagocytic leukocytes found in the blood, lymph, and lymphoid tissue. Divided into two classes, B and T lymphocytes, which are responsible for humoral and cellular immunity, respectively.

Lymphokines Cytokines produced by lymphocytes and capable of regulating the immune response. Examples are interleukin-2 and interferon.

Lymphoma Any neoplastic disorder of the lymphoid tissue, including Hodgkin's disease. Classifications are based on predominant cell type and degree of differentiation.

Macrophage Any of the large, mononuclear, highly phagocytic cells derived from monocytes; arise from stem cells in the bone marrow, develop into monocytes, circulate in the bloodstream for approximately 40 hours, and then enter various tissues, where they increase in size and phagocytic activity to become macrophages. They are usually immobile but become mobile when stimulated by inflammation. They have a vital role in the immune system.

Magnetic resonance imaging (MRI) A type of diagnostic radiography that visualizes soft tissues of the body by applying an external magnetic field that distinguishes between hydrogen atoms in different environments, producing an image. Provides information that allows the distinction between normal tissues versus cancerous, atherosclerotic, or traumatized tissues.

Maintenance chemotherapy This leukemia therapy begins when the marrow and peripheral blood have recovered, after either induction or consolidation therapy. Drug doses are chosen to cause significant, but not life-threatening, cytopenias. Not recommended to treat acute myelocytic leukemia.

Malignant Having the properties of anaplasia, invasiveness, and metastasis; referring to cancerous growths and tumors.

Malignant melanoma Least common form of skin cancer; it starts in the cells that produce skin coloring (melanocyte) and frequently metastasizes.

Malignant transformation Cellular transformation in which the cells take on properties of anaplasia, invasiveness, and metastasis; term used in conjunction with tumor development.

Meningioma Benign, slow-growing tumor that originates in the meninges, usually next to the dura mater; increased intercranial pressure is common.

Metastasis Secondary malignant lesions originating from the primary tumor but located in anatomically distant places.

Metastatic cascade A series of steps that, once initiated, continue to the end result of the transfer of abnormal cells to a site in the body that is distant from the site initially affected. The end result is the formation of a new focus of disease in a distant part of the body.

Micrometastases Formation of microscopic secondary tumors created by cancerous cells escaping into the lymphatic or vascular flow, where they can travel to distant sites.

Mohs surgery A technique for microscopically controlled serial excisions of fresh tissue used for microscopic analysis in the diagnosis and treatment of skin cancer.

Monoclonal antibodies (MoAbs) Antibodies formed through a special process of immunizing mice with a desired antigen, removing immunized lymphocytes from the mice, and fusing the lymphocytes with mouse myeloma cells to form a hybridoma, which is capable of unlimited cell division. Cells that produce the desired antibody are selected, and those are cloned to produce large amounts of uniform antibodies specific to the target antigen. These antibodies are still being tested in an attempt to find antibodies that are tumor cell specific for various cancers.

Monoclonal gammopathy of undetermined significance (MGUS) Pathological (immunoglobulin synthesis) condition of plasma cells; marked by excessive levels of paraproteins in the blood. In approximately 20% of cases, it is a precursor to multiple myeloma.

Mortality The number of deaths due to a disease, in this case, cancer.

Mortality rate The death rate; the ratio of total number of deaths from a particular disease (cancer) divided by the total number of people in the population during a given period of time (usually 1 year). The results are usually multiplied by 100,000 to express the rate more conveniently.

Mucositis Inflammation of a mucous membrane. Oral mucositis is a common side effect of some types of chemotherapy.

Mutation A change in genetic material; usually occurs in one gene; the change is transmissible.

Myelodysplastic syndrome Characterized by abnormal stem cells, anemia, neutropenia, and thrombocytopenia; a group of bone marrow disorders of varying duration preceding the onset of myelogenous leukemia.

Myelosuppression A reduction in bone marrow function, resulting in a reduced release of erythrocytes, leukocytes, and platelets into the peripheral circulation and/or a release of immature cells into the circulating blood.

Nadir The period of time when antineoplastic therapy has its most profound effects on the bone marrow; when the blood counts reach their lowest points.

Natural killer cells A group of large, granular lymphocytes that have the intrinsic ability to recognize and destroy some virally infected cells and some tumor cells.

Neoadjuvant therapy Preliminary cancer therapy (usually chemotherapy or radiation therapy) that precedes a necessary second modality of treatment (e.g., surgery).

Neuroblastoma Most common extracranial, solid malignant tumor in children; originates from neural crest cells of the sympathetic nervous system, with primary sites in the mediastinal and retroperitoneal regions.

Neutropenia Abnormally low number of white blood cells (neutrophils) in the blood.

Nonseminomatous tumors A histologic type of testicular cancer consisting of the embryonal (including yolk sac), teratocarcinoma, teratoma, and choriocarcinoma tumors, which can produce human chorionic gonadotropins.

Non-small cell carcinoma of the lung A broad term referring to all bronchogenic cancers that are not small cell; includes large-cell, adenocarcinoma, squamous cell, and epidermoid lung cancers.

Observed survival rate The proportion of a cohort of persons with cancer that are still alive after a given time interval.

Odynophagia Painful swallowing.

Oligodendroglioma Slow-growing brain tumor that presents as circumscribed, spongy, and vascular mass, usually located in the frontal lobes; fewer than 5% of primary brain tumors. Most commonly presents as a seizure disorder.

Ommaya reservoir This device is a subcutaneous cerebrospinal fluid (CSF) reservoir that is implanted surgically under the scalp and provides access to the CSF through a burr hole in the skull. Drugs are injected into the reservoir with a syringe, and the domed reservoir is then depressed manually to mix the drug within the CSF. This device eliminates the need for multiple lumbar punctures during repeated administration of intrathecal chemotherapy.

Oncogene Gene whose protein products may be involved in the processes of transformation of a normal cell to a malignant state. Classically, it is a normal cellular gene that has been incorporated into an RNA virus and causes the transformation when the virus infects the cell.

Opioids Natural, semisynthetic, and synthetic drugs that relieve pain by binding to opioid receptors in the nervous system. Opioids include all agonists and antagonists with morphine-like activity, as well as naturally occurring and synthetic opioid peptides.

Orchiectomy Surgical removal of one or both testes.

Osteoblast cells A cell arising from a fibroblast, which, as it matures, is associated with bone production.

Osteoradionecrosis Necrosis of bone, most commonly the mandible, resulting from high-dose radiation; occurs in treatment of head and neck cancer.

Osteosarcoma Most common primary bone cancer.

Pain The International Association for the Study of Pain defines it as an unpleasant sensory and emotional experience from actual or potential tissue damage; pain consists of not only the perception of an uncomfortable stimulus but also the response to that perception.

Acute pain Produced by a sudden illness or injury; is often accompanied by physiologic indicators, such as elevated blood pressure, tachycardia, papillary dilation, hyperventilation, and diaphoresis.

Breakthrough pain Intermittent exacerbations of pain in patients receiving opioid therapy for chronic cancer.

Chronic pain Long-lasting discomfort that may include episodic exacerbations; in cancer, clear distinctions between types of pain are not always possible; chronic pain may be due to tumor involvement and/or effects of cancer treatment.

Neuropathic pain A type of pain that occurs through abnormal processing of sensory input by the central or peripheral nervous system; it is distinctly different from nociceptive pain. Pain reports of people who have neuropathic pain may be disproportionate to physical findings.

Nociceptive pain Normal processing of stimuli (somatic and visceral) from damage to normal tissues or from prolonged exposure to an agent that has the potential to damage normal tissue; usually responsive to opioids and/or nonopioids.

Procedural pain A feeling of distress, suffering, or agony caused by the stimulation of nerve endings during a medical procedure. The distress may also be psychological and caused by fear of the known or the unknown.

Papanicolaou (Pap) test A technique that uses exfoliated cells and subjects them to cytologic staining for the purpose of detecting abnormal cells. Most commonly used to detect cancer of the cervix and uterus, but also may be used in the diagnosis of human papillovirus infection, lung, peritoneal, and genitourinary cancers and in the evaluation of endocrine function.

Paraneoplastic syndrome A collective term for disorders arising from metabolic effects of cancer on tissues remote from the tumor. These disorders may appear as primary endocrine, hematologic, or neuromuscular problems.

Pelvic exenteration Total pelvic exenteration includes a radical hysterectomy, pelvic lymph node dissection, and removal of the bladder and rectosigmoid. Occasionally, a posterior exenteration, which preserves the bladder, or an anterior exenteration, which preserves the rectum, can be performed.

Pericardial effusion Accumulation of fluid in the pericardial sac.

Peripheral blood stem cell transplantation Transplantation of stem cells harvested from the peripheral blood through a process called *aphoresis,* as compared with traditional bone marrow transplantation, in which stem cells are surgically harvested from the bone marrow.

Pheochromocytoma A usually benign tumor of the sympathoadrenal system that produces catecholamines; produces a hypertension that may have a sudden onset.

Philadelphia chromosome (Ph[1]) An abnormality of chromosome 22, characterized by shortening of its long arms. This chromosome is seen in the marrow cells of most patients with chronic myelogenous leukemia.

Plasma cells Descendants of B cells that are capable of producing antibodies; also called *plasmacyte*.

Plasmacytoma A malignant tumor of plasma cells occurring in the bone marrow; usually a discrete, presumably solitary, plasma cell tumor mass.

Ploidy In genetics, the number of chromosome sets in a cell.

Euploidy The state of having a complete set of chromosomes.

Diploidy The state of having two full sets of chromosomes.

Aneuplolidy The state of having an abnormal number of chromosomes.

Hyperdiploid A cell with more than two full sets of chromosomes.

Hypodiploid A cell with less than two full sets of chromosomes.

Pluripotent stem cell The cell that can generate all cell lineages in the bone marrow, such as red blood cells, white blood cells, and platelets (see *stem cell*).

Polyp Any growth or mass protruding from a mucous membrane. Polyps are usually an overgrowth of normal tissue, but sometimes they are true tumors.

Predictive value The percentage of persons with a positive screening test result who actually have cancer.

Prevalence The number of existing cases of a disease in a given population at a specific time.

Primary prevention Interventions aimed at protecting individuals from cancer before pathological changes have begun; includes both general health promotion and specific measures.

Prostate-specific antigen (PSA) Secreted by the epithelial cells of the prostate gland; a tumor marker that has been used to monitor tumor activity of prostate carcinomas. Serum levels are elevated in benign prostatic hyperplasia and prostate cancer; used as a screening test for prostate cancer.

Proto-oncogenes Genes in normal cells similar to viral-transforming genes. Some proto-oncogenes encode proteins that influence controlled cellular proliferation and differentiation. Mutations, amplifications, and rearrangements of proto-oncogenes allow them to function as oncogenes.

Purge To remove all tumor cells; as in purged bone marrow.

Radiofrequency ablation This technique uses high-energy radio waves to treat liver cancer. A thin, needle-like probe temporarily placed into the tumor releases high-frequency alternating current that creates frictional heating and destroys the cancer cells.

Radionuclide A type of atom that is radioactive and disintegrates with the emission of corpuscular or electromagnetic radiations; used in nuclear medicine scanning for diagnostic and evaluative purposes.

Relative risk A ratio comparing the rate of disease in exposed individuals with the rate of disease in unexposed individuals. This risk does not reveal probability of disease occurrence; rather, it measures the strength of the association between a factor and the outcome. The higher the relative risk, the greater the evidence for causation.

Relative survival rate The observed survival rate of cancer patients divided by the expected survival rate in the general population. This rate reflects the fact that some patients with cancer die of causes other than their cancer.

Response rate Percentage of patients showing some evidence of improvement after an intervention.

Retinoblastoma A malignant, congenital hereditary blastoma composed of retinal cells arising from retinoblasts; usually occurs in children younger than 5 years of age.

Risk The probability that an individual member of the population will develop or die of cancer in a given period of time; estimated by incidence and mortality rates.

Risk factor An element of personal behavior, genetic make-up, or exposure to a known cancer-causing agent that increases a person's chances of developing a particular form of cancer.

Sarcoma A tumor that is often highly malignant, composed of cells derived from connective tissue, such as bone and cartilage, muscle, blood vessel, lymphoid tissue, and epithelial tissue. These tumors usually develop rapidly and metastasize through the lymph channels. The different types of sarcomas are named for the different types of tissues they affect.

- **Ewing's sarcoma** A malignant tumor of bone that arises in medullary tissue, occurring more often in cylindrical bones, with pain, fever, and leukocytosis as prominent symptoms.
- **Fibrosarcoma** A sarcoma arising from collagen-producing fibroblasts.
- **Kaposi's sarcoma** Malignant neoplastic vascular proliferation characterized by the development of bluish red cutaneous nodules, usually on the lower extremities, which spread slowly, increase in size and number, and spread to more proximal sites. The tumors often remain confined to the skin and subcutaneous tissue, but widespread visceral involvement may occur.
- **Osteogenic sarcoma** Malignant primary tumor of the bone composed of a malignant connective tissue stroma with evidence of osteoid, bone, and/or cartilage formation.

Schwannomas A neoplasm originating from Schwann cells (of the myelin sheath) of neurons. These neoplasms include neurofibromas and neurilemomas.

Screening Tests that are systematically applied to defined populations for the detection of early and asymptomatic disease.

Secondary prevention Interventions aimed at detecting cancer early and treating it promptly.

Seed implant Small capsule made of radioactive iodine, iridium, or gold implanted at the location of the tumor; most commonly used in the treatment of prostate cancer.

SEER Surveillance, Epidemiology, and End Results Program of the National Cancer Institute. Maintains the statistical database of cancer in the United States.

Selective estrogen receptor modulators (SERMs) Estrogen analogue compounds that mimic the effects of estrogen; agents that activate some estrogen receptors, but not others, creating estrogen-like effects on target tissues while not affecting other tissues.

Seminoma A malignant tumor of the testes thought to arise from the primordial germ cells of the sexually undifferentiated embryonic gonad; accounts for half of all testicular malignancies.

Sensitivity The probability that a screening test will correctly classify an individual as positive for cancer when the individual has the disease.

Sexuality The collective characteristics of an individual related to sexual attitudes and activity.

Small-cell carcinoma of the lung A radiosensitive tumor composed of small, undifferentiated cells; includes oat-cell, intermediate, and mixed carcinomas; accounts for 25% of all lung cancers.

Specificity The probability that a person not having a disease will be correctly identified by a clinical/diagnostic test; the number of true negatives divided by the number of true negatives and false positives.

Specific immunity Antigen response that is recognized by lymphocytes, triggering a cascade of events to destroy the invader.

Spinal cord compression (SCC) Pressure on the spinal cord by a tumor, causing a medical emergency that can lead to paraplegia, quadriplegia, loss of bowel and bladder function, and possibly death. Usually seen in cancers that have a tendency toward bony metastasis, such as breast cancer.

Staging The classification of the severity of disease in distinct stages on the basis of established criteria.

Stem cell The hematopoietic pluripotent stem cell is the source of new cells in the blood. Stem cells are capable of self-replication and differentiation. Daughter cells of the pluripotent stem cell divide and differentiate to become lymphocytes, neutrophils, monocytes, macrophages, eosinophils, basophils, erythrocytes, and platelets.

Stereotactic radiosurgery Using a stereotactic frame to accurately deliver a high dose of ionizing radiation to a relatively small target area in one fraction; known as stereotactic radiotherapy when delivered in a fractionated manner. These methods offer patients with brain tumors and arteriovenous malformations an alternative to surgery.

Stereotactic surgery A surgical technique in which precise localization of the target tissue is accomplished through the use of three-dimensional coordinates; stereotactic techniques are used in breast biopsies, brain surgery, and procedures requiring precision to identify, cut, or remove tissue.

Superior vena cava syndrome (SVCS) An oncologic emergency that occurs when tumors of the superior mediastinum on the right obstruct the return of blood to the heart by the superior vena cava. This produces a characteristic syndrome of edema of the upper half of the body associated with prominent collateral circulation. This condition necessitates prompt therapy aimed at relieving the pressure on the superior vena cava.

Support Usually used in the term *social support,* defined as that situation in which ill persons believe they are loved, they are an important part of a network of communication, and they are esteemed and valued, and that a network of mutual obligations exists exclusive of tangible or material aid.

Survival rate Percentage of people with no trace of disease within a specific time frame after diagnosis or treatment; for example, 5-year survival rate.

Survivorship The state of living with cancer.

Syndrome of inappropriate secretion of antidiurectic hormone (SIADH) A disorder in which antidiuretic hormone (ADH, vasopressin) is continually released, resulting in persistent hyponatremia, hypovolemia, and elevated urine osmolality, leading to weakness, confusion, nausea, and vomiting. Causes include ADH-secreting tumor cells (especially pancreatic carcinoma or oat-cell lung carcinoma). Treatment aims to remove the underlying cause (the tumor), restrict fluid intake/output, and protect patients from injury.

Syngeneic bone marrow transplantation Transplanting bone marrow cells from an identical twin.

Targeted therapy New drugs that affect the cancer cell by inhibiting either angiogenesis or certain growth factors and their receptors.

T cells Thymus-dependent lymphocytes, also called *T lymphocytes,* which originate from stem cells and undergo differentiation in the thymus; lymphocytes that are primarily responsible for cell mediated immunity. Differentiated T cells play important roles in the immune system:

- **Cytotoxic T cells** Differentiated T lymphocytes capable of recognizing and lysing target/foreign cells.
- **Helper T cells** Differentiated T lymphocytes whose cooperation (help) is needed for the production of antibodies against most T-dependent antigens; stimulate T cells and B cells.

Tertiary prevention Interventions aimed at limitation of disability and rehabilitation of those with disability.

Thermography A technique in which an infrared camera photographically portrays the body's surface temperature, based on self-emanating infrared radiation; sometimes used in the diagnosis of pathological underlying processes, such as breast tumors.

Therapies Interventions designed to treat disease, illness, or disability.

Thrombocytopenia An abnormally low quantity of platelets in the circulating blood.

Thyroid cancer Because the thyroid contains a variety of cells, malignant tumors may arise within the thyroid from any of the following cells:

- **Anaplastic thyroid carcinoma** Resembles a variety of other tumors, such as sarcoma. Highly malignant and locally invasive. Invasion beyond the thyroid usually present at the time of diagnosis. Often presents with compression of the esophagus and trachea.
- **Follicular thyroid carcinoma** Usually solitary and encapsulated. May be well circumscribed and well differentiated.
- **Medullary thyroid carcinoma** Tends to be unencapsulated; cells vary in morphology but do not contain papillary or follicular cells.
- **Papillary thyroid carcinoma** Usually multifocal and unencapsulated. Pure papillary is uncommon; usually mixed with follicular.

TNM staging classification A system of cancer staging (determining how much and where cancer is present) in which *T* stands for the extent of the primary tumor, *N* stands for the presence or absence and extent of regional lymph node metastasis, and *M* stands for the presence or absence of distant metastasis. This is the staging system recommended by the American Joint Committee on Cancer.

Tolerance A reduced responsiveness to any effect of any drug/stimulus as a consequence of prolonged exposure to that drug/stimulus, necessitating larger doses of the drug/stimulus to produce an equivalent effect.

Total parenteral nutrition (TPN) Nutritional supplementation by peripheral intravenous or central intravenous line infusion; also known as *intravenous hyperalimentation.*

Transcutaneous electrical nerve stimulation (TENS) Mild electrical stimulation applied by electrodes in contact with the skin over a painful area. The stimulation interferes with the transmission of pain signals and helps suppress the sensation of pain in the area; current is supplied by a hand-held battery-operated pulse generator.

Tumor Neoplasm; a new growth of tissue in which cell growth is uncontrolled and progressive.

Tumor angiogenesis factor (TAF) A protein in cancer tumors thought to be essential to cancer growth; stimulates growth of new capillaries that provide nutrients and remove waste from the tumor.

Tumor-infiltrating lymphocytes (TILs) Lymphocytes collected from the site of a solid tumor and cultured in interleukin-2. When these cells are injected back into the tumor-bearing host, they display activity against the specific tumor from which they originated.

Tumor lysis syndrome (TLS) Severe hyperphosphatemia, hyperkalemia, hypocalcemia, and hyperuricemia occurring after effective induction chemotherapy of rapidly growing malignant tumors; thought to be due to release of intracellular products after cell lysis.

Tumor markers Proteins in the body that may be present in abnormal amounts in the presence of certain cancers. The most useful markers are specific, sensitive, and proportional to the tumor load, thereby being useful in the screening, diagnosis, and monitoring of recurrence or response to treatment.

Tumor necrosis factor (TNF) Either of two lymphokines capable of causing in vivo hemorrhagic necrosis of some tumor cells while not affecting normal cells.

Tumorocidal Destructive to cancer cells.

Tumor-suppressor genes Also known as *anti-oncogenes;* genes coding for proteins that "turn off" malignant growth by masking the phenotypic expression of a mutation by a suppressor (second mutation) at a different site than the first; the organism appears to be reverted but is actually doubly mutant.

Ultrasound Radiologic technique in which deep structures of the body are visualized via the reflections of ultrasonic waves directed into the tissues; uterine tumors and other pelvic masses can be detected with the use of this technique.

Ultraviolet radiation (UVR) The type of light that consists of electromagnetic radiation beyond the violet end of the spectrum, having wavelengths of 200—400 nanometers. These rays have powerful chemical and actinic properties, induce sunburn and tanning of the skin, and act on ergosterol in the skin, leading to the production of vitamin D_2 (ergocalciferol).

Underserved populations Populations of individuals who do not receive adequate services, in this case, health care services. This term is used in relation to people in certain geographic regions, individuals of low socioeconomic status, individuals of various racial/ethnic groups, or a combination of these characteristics.

Undifferentiated or anaplastic Characterized by a loss of differentiation of cells, an irreversible alteration in adult cells toward more primitive cell types; a characteristic of cancer cells.

Vascular access device (VAD) A device that provides intravascular access.

Tunneled catheter Single-, double-, or triple-lumen catheter with Dacron cuff that secures catheter within the subcutaneous tissue and minimizes the risk of ascending bacteria within the tunnel; peripherally inserted catheter.

PICC Single- or double-lumen catheters inserted intravenously, usually in the antecubital area.

Implantable port Provides access to peritoneal, arterial, venous, or epidural body systems through a portal septum.

Vector A plasmid or viral chromosome into whose genome a fragment of foreign DNA is inserted; used to introduce the foreign DNA into a host cell in the cloning of DNA.

Veno-occlusive disease An acute or chronic disease of the liver characterized by partial or complete occlusion of the branches of the hepatic veins by endophlebitis and thrombosis, leading to centrilobular necrosis, fibrosis, and ascites.

Watchful waiting/expectant management Observation of a cancer patient's disease through ongoing testing/follow-up rather than aggressive up-front therapy; this term is often used in relation to patients with prostate cancer.

Wilms' tumor A rapidly developing, malignant, mixed tumor of the kidneys; composed of embryonal elements; usually occurs before the age of 5.

Xeroderma pigmentosa A rare pigmentary, atrophic, autosomal recessive disease affecting all races in which the skin and eyes are extremely sensitive to light; it begins in childhood and progresses to early development of excessive freckling, keratosis, papillomas, carcinoma, and melanoma.

Xerostomia Dryness of the mouth from salivary gland dysfunction.

Index

(*Note:* Page numbers in *italics* indicate tables and figures.)

D

E

O